Artificial Intelligence in Healthcare: Current State and Future Perspectives

Artificial Intelligence in Healthcare: Current State and Future Perspectives

Editor

Tim Hulsen

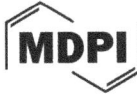

Basel • Beijing • Wuhan • Barcelona • Belgrade • Novi Sad • Cluj • Manchester

Editor
Tim Hulsen
Data Science & AI Engineering
Philips
Eindhoven
Netherlands

Editorial Office
MDPI
St. Alban-Anlage 66
4052 Basel, Switzerland

This is a reprint of articles from the Special Issue published online in the open access journal *AI* (ISSN 2673-2688) (available at: www.mdpi.com/journal/ai/special_issues/6NQ2431LZE).

For citation purposes, cite each article independently as indicated on the article page online and as indicated below:

Lastname, A.A.; Lastname, B.B. Article Title. *Journal Name* **Year**, *Volume Number*, Page Range.

ISBN 978-3-7258-1084-0 (Hbk)
ISBN 978-3-7258-1083-3 (PDF)
doi.org/10.3390/books978-3-7258-1083-3

Cover image courtesy of Tim Hulsen
Licensed by Panchenko Vladimir/Shutterstock

© 2024 by the authors. Articles in this book are Open Access and distributed under the Creative Commons Attribution (CC BY) license. The book as a whole is distributed by MDPI under the terms and conditions of the Creative Commons Attribution-NonCommercial-NoDerivs (CC BY-NC-ND) license.

Contents

About the Editor vii

Tim Hulsen
Artificial Intelligence in Healthcare: ChatGPT and Beyond
Reprinted from: *AI* **2024**, *5*, 550-554, doi:10.3390/ai5020028 1

Gerardo Cazzato, Marialessandra Capuzzolo, Paola Parente, Francesca Arezzo, Vera Loizzi and Enrica Macorano et al.
Chat GPT in Diagnostic Human Pathology: Will It Be Useful to Pathologists? A Preliminary Review with 'Query Session' and Future Perspectives
Reprinted from: *AI* **2023**, *4*, 1010-1022, doi:10.3390/ai4040051 6

James C. L. Chow, Leslie Sanders and Kay Li
Design of an Educational Chatbot Using Artificial Intelligence in Radiotherapy
Reprinted from: *AI* **2023**, *4*, 319-332, doi:10.3390/ai4010015 19

Adham H. El-Sherbini, Hafeez Ul Hassan Virk, Zhen Wang, Benjamin S. Glicksberg and Chayakrit Krittanawong
Machine-Learning-Based Prediction Modelling in Primary Care: State-of-the-Art Review
Reprinted from: *AI* **2023**, *4*, 437-460, doi:10.3390/ai4020024 33

Thomas T. H. Wan and Hunter S. Wan
Predictive Analytics with a Transdisciplinary Framework in Promoting Patient-Centric Care of Polychronic Conditions: Trends, Challenges, and Solutions
Reprinted from: *AI* **2023**, *4*, 482-490, doi:10.3390/ai4030026 57

Lauren M. Paladino, Alexander Hughes, Alexander Perera, Oguzhan Topsakal and Tahir Cetin Akinci
Evaluating the Performance of Automated Machine Learning (AutoML) Tools for Heart Disease Diagnosis and Prediction
Reprinted from: *AI* **2023**, *4*, 1036-1058, doi:10.3390/ai4040053 66

Marco Leo, Pierluigi Carcagnì, Luca Signore, Francesco Corcione, Giulio Benincasa and Mikko O. Laukkanen et al.
Convolutional Neural Networks in the Diagnosis of Colon Adenocarcinoma
Reprinted from: *AI* **2024**, *5*, 324-341, doi:10.3390/ai5010016 89

Md Easin Hasan and Amy Wagler
New Convolutional Neural Network and Graph Convolutional Network-Based Architecture for AI Applications in Alzheimer's Disease and Dementia-Stage Classification
Reprinted from: *AI* **2024**, *5*, 342-363, doi:10.3390/ai5010017 107

Juraj Tomášik, Márton Zsoldos, Ľubica Oravcová, Michaela Lifková, Gabriela Pavleová and Martin Strunga et al.
AI and Face-Driven Orthodontics: A Scoping Review of Digital Advances in Diagnosis and Treatment Planning
Reprinted from: *AI* **2024**, *5*, 158-176, doi:10.3390/ai5010009 129

Devika Rankhambe, Bharati Sanjay Ainapure, Bhargav Appasani and Amitkumar V. Jha
A Flower Pollination Algorithm-Optimized Wavelet Transform and Deep CNN for Analyzing Binaural Beats and Anxiety
Reprinted from: *AI* **2023**, *5*, 115-135, doi:10.3390/ai5010007 148

Tim Hulsen
Explainable Artificial Intelligence (XAI): Concepts and Challenges in Healthcare
Reprinted from: *AI* **2023**, *4*, 652-666, doi:10.3390/ai4030034 . . . . **169**

About the Editor

Tim Hulsen

Tim Hulsen is a senior data and AI scientist with broad experience in both academia and industry, working on a wide range of projects, mostly in oncology. After receiving his M.Sc. in biology in 2001, he obtained a Ph.D. in bioinformatics in 2007 from a collaboration between Radboud University Nijmegen and the pharma company N.V. Organon.

After two years post-doc at the Radboud University Nijmegen, he moved to Philips Research in 2009, where he worked on biomarker discovery for one year before moving to the data management and data science field, working on big data projects in oncology, such as Prostate Cancer Molecular Medicine (PCMM), Translational Research IT (TraIT), Movember Global Action Plan 3 (GAP3), the European Randomized Study of Screening for Prostate Cancer (ERSPC), and Liquid Biopsies and Imaging (LIMA).

His most recent projects are ReIMAGINE, which is about the use of imaging to prevent unnecessary biopsies in prostate cancer, and SMART-BEAR, which is about the development of an innovative platform to support the healthy and independent living of elderly people. He is the author of several publications on big data, data management, data science, and artificial intelligence in the context of healthcare and medicine.

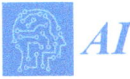

Editorial

Artificial Intelligence in Healthcare: ChatGPT and Beyond

Tim Hulsen

Data Science & AI Engineering, Philips, 5656 AE Eindhoven, The Netherlands; tim.hulsen@philips.com

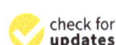

Citation: Hulsen, T. Artificial Intelligence in Healthcare: ChatGPT and Beyond. *AI* **2024**, *5*, 550–554. https://doi.org/10.3390/ai5020028

Received: 29 February 2024
Accepted: 17 April 2024
Published: 19 April 2024

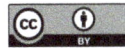

Copyright: © 2024 by the author. Licensee MDPI, Basel, Switzerland. This article is an open access article distributed under the terms and conditions of the Creative Commons Attribution (CC BY) license (https://creativecommons.org/licenses/by/4.0/).

Artificial intelligence (AI), the simulation of human intelligence processes by machines, is having a growing impact on healthcare [1]. As healthcare all around the globe is suffering from personnel shortages [2], AI can be of crucial importance. It can help in three ways: by helping health researchers, by helping medical staff, and by helping patients. Via AI, researchers can provide new approaches to merge, analyze, and process complex "big data" and gain more actionable insights, understanding, and knowledge at an individual and population level [3]. Medical staff can be helped by AI-assisted clinical decision support (CDS), by machine learning (ML) and deep learning (DL) models analyzing large medical datasets, by summarizing radiology and pathology reports using Natural Language Processing (NLP), by automating repetitive but time-consuming tasks, and much more [4]. Patients can talk to chatbots who have access to all medical knowledge in the world, including the patient's medical history, and provide personalized advice [5]. The increasing use of AI in healthcare provides many new and interesting possibilities but also causes issues around trust (the "black box" problem: what does the AI algorithm actually do? [6]) and privacy. This Special Issue intends to show some examples of how AI impacts healthcare, with some discussion on potential future developments as well as challenges. Since this Special Issue contains papers from 2023 and 2024, the era of Generative AI (GenAI) [7], naturally there are papers related to ChatGPT and chatbots. There are also papers on prediction modeling in primary care, polychronic conditions, and heart disease. Other papers focus on the classification of colon cancer and Alzheimer's disease. Finally, there are papers on orthodontic diagnosis and treatment planning, anxiety treatment, and explainable AI (XAI).

"Chat GPT in Diagnostic Human Pathology: Will It Be Useful to Pathologists? A Preliminary Review with 'Query Session' and Future Perspectives" by Cazzato et al. (contribution 1) conducts a systematic review on the use of ChatGPT in pathology. It follows the PRISMA guidelines and uses literature from the PubMed, Scopus, and Web of Science (WoS) databases. Five publications were included after screening for eligibility and inclusion criteria. They also performed a 'query session' with ChatGPT regarding pathologies such as pigmented skin lesions, malignant melanomas and variants, and Gleason's score of prostate adenocarcinomas. ChatGPT is shown to be able to advise the pathologist by providing large amounts of scientific data for use in routine microscopic diagnostic practice. However, there are certain limitations that need to be addressed and resolved, such as bias in the training data, the amount of data available, and 'hallucination' phenomena. The authors also stress that an AI-driven system should always provide support and never have a decision-making motive during the histopathological diagnostic process.

"Design of an Educational Chatbot Using Artificial Intelligence in Radiotherapy" by Chow et al. (contribution 2) shows how to design an AI-enabled chatbot for educational purposes in radiotherapy, using the dialogue tree and layered structure with AI features such as NLP. The chatbot can provide humanlike communication to users requesting information on radiotherapy, based on the question-and-answer approach. When the user may not be able to pinpoint the question exactly, it will be user-friendly and reassuring, offering a list of questions for the user to select. The NLP system helps the chatbot predict the intent of the user and provide the most accurate and precise response. Preferred educational features in a chatbot are functional features such as mathematical operations, which should be modified and updated regularly. The authors conclude that an AI-enabled educational chatbot can be created to provide information transfer to users with different levels of radiotherapy knowledge (e.g., patients, the general public, or radiation staff). The chatbot should be upgraded and fine-tuned regularly, while its performance should be tested and evaluated.

"Machine-Learning-Based Prediction Modelling in Primary Care: State-of-the-Art Review" by El-Sherbini et al. (contribution 3) summarizes the potential of ML and its subsets in influencing two domains of primary care: pre-operative care and screening. ML can be utilized in preoperative treatment to predict postoperative results and assist physicians in selecting surgical interventions. Clinicians can reduce risk and improve patient outcomes using ML algorithms. ML can also improve the precision and effectiveness of screening tests. Healthcare professionals can identify diseases at an early and curable stage by using ML models to scan medical images for diseases or anomalies. ML can be used to identify people at an increased risk of developing specific disorders or diseases, even before any symptoms are visible. It can assess patient data such as medical history, genetics, and lifestyle factors to identify patients at higher risk, enabling targeted interventions such as lifestyle adjustments or early screening. In conclusion, the use of ML in primary care can potentially improve patient outcomes, reduce healthcare costs, and boost the productivity of healthcare personnel.

"Predictive Analytics with a Transdisciplinary Framework in Promoting Patient-Centric Care of Polychronic Conditions: Trends, Challenges, and Solutions" by Wan and Wan (contribution 4) comments on an innovative approach to the development of predictive analytics, which is centered on the development of predictive models for varying stages of chronic disease through integrating all types of datasets, adding various new features to a theoretically driven data warehousing, creating purpose-specific prediction models, and integrating multi-criteria predictions of chronic disease progression based on a biomedical evolutionary learning platform. This commentary identifies trends, challenges, and solutions in conducting innovative AI-based healthcare research, improving understandings of disease-state transitions from diabetes to other chronic polychronic conditions. Therefore, better predictive models could be further formulated to expand from inductive to deductive inquiries in care management research.

"Evaluating the Performance of Automated Machine Learning (AutoML) Tools for Heart Disease Diagnosis and Prediction" by Paladino et al. (contribution 5) discusses the creation of ten machine learning models using the standard practices of exploratory data analysis (EDA), data cleansing, feature engineering, and others, utilizing the Python "sklearn" library. Their toolkit included an array of models: logistic regression, support vector machines, decision trees, random forest, and various ensemble models. Employing five-fold cross-validation, these traditionally developed models demonstrated accuracy rates spanning from 55% to 60%. Automated machine learning (AutoML) tools perform better and have superior capability in generating predictive models. Their findings suggest that AutoML tools can simplify the generation of robust ML models with higher performance than models created by traditional ML methodologies. However, the limitations of AutoML tools must be considered, and strategies need to be developed to overcome them. The successful deployment of ML models designed via AutoML could revolutionize the treatment and prevention of heart disease globally.

"Convolutional Neural Networks in the Diagnosis of Colon Adenocarcinoma" by Leo et al. (contribution 6) analyzes different architectures and ensembling strategies to develop the most efficient network combinations to improve binary and ternary classification of colorectal cancer. They propose a two-stage pipeline approach to diagnose colon adenocarcinoma grading from histological images in a similar manner to that of a pathologist, using a transformer architecture with subsequent classification using a convolutional neural network (CNN) ensemble, which improved the learning efficiency and shortened the learning time. Moreover, they prepared and published a dataset for clinical validation of the developed artificial neural network, which suggested the discovery of novel histological phenotypic alterations in adenocarcinoma sections that could have prognostic value. They conclude that AI can significantly improve the reproducibility, efficiency, and accuracy of colon cancer diagnosis, which are required for precision medicine to personalize cancer treatment.

"A new Convolution Neural Networks and Graph Convolution Networks-based architecture for AI applications in Alzheimer's Disease Stages Classification" by Hasan and Wagler (contribution 7) proposes a computer-assisted method based on an advanced DL algorithm to differentiate between people with varying degrees of dementia. They developed the following four separate models for classifying different dementia stages: (1) CNNs built from scratch; (2) pre-trained VGG16 with additional convolutional layers; (3) graph convolutional networks (GCNs); and (4) CNN-GCN fusion models. These models were trained and evaluated using 6,400 whole-brain magnetic resonance imaging (MRI) scans obtained from the Alzheimer's Disease Neuroimaging Initiative (ADNI). A five-fold cross-validation technique was applied to all the models. Particularly, the CNN-GCN model shows excellent performance in classifying different stages of dementia. Understanding the stages of dementia can assist researchers in uncovering molecular markers and pathways connected with each stage.

"AI and Face-Driven Orthodontics: A Scoping Review of Digital Advances in Diagnosis and Treatment Planning" by Tomášik et al. (contribution 8) highlights the current digital advances that, thanks to AI tools, allow us to implement facial features beyond symmetry and proportionality and incorporate facial analysis into diagnosis and treatment planning in orthodontics. The topics with the greatest research potential within digital orthodontics over the last five years were identified. The most researched and cited topic was AI and its applications in orthodontics. AI can be applied in automated 2D or 3D cephalometric analysis, facial analysis, decision-making algorithms, and the evaluation of treatment progress and retention.

"A Flower Pollination Algorithm-Optimized Wavelet Transform and Deep CNN for Analyzing Binaural Beats and Anxiety" by Rankhambe et al. (contribution 9) discusses binaural beats, a low-frequency form of acoustic stimulation that can help reduce anxiety as well as alter other psychological situations and states by affecting mood and cognitive function. They analyzed the level of anxiety when hearing binaural beats using a novel optimized wavelet transform in which optimized wavelet parameters are extracted from the electroencephalogram (EEG) signal using the flower pollination algorithm, whereby artifacts are effectively removed from the EEG signal. They applied deep CNN-based signal processing, in which deep features are extracted from optimized EEG signal parameters. The proposed model outperforms existing techniques. Therefore, the optimized wavelet transform with a deep CNN can perform an effective decomposition of EEG data and extract deep features related to anxiety to analyze the effect of binaural beats on anxiety levels.

Finally, "Explainable Artificial Intelligence (XAI): Concepts and Challenges in Healthcare" by Hulsen (contribution 10) discusses the term XAI, which has been gaining momentum recently. XAI tries to ensure that AI algorithms (as well as their decisions) can be understood by humans, transforming "black box" algorithms to more transparent "glass box" algorithms. The paper mentions some central concepts in XAI, such as transparent and post-hoc models, AI-assisted decision-making, and explanation methods. It also describes several challenges around XAI in healthcare, such as legal and regulatory compliance, privacy and security, the balance between explainability and accuracy/performance, and explainability metrics. It provides discussion on whether XAI can really help healthcare advance, for example, by increasing understanding and trust, and offers future research possibilities in the area of XAI.

The manuscripts in this Special Issue give us only a brief overview of the wide use of AI in healthcare. It shows how Generative AI can help pathologists and educate patients, how AI can help build predictive models based on medical data, how it can help classify diseases, how it can assist with treatments, and it explains the concept of XAI. As the importance of

AI, and specifically Generative AI with its Large Language Models (LLMs) consuming TBs of data and using many MWhs of electricity during training [8], is growing, data quality as well as sustainability are becoming more prominent as well. LLMs in the healthcare arena need high-quality, reliable medical data to work with. The large computing power needed to run LLMs causes sustainability issues in a world that is already heading towards an energy crisis. Luckily, researchers are working on ways to minimize computation power by inventing methods to reduce computations while preserving model accuracy [9]. While AI is gaining importance, there is also more focus on responsible AI (RAI) [10], which tries to prevent negative effects, especially in Generative AI, such as toxicity and hallucinations. AI in healthcare needs to be both explainable and responsible to make sure that clinical decisions are fully transparent and ethical. In the future, AI might also converge with other technological trends such as the Digital Twin [11] and the Metaverse [12], offering many opportunities to improve healthcare.

Conflicts of Interest: The author is an employee of Philips.

List of Contributions:

1. Cazzato, G.; Capuzzolo, M.; Parente, P.; Arezzo, F.; Loizzi, V.; Macorano, E.; Marzullo, A.; Cormio, G.; Ingravallo, G. Chat GPT in Diagnostic Human Pathology: Will It Be Useful to Pathologists? A Preliminary Review with ‘Query Session’ and Future Perspectives. *AI* **2023**, *4*, 1010–1022.
2. Chow, J.C.L.; Sanders, L.; Li, K. Design of an Educational Chatbot Using Artificial Intelligence in Radiotherapy. *AI* **2023**, *4*, 319–332.
3. El-Sherbini, A.H.; Hassan Virk, H.U.; Wang, Z.; Glicksberg, B.S.; Krittanawong, C. Machine-Learning-Based Prediction Modelling in Primary Care: State-of-the-Art Review. *AI* **2023**, *4*, 437–460.
4. Wan, T.T.H.; Wan, H.S. Predictive Analytics with a Transdisciplinary Framework in Promoting Patient-Centric Care of Polychronic Conditions: Trends, Challenges, and Solutions. *AI* **2023**, *4*, 482–490.
5. Paladino, L.M.; Hughes, A.; Perera, A.; Topsakal, O.; Akinci, T.C. Evaluating the Performance of Automated Machine Learning (AutoML) Tools for Heart Disease Diagnosis and Prediction. *AI* **2023**, *4*, 1036–1058.
6. Leo, M.; Carcagnì, P.; Signore, L.; Corcione, F.; Benincasa, G.; Laukkanen, M.O.; Distante, C. Convolutional Neural Networks in the Diagnosis of Colon Adenocarcinoma. *AI* **2024**, *5*, 324–341.
7. Hasan, M.E.; Wagler, A. New Convolutional Neural Network and Graph Convolutional Network-Based Architecture for AI Applications in Alzheimer’s Disease and Dementia-Stage Classification. *AI* **2024**, *5*, 342–363.
8. Tomášik, J.; Zsoldos, M.; Oravcová, Ľ.; Lifková, M.; Pavleová, G.; Strunga, M.; Thurzo, A. AI and Face-Driven Orthodontics: A Scoping Review of Digital Advances in Diagnosis and Treatment Planning. *AI* **2024**, *5*, 158–176.
9. Rankhambe, D.; Ainapure, B.S.; Appasani, B.; Jha, A.V. A Flower Pollination Algorithm-Optimized Wavelet Transform and Deep CNN for Analyzing Binaural Beats and Anxiety. *AI* **2024**, *5*, 115–135.
10. Hulsen, T. Explainable Artificial Intelligence (XAI): Concepts and Challenges in Healthcare. *AI* **2023**, *4*, 652–666.

References

1. Hulsen, T. Literature analysis of artificial intelligence in biomedicine. *Pharmacogenomics Res. Pers. Med.* **2021**, *8* (Suppl. S1), S64–S77. [CrossRef]
2. Winter, V.; Schreyögg, J.; Thiel, A. Hospital staff shortages: Environmental and organizational determinants and implications for patient satisfaction. *Health Policy* **2020**, *124*, 380–388. [CrossRef] [PubMed]
3. Hulsen, T.; Friedecký, D.; Renz, H.; Melis, E.; Vermeersch, P.; Fernandez-Calle, P. From big data to better patient outcomes. *Clin. Chem. Lab. Med. (CCLM)* **2023**, *61*, 580–586. [CrossRef] [PubMed]
4. Lin, S. A Clinician's Guide to Artificial Intelligence (AI): Why and How Primary Care Should Lead the Health Care AI Revolution. *J. Am. Board Fam. Med.* **2022**, *35*, 175–184. [CrossRef] [PubMed]
5. King, M.R. The future of AI in medicine: A perspective from a Chatbot. *Ann. Biomed. Eng.* **2023**, *51*, 291–295. [CrossRef] [PubMed]

6. Wadden, J.J. Defining the undefinable: The black box problem in healthcare artificial intelligence. *J. Med. Ethics* **2022**, *48*, 764–768. [CrossRef] [PubMed]
7. Kuzlu, M.; Xiao, Z.; Sarp, S.; Catak, F.O.; Gurler, N.; Guler, O. The Rise of Generative Artificial Intelligence in Healthcare. In Proceedings of the 2023 12th Mediterranean Conference on Embedded Computing (MECO), Budva, Montenegro, 6–10 June 2023; pp. 1–4. [CrossRef]
8. de Vries, A. The growing energy footprint of artificial intelligence. *Joule* **2023**, *7*, 2191–2194. [CrossRef]
9. Ma, X.; Fang, G.; Wang, X. LLM-Pruner: On the Structural Pruning of Large Language Models. *arXiv* **2023**, arXiv:2305.11627. [CrossRef]
10. Trocin, C.; Mikalef, P.; Papamitsiou, Z.; Conboy, K. Responsible AI for digital health: A synthesis and a research agenda. *Inf. Syst. Front.* **2023**, *25*, 2139–2157. [CrossRef]
11. Erol, T.; Mendi, A.F.; Doğan, D. The digital twin revolution in healthcare. In Proceedings of the 2020 4th International Symposium on Multidisciplinary Studies and Innovative Technologies (ISMSIT), Istanbul, Turkey, 22–24 October 2020; pp. 1–7. [CrossRef]
12. Hulsen, T. Applications of the metaverse in medicine and healthcare. *Adv. Lab. Med./Av. En Med. De Lab.* **2023**. [CrossRef]

Disclaimer/Publisher's Note: The statements, opinions and data contained in all publications are solely those of the individual author(s) and contributor(s) and not of MDPI and/or the editor(s). MDPI and/or the editor(s) disclaim responsibility for any injury to people or property resulting from any ideas, methods, instructions or products referred to in the content.

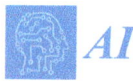

Review

Chat GPT in Diagnostic Human Pathology: Will It Be Useful to Pathologists? A Preliminary Review with 'Query Session' and Future Perspectives

Gerardo Cazzato [1,*], Marialessandra Capuzzolo [1], Paola Parente [2], Francesca Arezzo [3], Vera Loizzi [3], Enrica Macorano [4], Andrea Marzullo [1], Gennaro Cormio [3] and Giuseppe Ingravallo [1]

1. Section of Molecular Pathology, Department of Precision and Regenerative Medicine and Ionian Area (DiMePRe-J), University of Bari "Aldo Moro", 70124 Bari, Italy; m.capuzzolo@studenti.uniba.it (M.C.); andrea.marzullo@uniba.it (A.M.); giuseppe.ingravallo@uniba.it (G.I.)
2. Pathology Unit, Fondazione IRCCS Ospedale Casa Sollievo della Sofferenza, 71013 San Giovanni Rotondo, Italy; paolaparente77@gmail.com
3. IRCCS Istituto Tumori "Giovanni Paolo II", 70124 Bari, Italy; francesca.arezzo@uniba.it (F.A.); vera.loizzi@uniba.it (V.L.); gennaro.cormio@uniba.it (G.C.)
4. Section of Legal Medicine, Interdisciplinary Department of Medicine, University of Bari "Aldo Moro", 70124 Bari, Italy; enricamacorano@gmail.com
* Correspondence: gerardo.cazzato@uniba.it; Tel.: +39-340-520-3641

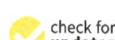

Citation: Cazzato, G.; Capuzzolo, M.; Parente, P.; Arezzo, F.; Loizzi, V.; Macorano, E.; Marzullo, A.; Cormio, G.; Ingravallo, G. Chat GPT in Diagnostic Human Pathology: Will It Be Useful to Pathologists? A Preliminary Review with 'Query Session' and Future Perspectives. *AI* **2023**, *4*, 1010–1022. https://doi.org/10.3390/ai4040051

Academic Editor: Tim Hulsen

Received: 9 October 2023
Revised: 30 October 2023
Accepted: 6 November 2023
Published: 22 November 2023

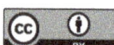

Copyright: © 2023 by the authors. Licensee MDPI, Basel, Switzerland. This article is an open access article distributed under the terms and conditions of the Creative Commons Attribution (CC BY) license (https://creativecommons.org/licenses/by/4.0/).

Abstract: The advent of Artificial Intelligence (AI) has in just a few years supplied multiple areas of knowledge, including in the medical and scientific fields. An increasing number of AI-based applications have been developed, among which conversational AI has emerged. Regarding the latter, ChatGPT has risen to the headlines, scientific and otherwise, for its distinct propensity to simulate a 'real' discussion with its interlocutor, based on appropriate prompts. Although several clinical studies using ChatGPT have already been published in the literature, very little has yet been written about its potential application in human pathology. We conduct a systematic review following the Preferred Reporting Items for Systematic Reviews and Meta-Analyses (PRISMA) guidelines, using PubMed, Scopus and the Web of Science (WoS) as databases, with the following keywords: ChatGPT OR Chat GPT, in combination with each of the following: pathology, diagnostic pathology, anatomic pathology, before 31 July 2023. A total of 103 records were initially identified in the literature search, of which 19 were duplicates. After screening for eligibility and inclusion criteria, only five publications were ultimately included. The majority of publications were original articles ($n = 2$), followed by a case report ($n = 1$), letter to the editor ($n = 1$) and review ($n = 1$). Furthermore, we performed a 'query session' with ChatGPT regarding pathologies such as pigmented skin lesions, malignant melanoma and variants, Gleason's score of prostate adenocarcinoma, differential diagnosis between germ cell tumors and high grade serous carcinoma of the ovary, pleural mesothelioma and pediatric diffuse midline glioma. Although the premises are exciting and ChatGPT is able to co-advise the pathologist in providing large amounts of scientific data for use in routine microscopic diagnostic practice, there are many limitations (such as data of training, amount of data available, 'hallucination' phenomena) that need to be addressed and resolved, with the caveat that an AI-driven system should always provide support and never a decision-making motive during the histopathological diagnostic process.

Keywords: ChatGPT; chatbot; artificial intelligence; AI; pathology; histology

1. Introduction

Artificial Intelligence (AI) has revolutionized medical and scientific fields in just a few years, allowing for significant changes and the integration of diagnostic, therapeutic and patient care pathways [1]. Although at first it was mainly represented by the development of Machine Learning (ML) models [2], further advances such as Deep Learning (DL) with, among others, Convolutional Neural Networks (CNN) soon came to the fore [3]. A branch of AI includes conversational artificial intelligence, which has experienced unprecedented development in recent years, with numerous models and platforms developed to enable machines to understand and respond to natural language input [4]. In more detail, a chatbot is an item of software that simulates and develops human conversations (spoken or written), allowing users to interact with digital devices as though they were speaking with real people [5]. Chatbot might be as basic as a program that responds to a single enquiry or as complex as a digital assistant that learns and develops as it gathers and elaborates information to provide higher levels of personalization [6]. The chatbots designed specifically for activities (declarational) are 'single-purpose' software that focus on carrying out a certain function; regulated responses to user requests are generated using Natural Language Process (NLP) and very little machine learning [7]. The interactions with these chatbots are quite particular and structured, and they are best suited for assistance and service functions like frequently asked and consolidated questions. Common questions can be managed by activity-specific chatbots, such as inquiries about working hours or straightforward transactions that do not involve many variables. Even while they employ NLP in a way that allows users to experiment with it easily, their capabilities are still somewhat limited. These are the most popular chatbots right now [7,8]. Virtual assistants, also known as digital assistants or data-driven predictive (conversational) chatbots, are significantly more advanced, interactive and customized than task-specific chatbots. These chatbots use ML, NLP and context awareness to learn. They employ data analysis and predictive intelligence to offer customization based on user profiles and past user behavior. Digital assistants can gradually learn a user's preferences, make suggestions and even foresee needs. They can start talks in addition to monitoring data and rules. Predictive chatbots that focus on the needs of the user and are data-driven include Apple's Siri and Amazon's Alexa [9].

A clear example of such an approach is ChatGPT, an acronym for Generative Pretrained Transformer, which is a powerful and versatile NLP tool that uses advanced machine learning algorithms to generate human-like responses within a conversation (https://chat.openai.com, accessed on 1 July 2023). Released on 30 November 2022 by OpenAI, ChatGPT (version 3.5) was trained until the end of 2021 on more than 300 billion words, with the ability to respond to a huge variety of topics and with the ability to learn from its human interlocutor [10]. In the first few months after its official launch, many papers were published in the purely informatic field, but, as the weeks went by, the medical and scientific fields were also interested, with a particular interest in the education, research and simulation of clinical pictures of patients, as well as applications in hygiene and public health, clinical medicine, oncology and surgery [11].

On the other hand, in the literature there is a paucity of information regarding the reliability of ChatGPT in assisting the routine activity of the pathologist [12]; among other papers, a recent manuscript by Schukow C. et al. [12,13] underlined the lack of studies that evaluate this relationship, focusing more on the three fundamental criteria on which a potential use of ChatGPT should be based: (1) a chatbot should have a strong performance; (2) an ideal chatbot should be freely accessible for public use; (3) it should be trained on known and recoverable data.

In this review paper, we will try to summarize the potential use of ChatGPT in pathological anatomy, discuss the fields of application studied so far, perform some 'query sessions' about pathological topics that could help the pathologist and try to outline future perspectives, with particular regard to present limitations.

2. Materials and Methods

A systematic review was elaborated following the Preferred Reporting Items for Systematic Reviews and Meta-Analyses (PRISMA) guidelines, using PubMed, Scopus and Web of Science (WoS) databases before 31 July 2023 with the following terms: ChatGPT OR Chat GPT, in combination with each of the following: pathology, diagnostic pathology, anatomic pathology. Only articles in English were recorded. Review articles, meta-analyses, observational studies, case reports, survey snapshot studies, letters to the editor and comments to the letters were all included. Other potentially relevant articles were identified by manually checking the references of the included literature. The articles all had to meet the following inclusion criteria: (1) covering pathological anatomy topics in light of the use of ChatGPT, with the opportunity to discuss strengths and/or limitations; (2) the articles had to necessarily relate ChatGPT to pathology. Exclusion criteria were articles that talked about ChatGPT in general or relating it to other aspects not pertaining to pathological anatomy.

An independent extraction of articles was performed by two investigators (G.C. and M.C.) according to the inclusion criteria, before 31 July 2023. Disagreement was resolved by discussion between the two review authors (Figure 1).

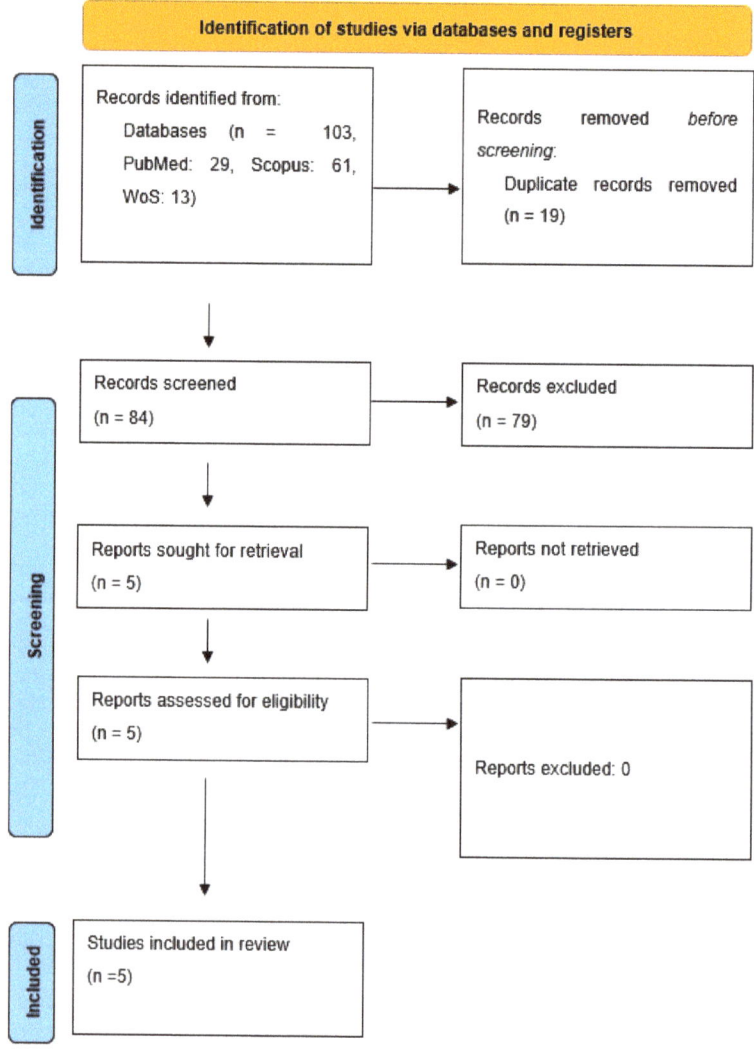

Figure 1. PRISMA flow-chart using in this review.

Furthermore, to explore the reliability of ChatGPT in potentially supporting the pathologist's routine diagnostic activity, we developed questions (G.C. and M.C.) that we asked ChatGPT regarding examples of diagnostic approaches in real-life patient cases. Specifically, the first author (G.C.) created a free account on the Open AI site and conducted the conversations with the chatbot. No plugins or other accessories were used in the platform, and all results presented were obtained with ChatGPT version 3.5 and the query sessions were performed between 1 October and 30 October 2023. Some examples of the conversations are summarized in Figures 2–6.

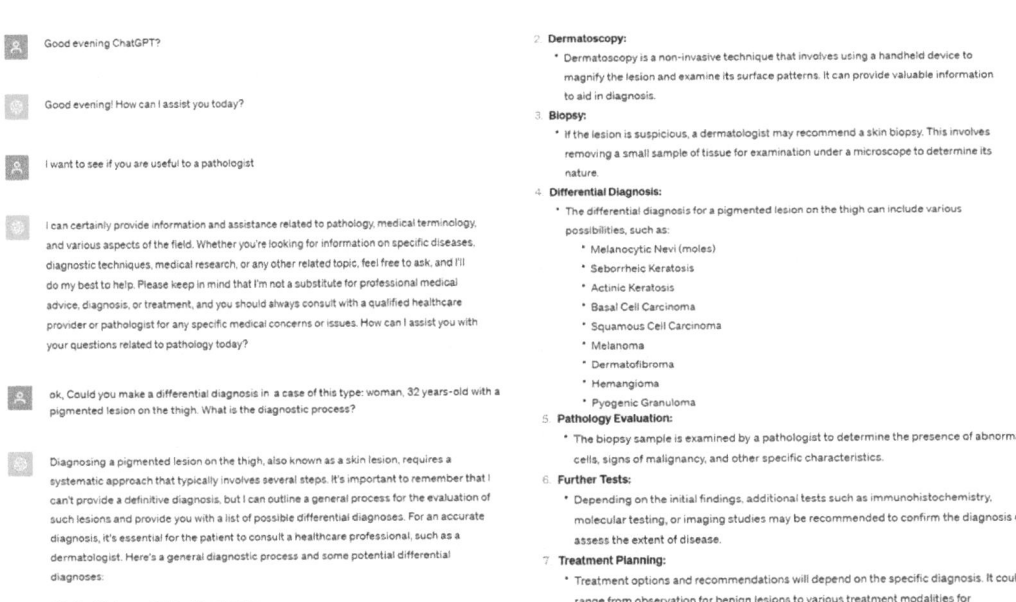

Figure 2. The first author (G.C.) posted a request to ChatGPT: "Could you make a differential diagnosis in a case of this type: woman, 32 years-old with a pigmented lesion on the thigh. What is the diagnostic process?" ChatGPT replied, "Diagnosing a pigmented lesion on the thigh, also known as a skin lesion, requires a systematic approach that typically involves several steps. It is important to remember that I cannot provide a definitive diagnosis, but I can outline a general process for the evaluation of such lesions and provide a list of possible differential diagnoses. For an accurate diagnosis, it is essential for the patient to consult a healthcare professional, such as a dermatologist. Here is a general diagnostic process and some potential differential diagnoses [...]" (see Figure 2 for the rest). The version of ChatGPT used was dated 25 September 2023, and the average time taken from request entry was about 23.43 s.

OK, thank you ChatGPT. Now, could you explain to me the clinical criteria for suspecting malignant melanoma?

Certainly, I can provide you with an overview of the clinical criteria for suspecting malignant melanoma, but please keep in mind that I am not a medical professional, and you should consult with a healthcare professional for personalized advice. The diagnosis and evaluation of skin lesions should be done by a qualified dermatologist or healthcare provider.

Malignant melanoma is a type of skin cancer that arises from melanocytes, the pigment-producing cells in the skin. Detecting melanoma involves assessing various clinical features, often using the ABCDE criteria:

1. **Asymmetry:** One half of the mole does not match the other half in terms of shape, size, or color.
2. **Border Irregularity:** The edges of the mole are not well-defined; they may be uneven, notched, or blurred.
3. **Color variations:** Melanomas often have uneven coloring, with different shades of brown, black, or even red, white, or blue.
4. **Diameter:** Melanomas are typically larger than common moles. While size alone is not a definitive indicator, moles larger than 6 millimeters (about the size of a pencil eraser) should be examined.
5. **Evolution or change in appearance:** Any change in size, shape, color, or elevation, or the development of new symptoms such as bleeding or itching, should be carefully evaluated.

In addition to the ABCDE criteria, the "EFG" rule is sometimes used:

1. **Evolving:** The mole is changing in size, shape, or color.
2. **Firm:** The mole feels hard or lumpy.
3. **Growing:** The mole is increasing in size.

It's important to note that while these criteria are helpful, not all melanomas exhibit all these characteristics, and some benign moles may exhibit similar features. Regular skin self-exams and professional skin checks are crucial for early detection.

If you have concerns about a mole or skin lesion, it's essential to consult with a healthcare professional, preferably a dermatologist, who can perform a thorough examination and, if necessary, order additional tests such as a biopsy for a definitive diagnosis. Early detection and treatment of melanoma are crucial for a better prognosis.

Figure 3. The first author (G.C.) followed up the initial enquiry with another question concerning clinical features useful for suspecting malignant melanoma. ChatGPT provided the ABCDE criteria together with other parameters (detectability, hardness/compactness and lesion growth). The version used was always that of 25 September 2023. ChatGPT had an average response time of 44.32 s.

OK, thank you very much ChatGPT. Now could you please explain to me the histological features of Malignant Melanoma?

Certainly. Malignant melanoma is diagnosed through a biopsy, where a small sample of the suspicious skin lesion is removed and examined under a microscope. The histological features, or the characteristics observed in the tissue at a microscopic level, play a crucial role in confirming the diagnosis of malignant melanoma. Here are some key histological features associated with malignant melanoma:

1. **Nesting and Invasion:** Malignant melanoma often exhibits a nested or "nest within a nest" growth pattern. Melanoma cells can invade surrounding tissues, including the epidermis (the outer layer of the skin) and the dermis (the deeper layer of the skin).
2. **Asymmetry of Melanocytes:** The melanocytes in melanoma are often irregularly distributed and asymmetrical in shape and size. This is in contrast to normal skin, where melanocytes are more evenly distributed.
3. **Cytological Atypia:** Melanoma cells typically show significant variation in size and shape, a feature known as cytological atypia. This atypical appearance is one of the hallmarks of melanoma.
4. **Mitotic Figures:** Mitotic figures, which are indicators of cell division, are often increased in melanoma. The presence of a higher number of mitotic figures suggests a more aggressive and rapidly growing tumor.
5. **Pigment Variation:** Melanomas can exhibit variable pigmentation within the tumor, resulting in areas of dark and light pigmentation. This can be seen on microscopic examination.
6. **Inflammatory Infiltrate:** Inflammatory cells may be present around and within the tumor, reflecting the body's immune response to the malignant cells.
7. **Ulceration:** In some cases, melanomas may ulcerate, meaning there is a breakdown of the overlying skin. Ulceration is associated with a poorer prognosis.

It's important to note that there are different subtypes of malignant melanoma, each with its own histological characteristics. The subtypes include superficial spreading melanoma, nodular melanoma, lentigo maligna melanoma, and acral lentiginous melanoma, among others.

The histological examination is a critical component of the diagnostic process and provides valuable information about the nature of the melanoma, its aggressiveness, and the appropriate course of treatment. If you have concerns about a suspicious skin lesion, it's crucial to consult with a dermatologist or healthcare provider for a thorough evaluation and biopsy if necessary.

Perfect ChatGPT, and could you explain me "balloon cell melanoma"?

"Balloon cell melanoma" is a rare and distinct variant of malignant melanoma characterized by the presence of balloon cells within the tumor. Balloon cells are large, rounded or oval-shaped cells with clear cytoplasm, giving them a balloon-like appearance under the microscope.

Here are some key features associated with balloon cell melanoma:

1. **Cellular Morphology:** The hallmark feature of balloon cell melanoma is the presence of balloon cells, which are large and have a clear or vacuolated cytoplasm. These cells can sometimes be mistaken for other cell types due to their distinctive appearance.
2. **Melanocytic Origin:** Despite the unusual morphology, balloon cell melanoma is still considered a type of malignant melanoma. The tumor arises from melanocytes, the pigment-producing cells in the skin.
3. **Histological Examination:** Diagnosis is confirmed through histological examination of a biopsy specimen. The biopsy allows pathologists to analyze the cellular characteristics,
4. **Clinical Presentation:** Balloon cell melanoma may present as a pigmented lesion on the skin, similar to other forms of melanoma. It can occur in sun-exposed areas or less commonly in areas not typically exposed to sunlight.
5. **Immunohistochemistry:** Special staining techniques, such as immunohistochemistry, may be used to further characterize the tumor cells and confirm their melanocytic origin. Immunohistochemistry involves using antibodies to detect specific proteins, helping to identify the type of cells present in the tissue.

Figure 4. Other answers of ChatGPT to questions proposed by authors.

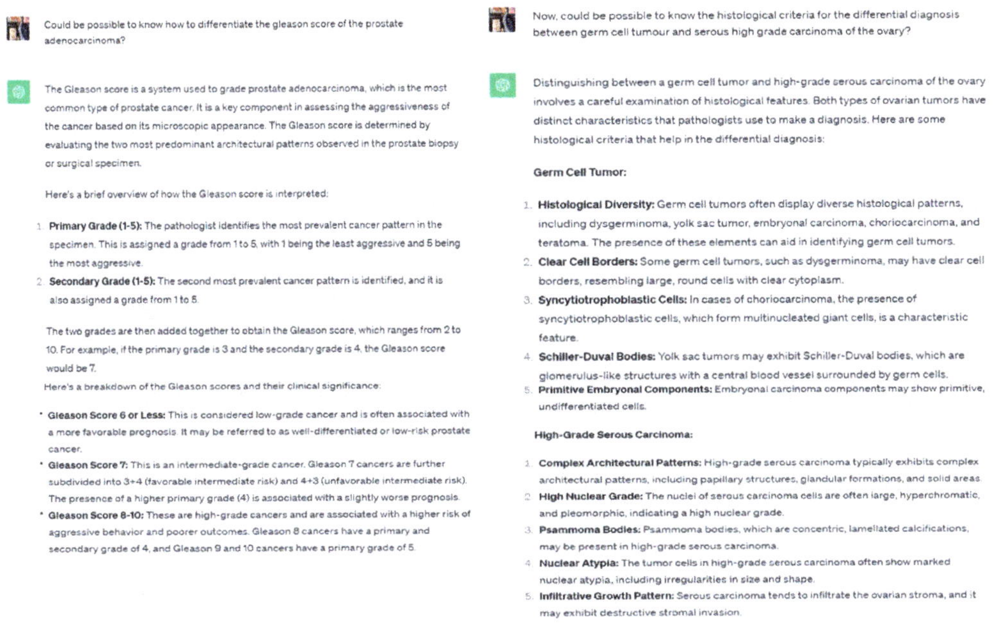
Could be possible to know how to differentiate the gleason score of the prostate adenocarcinoma?

The Gleason score is a system used to grade prostate adenocarcinoma, which is the most common type of prostate cancer. It is a key component in assessing the aggressiveness of the cancer based on its microscopic appearance. The Gleason score is determined by evaluating the two most predominant architectural patterns observed in the prostate biopsy or surgical specimen.

Here's a brief overview of how the Gleason score is interpreted:

1. **Primary Grade (1-5):** The pathologist identifies the most prevalent cancer pattern in the specimen. This is assigned a grade from 1 to 5, with 1 being the least aggressive and 5 being the most aggressive.
2. **Secondary Grade (1-5):** The second most prevalent cancer pattern is identified, and it is also assigned a grade from 1 to 5.

The two grades are then added together to obtain the Gleason score, which ranges from 2 to 10. For example, if the primary grade is 3 and the secondary grade is 4, the Gleason score would be 7.

Here's a breakdown of the Gleason scores and their clinical significance:

- **Gleason Score 6 or Less:** This is considered low-grade cancer and is often associated with a more favorable prognosis. It may be referred to as well-differentiated or low-risk prostate cancer.
- **Gleason Score 7:** This is an intermediate-grade cancer. Gleason 7 cancers are further subdivided into 3+4 (favorable intermediate risk) and 4+3 (unfavorable intermediate risk). The presence of a higher primary grade (4) is associated with a slightly worse prognosis.
- **Gleason Score 8-10:** These are high-grade cancers and are associated with a higher risk of aggressive behavior and poorer outcomes. Gleason 8 cancers have a primary and secondary grade of 4, and Gleason 9 and 10 cancers have a primary grade of 5.

Now, could be possible to know the histological criteria for the differential diagnosis between germ cell tumour and serous high grade carcinoma of the ovary?

Distinguishing between a germ cell tumor and high-grade serous carcinoma of the ovary involves a careful examination of histological features. Both types of ovarian tumors have distinct characteristics that pathologists use to make a diagnosis. Here are some histological criteria that help in the differential diagnosis:

Germ Cell Tumor:

1. **Histological Diversity:** Germ cell tumors often display diverse histological patterns, including dysgerminoma, yolk sac tumor, embryonal carcinoma, choriocarcinoma, and teratoma. The presence of these elements can aid in identifying germ cell tumors.
2. **Clear Cell Borders:** Some germ cell tumors, such as dysgerminoma, may have clear cell borders, resembling large, round cells with clear cytoplasm.
3. **Syncytiotrophoblastic Cells:** In cases of choriocarcinoma, the presence of syncytiotrophoblastic cells, which form multinucleated giant cells, is a characteristic feature.
4. **Schiller-Duval Bodies:** Yolk sac tumors may exhibit Schiller-Duval bodies, which are glomerulus-like structures with a central blood vessel surrounded by germ cells.
5. **Primitive Embryonal Components:** Embryonal carcinoma components may show primitive, undifferentiated cells.

High-Grade Serous Carcinoma:

1. **Complex Architectural Patterns:** High-grade serous carcinoma typically exhibits complex architectural patterns, including papillary structures, glandular formations, and solid areas.
2. **High Nuclear Grade:** The nuclei of serous carcinoma cells are often large, hyperchromatic, and pleomorphic, indicating a high nuclear grade.
3. **Psammoma Bodies:** Psammoma bodies, which are concentric, lamellated calcifications, may be present in high-grade serous carcinoma.
4. **Nuclear Atypia:** The tumor cells in high-grade serous carcinoma often show marked nuclear atypia, including irregularities in size and shape.
5. **Infiltrative Growth Pattern:** Serous carcinoma tends to infiltrate the ovarian stroma, and it may exhibit destructive stromal invasion.

Figure 5. Other query sessions in which the first author (G.C.) ask to ChatGPT "..how to differentiate the gleason score of the prostate adenocarcinoma" and "..to know the histological criteria for the differential diagnosis between germ cell tumour and serous high grade carcinoma of the ovary".

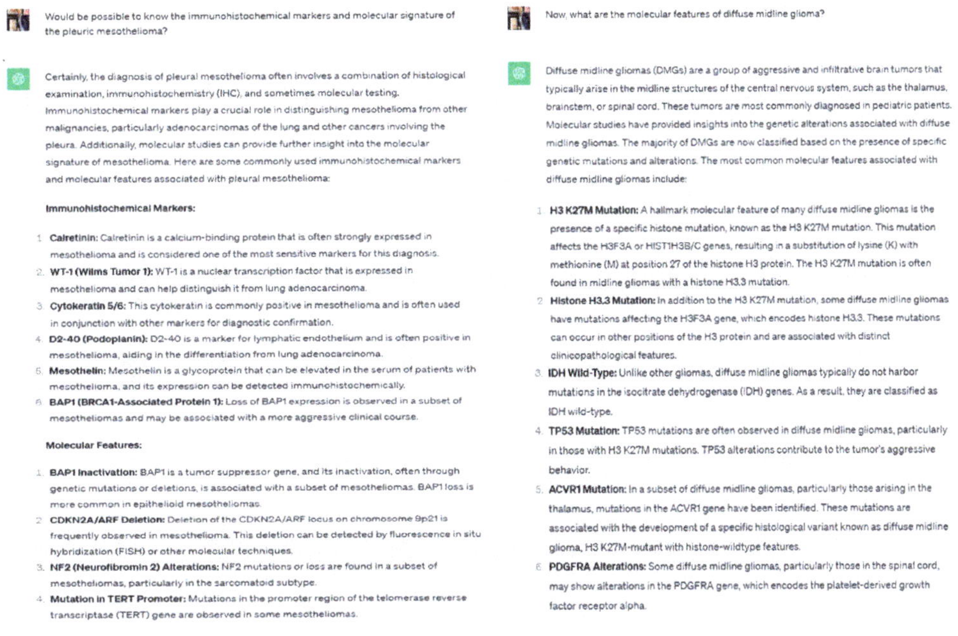
Would be possible to know the immunohistochemical markers and molecular signature of the pleuric mesothelioma?

Certainly, the diagnosis of pleural mesothelioma often involves a combination of histological examination, immunohistochemistry (IHC), and sometimes molecular testing. Immunohistochemical markers play a crucial role in distinguishing mesothelioma from other malignancies, particularly adenocarcinomas of the lung and other cancers involving the pleura. Additionally, molecular studies can provide further insight into the molecular signature of mesothelioma. Here are some commonly used immunohistochemical markers and molecular features associated with pleural mesothelioma:

Immunohistochemical Markers:

1. **Calretinin:** Calretinin is a calcium-binding protein that is often strongly expressed in mesothelioma and is considered one of the most sensitive markers for this diagnosis.
2. **WT-1 (Wilms Tumor 1):** WT-1 is a nuclear transcription factor that is expressed in mesothelioma and can help distinguish it from lung adenocarcinoma.
3. **Cytokeratin 5/6:** This cytokeratin is commonly positive in mesothelioma and is often used in conjunction with other markers for diagnostic confirmation.
4. **D2-40 (Podoplanin):** D2-40 is a marker for lymphatic endothelium and is often positive in mesothelioma, aiding in the differentiation from lung adenocarcinoma.
5. **Mesothelin:** Mesothelin is a glycoprotein that can be elevated in the serum of patients with mesothelioma, and its expression can be detected immunohistochemically.
6. **BAP1 (BRCA1-Associated Protein 1):** Loss of BAP1 expression is observed in a subset of mesotheliomas and may be associated with a more aggressive clinical course.

Molecular Features:

1. **BAP1 Inactivation:** BAP1 is a tumor suppressor gene, and its inactivation, often through genetic mutations or deletions, is associated with a subset of mesotheliomas. BAP1 loss is more common in epithelioid mesotheliomas.
2. **CDKN2A/ARF Deletion:** Deletion of the CDKN2A/ARF locus on chromosome 9p21 is frequently observed in mesothelioma. This deletion can be detected by fluorescence in situ hybridization (FISH) or other molecular techniques.
3. **NF2 (Neurofibromin 2) Alterations:** NF2 mutations or loss are found in a subset of mesotheliomas, particularly in the sarcomatoid subtype.
4. **Mutation in TERT Promoter:** Mutations in the promoter region of the telomerase reverse transcriptase (TERT) gene are observed in some mesotheliomas.

Now, what are the molecular features of diffuse midline glioma?

Diffuse midline gliomas (DMGs) are a group of aggressive and infiltrative brain tumors that typically arise in the midline structures of the central nervous system, such as the thalamus, brainstem, or spinal cord. These tumors are most commonly diagnosed in pediatric patients. Molecular studies have provided insights into the genetic alterations associated with diffuse midline gliomas. The majority of DMGs are now classified based on the presence of specific genetic mutations and alterations. The most common molecular features associated with diffuse midline gliomas include:

1. **H3 K27M Mutation:** A hallmark molecular feature of many diffuse midline gliomas is the presence of a specific histone mutation, known as the H3 K27M mutation. This mutation affects the H3F3A or HIST1H3B/C genes, resulting in a substitution of lysine (K) with methionine (M) at position 27 of the histone H3 protein. The H3 K27M mutation is often found in midline gliomas with a histone H3.3 mutation.
2. **Histone H3.3 Mutation:** In addition to the H3 K27M mutation, some diffuse midline gliomas have mutations affecting the H3F3A gene, which encodes histone H3.3. These mutations can occur in other positions of the H3 protein and are associated with distinct clinicopathological features.
3. **IDH Wild-Type:** Unlike other gliomas, diffuse midline gliomas typically do not harbor mutations in the isocitrate dehydrogenase (IDH) genes. As a result, they are classified as IDH wild-type.
4. **TP53 Mutation:** TP53 mutations are often observed in diffuse midline gliomas, particularly in those with H3 K27M mutations. TP53 alterations contribute to the tumor's aggressive behavior.
5. **ACVR1 Mutation:** In a subset of diffuse midline gliomas, particularly those arising in the thalamus, mutations in the ACVR1 gene have been identified. These mutations are associated with the development of a specific histological variant known as diffuse midline glioma, H3 K27M-mutant with histone-wildtype features.
6. **PDGFRA Alterations:** Some diffuse midline gliomas, particularly those in the spinal cord, may show alterations in the PDGFRA gene, which encodes the platelet-derived growth factor receptor alpha.

Figure 6. Another query session related to immunohistochemical features and molecular characteristics of pleural mesothelioma and to molecular features of pediatric diffuse midline glioma (diffuse intrinsic pontine glioma).

3. Results

A total of 103 records were initially identified in the literature search, of which 19 were duplicates. After screening for eligibility and inclusion criteria, only five publications were ultimately included (Figure 1). The majority of publications were original articles ($n = 2$), followed by a case report ($n = 1$), letter to the editor ($n = 1$) and review ($n = 1$).

Figure 1 summarizes the review process following PRISMA guidelines and Table 1 summarizes the features of the five studies included in our review.

Table 1. Features (name of author, year, number of reference, type of application of ChatGPT, strengths and weaknesses) of ChatGPT in the publication analyzed in our literature review.

Year Authors	Type of Paper	Application of ChatGPT	Strengths	Weakness
Sallam 2023 [12]	Review	Scientific research	Speeding of the review	Erroneous contents
			Computer code generation	Hallucination phenomena
		Medical practice	Simplification of the workflow	Risk of incorrect/inaccurate information
			Improved diagnostics, cost savings, improved health literacy	Transparency and legal issues
				Limited knowledge before 2021
		Health education		Risk of spreading misinformation
				Copyright issues
				Lack of originality
Sinha [14] 2023	Article	Query session of 100 questions	Reasonable level of rationality	Lack of true understanding of the underlying significance and context of the information
Sorin [15] 2023	Article	ChatGPT in a molecular tumor board	Clinical recommendations of ChatGPT in line with those of the oncology committee in 70% of the cases	High difficulty in providing empirical decisions on the therapeutic path
Naik [16] 2023	Case Report	ChatGPT in the setting of clinical management	Provide clinical and pathological information	Allucination phenomena
Yamin MA [17] 2023	Article	ChatGPT in gastrointestinal pathology	Summarize patient records	Risk of inaccurate information
			Incorporation into digital pathology	Allucination phenomena
			Education and research	

Regarding the 'query session', the first question was related to the diagnostical and therapeutical approach in a clinical case of a '32 years-old woman with a pigmented lesion on the thigh'. ChatGPT was able to answer correctly and comprehensively, summarizing the different anamnestic stages peculiar to the case, with a satisfactory explanation of concepts such as dermoscopy, biopsy and main differential diagnosis. Furthermore, ChatGPT cautioned against using this information without proper vetting and validation by an experienced pathologist. We consider this first step very satisfactory (ChatGPT's responses were assessed individually by three reviewers who checked each response to the standardized responses to evaluate the response's consistency. Based on their ranking, responses were classified as either "consistent" or "inconsistent." Throughout the evaluation process, there was strong agreement amongst the three reviewers, guaranteeing a consistent and unbiased assessment of the responses).

Going into more detail, the first author went on to ask ChatGPT: "OK, thank you ChatGPT. Now, could you please explain to me the clinical criteria for suspecting malignant melanoma?" and ChatGPT, in a very performant and correct manner, replied: "Certainly, I can provide you with an overview of the clinical criteria for suspecting malignant melanoma, but please keep in mind that I am not a medical professional, and you should consult with a healthcare professional for personalized advice. The diagnosis and evaluation of skin lesions should be done by a qualified dermatologist or healthcare provider.

Malignant melanoma is a type of skin cancer that arises from melanocytes, the pigment-producing cells in the skin. Detecting melanoma involves assessing various clinical features, often using the ABCDE criteria:

Asymmetry: One half of the mole does not match the other half in terms of shape, size, or color.

Border irregularity: The edges of the mole are not well-defined; they may be uneven, notched, or blurred.

Color variations: Melanomas often have uneven coloring, with different shades of brown, black, or even red, white, or blue.

Diameter: Melanomas are typically larger than common moles. While size alone is not a definitive indicator, moles larger than 6 millimeters (about the size of a pencil eraser) should be examined.

Evolution or change in appearance: Any change in size, shape, color, or elevation, or the development of new symptoms such as bleeding or itching, should be carefully evaluated.

In addition to the ABCDE criteria, the "EFG" rule is sometimes used:

Evolving: The mole is changing in size, shape, or color.

Firm: The mole feels hard or lumpy.

Growing: The mole is increasing in size.

It's important to note that while these criteria are helpful, not all melanomas exhibit all these characteristics, and some benign moles may exhibit similar features. Regular skin self-exams and professional skin checks are crucial for early detection". (see Figure 3 for the rest of ChatGPT's response).

Again, ChatGPT proved to be quite performant and was able to provide correct answers to the appropriate questions (Figure 3).

Finally, the first author asked ChatGPT: "OK, thank you very much ChatGPT. Now could you please explain to me the histological features of Malignant Melanoma?" and ChatGPT replied: "Certainly. Malignant melanoma is diagnosed through a biopsy, where a small sample of the suspicious skin lesion is removed and examined under a microscope. The histological features, or the characteristics observed in the tissue at a microscopic level, play a crucial role in confirming the diagnosis of malignant melanoma. Here are some key histological features associated with malignant melanoma:

Nesting and Invasion: Malignant melanoma often exhibits a nested or "nest within a nest" growth pattern. Melanoma cells can invade surrounding tissues, including the epidermis (the outer layer of the skin) and the dermis (the deeper layer of the skin).

Asymmetry of Melanocytes: The melanocytes in melanoma are often irregularly distributed and asymmetrical in shape and size. This is in contrast to normal skin, where melanocytes are more evenly distributed.

Cytological Atypia: Melanoma cells typically show significant variation in size and shape, a feature known as cytological atypia. This atypical appearance is one of the hallmarks of malignant cells.

Mitotic Figures: Mitotic figures, which are indicators of cell division, are often increased in melanoma. The presence of a higher number of mitotic figures suggests a more aggressive and rapidly growing tumor.

Pigment Variation: Melanomas can exhibit variable pigmentation within the tumor, resulting in areas of dark and light pigmentation. This can be seen on microscopic examination.

Inflammatory Infiltrate: Inflammatory cells may be present around and within the tumor, reflecting the body's immune response to the malignant cells.

Ulceration: In some cases, melanomas may ulcerate, meaning there is a breakdown of the overlying skin. Ulceration is associated with a poorer prognosis.

It's important to note that there are different subtypes of malignant melanoma, each with its own histological characteristics. The subtypes include superficial spreading melanoma, nodular melanoma, lentigo maligna melanoma, and acral lentiginous melanoma, among others.

The histological examination is a critical component of the diagnostic process and provides valuable information about the nature of the melanoma, its aggressiveness, and the appropriate course of treatment. If you have concerns about a suspicious skin lesion, it's crucial to consult with a dermatologist or healthcare provider for a thorough evaluation and biopsy if necessary". Then, G.C. ask to ChatGPT: "Perfect ChatGPT, and could you explain me "balloon cell melanoma"?

ChatGPT

"Balloon cell melanoma" is a rare and distinct variant of malignant melanoma characterized by the presence of balloon cells within the tumor. Balloon cells are large, rounded or oval-shaped cells with clear cytoplasm, giving them a balloon-like appearance under the microscope.

Here are some key features associated with balloon cell melanoma:

Cellular Morphology: The hallmark feature of balloon cell melanoma is the presence of balloon cells, which are large and have a clear or vacuolated cytoplasm. These cells can sometimes be mistaken for other cell types due to their distinctive appearance.

Melanocytic Origin: Despite the unusual morphology, balloon cell melanoma is still considered a type of malignant melanoma. The tumor arises from melanocytes, the pigment-producing cells in the skin.

Histological Examination: Diagnosis is confirmed through histological examination of a biopsy specimen. The biopsy allows pathologists to analyze the cellular characteristics, including the presence of balloon cells, and determine the malignancy of the lesion.

Clinical Presentation: Balloon cell melanoma may present as a pigmented lesion on the skin, similar to other forms of melanoma. It can occur in sun-exposed areas or less commonly in areas not typically exposed to sunlight.

Immunohistochemistry: Special staining techniques, such as immunohistochemistry, may be used to further characterize the tumor cells and confirm their melanocytic origin. Immunohistochemistry involves using antibodies to detect specific proteins, helping to identify the type of cells present in the tissue (Figure 4).

Further, when ChatGPT was asked to provide references on balloon cell melanoma, two non-existent papers were provided (hallucination phenomenon), confirming what had already been reported by several papers previously.

4. Discussion

The application of AI to medicine has significantly co-assisted physicians' therapeutic decision-making processes, not replacing but instead complementing and enhancing the indispensable figure of the human [8]. The advent of ChatGPT has further enabled a breakthrough in Large Language Models (LLM) that enable the simulation of a real conversation on a wide variety of topics, including medical and scientific notions [11].

In a recent paper by Sallam [12], the various advantages and limitations of using ChatGPT in areas such as scientific research, practice and health education were analyzed. In particular, scientific research could really benefit from a useful and powerful tool such as ChatGPT by speeding up the process of literature reviews and computer code generation, allowing the human user to focus more on experimental design [13,18–21]; on the other hand, several authors [13,19,22] have highlighted issues of reliability of the data provided by ChatGPT with the generation of erroneous and/or inaccurate content, phenomena of 'hallucination' (by which is meant the generation of erroneous content but which can be considered plausible from a scientific point of view [23]) and the bias of the answers provided by ChatGPT, which is a reflection of the dataset used in training [12]. Finally, it is important to consider that ChatGPT may generate nonexistent references, as pointed out by Chen T.J. [24] and Lubowitz [25].

If in the early months the field of application was mostly restricted to clinical medicine, in recent times a number of papers have studied, tested and commented on the applicability of Chat GPT in the field of human pathology, making it possible to outline its real usefulness and current limitations.

The article by Sinha et al. [14] describes a study conducted on ChatGPT's ability to resolve complex rationality problems in the area of human pathology. Based on the clear finding that AI is used to analyze medical images, such as histopathologic slides, in order to identify and diagnose diseases with high precision, the authors take a cautious approach to the fact that NLP algorithms are used to analyze the relationships between pathologies, extract relevant information and aid in disease diagnosis. The goal of the study was to assess ChatGPT's ability to address high-level rational questions in the field of pathology. One hundred questions that were randomly chosen from a bank of inquiries regarding diseases and divided into 11 different systems of pathology were used. Experts have evaluated the responses provided by ChatGPT using both a scale of 0 to 5 and the tassonomy SOLE to assess the depth of understanding demonstrated in the responses.

The outcomes have shown that the responses provided by ChatGPT achieve a reasonable level of rationality, with a score of four or five. This means that AI is capable of correctly responding to high-level inquiries requiring in-depth knowledge of the subject. The report also highlights the limitations of AI in diagnosing diseases. Although it is possible to recognize schemes and categorize data, a true understanding of the underlying significance and context of the information is lacking. AI is unable to make logical judgements or evaluative decisions because it lacks the ability to comprehend personal values and judgements. Therefore, it is suggested that careful consideration should be given to the use of AI in medical education, with the goal of assisting human judgement rather than replacing it.

There are some limitations to the study, including the subjective nature of the evaluation procedure and the selection of particular questions from a single bank of data. The authors suggest that in order to obtain results that are more generally applicable, future studies may be conducted on a larger sample size and by a variety of institutions.

In the paper by Sorin V. et al. [15], the authors discuss how ChatGPT 3.5 can also operate within the molecular tumor board, not only starting from histopathological/diagnostic data, but also integrating other key components such as the genetic or molecular response and/or prediction of treatment response and prognosis data. Ten consecutive cases of women with breast cancer were considered and an attempt was made to assess how consistent the recommendations provided by the chatbot were with those of the tumor board. The results showed that ChatGPT's clinical recommendations were in line with those of the oncology committee in 70% of the cases, with concise clinical case summaries and explained and reasoned conclusions. However, the lowest scores (which were given by the second reviewer) were for the clinical recommendations of the chatbot, suggesting that deciding on clinical treatment from pathological/molecular data is highly challenging, requiring medical understanding and experience in the field. Furthermore, it was curious to note that ChatGPT never mentioned the role of medical radiologists, suggesting that incomplete training (and the consequent risk of bias) may influence the performance, and thus the responses, of the chatbot.

In another recent paper by Naik H.R. et al. [16], the authors described the case of a 58-year-old woman with bilateral synchronous breast cancer (s-BBC) who underwent bilateral mastectomy, sentinel lymph node biopsy (BLS), axillary lymphadenectomy with adjuvant radiotherapy and chemo/hormonotherapy. The particularity of the paper was related to the so-called 'hallucination phenomenon', i.e., a clear and confident response from ChatGPT but which is not real. One of the authors of the paper (Dr. Gurda), when asking the chatbot about s-BBC, noted that although the answer was plausible, the reference provided did not exist, although there were articles with similar information and authors.

This aspect is well addressed by the paper by Metze K. et al. [26], who conducted a study to assess the ability of ChatGPT to contribute to a review on Chagas disease, focusing on the role of individual researchers. Therefore, 50 names of researchers with at least four publications on Chagas disease were selected from Clarivate's Web of Science (WoS) database and for each researcher, the chatbot was asked to provide conceptual contributions related to the study of the disease. The answers were checked by two observers against the literature and incorrect information was removed. The percentage of correct words in the text generated by ChatGPT was calculated and the literature references were classified into three categories: completely correct, minor errors and major errors.

The results showed that the average percentage of correct words in the text generated by ChatGPT was 59.4% but the variation was wide, ranging from 10.0% to 100.0%. A positive correlation was observed between the percentage of correct words and the number of indexed publications of each author of interest, as well as with the number of citations and the author's H-index. However, the percentage of correct references was very low, averaging 7.07%, and both minor and major errors were found in the references.

In conclusion, the results of this study suggest that ChatGPT is still not a reliable source for literature reviews, especially in more specific areas with a relatively low number of publications, as there are still accuracy and misinformation issues to be addressed, especially in the field of medicine.

Yamin Ma [17], in a paper of July 2023, discusses the application of ChatGPT in the context of gastrointestinal pathology, hypothesizing three possible applications for ChatGPT:

(1) Ability to summarize patient records: ChatGPT could be integrated into the patent table to summarize patients' previous clinical information, helping pathologists better understand patients' current health status and saving time before case reviews.
(2) Incorporation into digital pathology: ChatGPT could improve the interpretation of computer-aided diagnosis (CAD) systems in gastrointestinal pathology. It would enable pathologists to ask specific questions on digitized images and obtain knowledge-based answers associated with diagnostic criteria and differential diagnosis.
(3) Role in education and research: ChatGPT could be used for health education, offering scientific explanations associated with medical terms in pathology. However, attention should be paid to the quality of the training data to avoid biased content and inaccurate information. The use of ChatGPT in research also requires caution as it may be insufficient or misleading.

Finally, the paper emphasizes that while recognizing the potential of ChatGPT, it is important to proceed with caution when using artificial intelligence-based technologies such as ChatGPT in gastrointestinal pathology. The aim should be to integrate such language models in a regulated and appropriate manner, exploiting their advantages to improve the quality of healthcare without replacing human expertise and without ignoring expert consultation in particular cases.

From what has been discussed so far and bearing in mind a paper published a few days ago [13], it would appear that at present, the use of ChatGPT in pathology is still in its early stages. In particular, with regard to ChatGPT version 3.5, it seems clear that the amount of data on which the algorithm has been trained plays a key role in its ability to provide correct answers to certain prompts. In particular, several papers have warned of the risk of possible bias and transparency issues [27,28] and of damage resulting from inaccurate or outright incorrect content [29–32]. One of the most problematic phenomena is hallucination, as ChatGPT seems, at present, to produce correct scientific content but not to direct the content itself to a real source/reference. Therefore, its use in pathology and, more generally, in scientific research must necessarily take these limitations into account [33].

Furthermore, it is important to say that there is need for a new framework on publication/authorship ethics in a new age of AI-sourced digital composition; it is always important to address the hallucination phenomena with a check of the user.

From an ethical point of view, it is very important to understand the issue of patients' private data, and if the use of medical clinical records is necessary, it will be important to find a way of protecting patient information.

Future Roadmaps

As highlighted in the work of Schukow et al. [13], it is imperative to outline future perspectives that the implementation of AI models will bring to the fore; first of all, it is important to consider how the use of AI methods applied to the writing of scientific articles will be managed, how to address the issue of consent and whether to modify the editorial lines of journals taking into account the use of chatbots. Secondly, it is very important to understand how ChatGPT can impact the possible option of specialization in pathological anatomy (increase or reduction) and how and to what extent there will be a need for a critical review of AI-generated content and whether or not the role of teacher/mentor can be delegated to ChatGPT.

Projecting to a future in which such systems may become more active, their integration with clinical, genetic, anamnestic, morphological and immunohistochemical data, which have always been key to pathologists' roles, will have to be screened by professionals with medical experience and knowledge, which are areas in which ChatGPT struggles the most.

Author Contributions: Conceptualization, G.C. (Gerardo Cazzato) and M.C.; methodology, G.C. (Gerardo Cazzato), F.A. and E.M.; software, G.C. (Gerardo Cazzato), F.A. and V.L.; validation, G.C. (Gerardo Cazzato), M.C., A.M. and G.I.; formal analysis, P.P. and A.M.; investigation, G.C. (Gerardo Cazzato); resources, G.C. (Gerardo Cazzato); data curation, G.C. (Gerardo Cazzato); writing—original draft preparation, G.C. (Gerardo Cazzato); writing—review and editing, G.C. (Gerardo Cazzato) and G.C. (Gennaro Cormio); visualization, G.I.; supervision, P.P., G.C. (Gennaro Cormio) and G.I. All authors have read and agreed to the published version of the manuscript.

Funding: This research received no external funding.

Institutional Review Board Statement: Not applicable.

Informed Consent Statement: Not applicable.

Data Availability Statement: Not applicable.

Conflicts of Interest: The authors declare no conflict of interest.

References

1. Xiang, Y.; Zhao, L.; Liu, Z.; Wu, X.; Chen, J.; Long, E.; Lin, D.; Zhu, Y.; Chen, C.; Lin, Z.; et al. Implementation of artificial intelligence in medicine: Status analysis and development suggestions. *Artif. Intell. Med.* **2020**, *102*, 101780. [CrossRef]
2. Haug, C.J.; Drazen, J.M. Artificial Intelligence and Machine Learning in Clinical Medicine, 2023. *N. Engl. J. Med.* **2023**, *30*, 1201–1208. [CrossRef] [PubMed]
3. Venerito, V.; Angelini, O.; Cazzato, G.; Lopalco, G.; Maiorano, E.; Cimmino, A.; Iannone, F. A convolutional neural network with transfer learning for automatic discrimination between low and high-grade synovitis: A pilot study. *Intern. Emerg. Med.* **2021**, *16*, 1457–1465. [CrossRef] [PubMed]
4. Eysenbach, G. The Role of ChatGPT, Generative Language Models, and Artificial Intelligence in Medical Education: A Conversation with ChatGPT and a Call for Papers. *JMIR Med. Educ.* **2023**, *9*, e46885. [CrossRef]
5. Bozic, J.; Tazl, O.A.; Wotawa, F. Chatbot Testing Using AI Planning. In Proceedings of the 2019 IEEE International Conference on Artificial Intelligence Testing (AITest), Newark, CA, USA, 4–9 April 2019; pp. 37–44. [CrossRef]
6. Adamopoulou, E.; Moussiades, L. An Overview of Chatbot Technology. *Artif. Intell. Appl. Innov.* **2020**, *584*, 373–383. [CrossRef]
7. Okonkwo, C.W.; Ade-Ibijola, A. Chatbots applications in education: A systematic review. *Comput. Educ. Artif. Intell.* **2021**, *2*, 100033. [CrossRef]
8. Khan, R.A.; Jawaid, M.; Khan, A.R.; Sajjad, M. ChatGPT-Reshaping medical education and clinical management. *Pak. J. Med. Sci.* **2023**, *39*, 605–607. [CrossRef]
9. Caldarini, G.; Jaf, S.; McGarry, K. A Literature Survey of Recent Advances in Chatbots. *Information* **2022**, *13*, 41. [CrossRef]

10. Panch, T.; Pearson-Stuttard, J.; Greaves, F.; Atun, R. Artificial intelligence: Opportunities and risks for public health. *Lancet Digit. Health* **2019**, *1*, e13–e14, Erratum in *Lancet Digit. Health* **2019**, *1*, e113. [CrossRef]
11. Mago, J.; Sharma, M. The Potential Usefulness of ChatGPT in Oral and Maxillofacial Radiology. *Cureus* **2023**, *15*, e42133. [CrossRef]
12. Sallam, M. ChatGPT Utility in Healthcare Education, Research, and Practice: Systematic Review on the Promising Perspectives and Valid Concerns. *Healthcare* **2023**, *11*, 887. [CrossRef] [PubMed]
13. Schukow, C.; Smith, S.C.; Landgrebe, E.; Parasuraman, S.; Folaranmi, O.O.; Paner, G.P.; Amin, M.B. Application of ChatGPT in Routine Diagnostic Pathology: Promises, Pitfalls, and Potential Future Directions. *Adv. Anat. Pathol.* **2023**, *27*, 406. [CrossRef] [PubMed]
14. Sinha, R.K.; Deb Roy, A.; Kumar, N.; Mondal, H. Applicability of ChatGPT in Assisting to Solve Higher Order Problems in Pathology. *Cureus* **2023**, *15*, e35237. [CrossRef] [PubMed]
15. Sorin, V.; Klang, E.; Sklair-Levy, M.; Cohen, I.; Zippel, D.B.; Balint Lahat, N.; Konen, E.; Barash, Y. Large language model (ChatGPT) as a support tool for breast tumor board. *NPJ Breast Cancer* **2023**, *9*, 44. [CrossRef] [PubMed]
16. Naik, H.R.; Prather, A.D.; Gurda, G.T. Synchronous Bilateral Breast Cancer: A Case Report Piloting and Evaluating the Implementation of the AI-Powered Large Language Model (LLM) ChatGPT. *Cureus* **2023**, *15*, e37587. [CrossRef]
17. Ma, Y. The potential application of ChatGPT in gastrointestinal pathology. *Gastroenterol. Endosc.* **2023**, *1*, 130–131. [CrossRef]
18. Nature editorial Tools such as ChatGPT threaten transparent science; here are our ground rules for their use. *Nature* **2023**, *613*, 612. [CrossRef]
19. Moons, P.; Van Bulck, L. ChatGPT: Can artificial intelligence language models be of value for cardiovascular nurses and allied health professionals. *Eur. J. Cardiovasc. Nurs.* **2023**, *22*, e55–e59. [CrossRef]
20. Biswas, S. ChatGPT and the Future of Medical Writing. *Radiology* **2023**, *307*, e223312. [CrossRef]
21. Lund, B.; Wang, S. Chatting about ChatGPT: How may AI and GPT impact academia and libraries? *Library Hi Tech News* **2023**, *40*, 26–29. [CrossRef]
22. The Lancet Digital Health. ChatGPT: Friend or foe? *Lancet Digit. Health* **2023**, *5*, e112–e114. [CrossRef]
23. Cascella, M.; Montomoli, J.; Bellini, V.; Bignami, E. Evaluating the Feasibility of ChatGPT in Healthcare: An Analysis of Multiple Clinical and Research Scenarios. *J. Med. Syst.* **2023**, *47*, 33. [CrossRef] [PubMed]
24. Chen, T.J. ChatGPT and Other Artificial Intelligence Applications Speed up Scientific Writing. *J. Chin. Med. Assoc.* **2023**, *86*, 351–353. [CrossRef] [PubMed]
25. Lubowitz, J. ChatGPT, An Artificial Intelligence Chatbot, Is Impacting Medical Literature. *Arthroscopy* **2023**, *39*, 1121–1122. [CrossRef]
26. Metze, K.; Morandin-Reis, R.C.; Lorand-Metze, I.; Florindo, J.B. The Amount of Errors in ChatGPT's Responses is Indirectly Correlated with the Number of Publications Related to the Topic Under Investigation. *Ann. Biomed. Eng.* **2023**, *51*, 1360–1361. [CrossRef]
27. Holzinger, A.; Keiblinger, K.; Holub, P.; Zatloukal, K.; Müller, H. AI for life: Trends in artificial intelligence for biotechnology. *New Biotechnol.* **2023**, *74*, 16–24. [CrossRef]
28. Jeblick, K.; Schachtner, B.; Dexl, J.; Mittermeier, A.; Stuber, A.T.; Topalis, J.; Weber, T.; Wesp, P.; Sabel, B.; Ricke, J.; et al. ChatGPT Makes Medicine Easy to Swallow: An Exploratory Case Study on Simplified Radiology Reports. *arXiv* **2022**, arXiv:2212.14882. [CrossRef]
29. Ahn, C. Exploring ChatGPT for information of cardiopulmonary resuscitation. *Resuscitation* **2023**, *185*, 109729. [CrossRef]
30. D'Amico, R.S.; White, T.G.; Shah, H.A.; Langer, D.J. I Asked a ChatGPT to Write an Editorial About How We Can Incorporate Chatbots into Neurosurgical Research and Patient Care. *Neurosurgery* **2023**, *92*, 663–664. [CrossRef]
31. Patel, S.B.; Lam, K. ChatGPT: The future of discharge summaries? *Lancet Digit. Health* **2023**, *5*, e107–e108. [CrossRef]
32. Ali, S.R.; Dobbs, T.D.; Hutchings, H.A.; Whitaker, I.S. Using ChatGPT to write patient clinic letters. *Lancet Digit. Health* **2023**, *5*, e179–e181. [CrossRef] [PubMed]
33. Goddard, J. Hallucinations in ChatGPT: A Cautionary Tale for Biomedical Researchers. *Am. J. Med.* **2023**, *136*, 1059–1060. [CrossRef] [PubMed]

Disclaimer/Publisher's Note: The statements, opinions and data contained in all publications are solely those of the individual author(s) and contributor(s) and not of MDPI and/or the editor(s). MDPI and/or the editor(s) disclaim responsibility for any injury to people or property resulting from any ideas, methods, instructions or products referred to in the content.

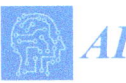

Article

Design of an Educational Chatbot Using Artificial Intelligence in Radiotherapy

James C. L. Chow [1,2,*], Leslie Sanders [3] and Kay Li [4]

1. Radiation Medicine Program, Princess Margaret Cancer Centre, University Health Network, Toronto, ON M5G 1X6, Canada
2. Department of Radiation Oncology, University of Toronto, Toronto, ON M5T 1P5, Canada
3. Department of Humanities, York University, Toronto, ON M3J 1P3, Canada
4. Department of English, University of Toronto, Toronto, ON M5R 0A3, Canada
* Correspondence: james.chow@rmp.uhn.ca; Tel.: +1-416-946-4501

Abstract: *Context*: In cancer centres and hospitals particularly during the pandemic, there was a great demand for information, which could hardly be handled by the limited manpower available. This necessitated the development of an educational chatbot to disseminate topics in radiotherapy customized for various user groups, such as patients and their families, the general public and radiation staff. *Objective*: In response to the clinical demands, the objective of this work is to explore how to design a chatbot for educational purposes in radiotherapy using artificial intelligence. *Methods*: The chatbot is designed using the dialogue tree and layered structure, incorporated with artificial intelligence features such as natural language processing (NLP). This chatbot can be created in most platforms such as the IBM Watson Assistant and deposited in a website or various social media. *Results*: Based on the question-and-answer approach, the chatbot can provide humanlike communication to users requesting information on radiotherapy. At times, the user, often worried, may not be able to pinpoint the question exactly. Thus, the chatbot will be user friendly and reassuring, offering a list of questions for the user to select. The NLP system helps the chatbot to predict the intent of the user so as to provide the most accurate and precise response to him or her. It is found that the preferred educational features in a chatbot are functional features such as mathematical operations, which should be updated and modified routinely to provide new contents and features. *Conclusions*: It is concluded that an educational chatbot can be created using artificial intelligence to provide information transfer to users with different backgrounds in radiotherapy. In addition, testing and evaluating the performance of the chatbot is important, in response to user's feedback to further upgrade and fine-tune the chatbot.

Keywords: artificial intelligence; machine learning; natural language processing; chatbot; radiotherapy; Internet of Things; healthcare

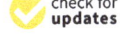

Citation: Chow, J.C.L.; Sanders, L.; Li, K. Design of an Educational Chatbot Using Artificial Intelligence in Radiotherapy. *AI* **2023**, *4*, 319–332. https://doi.org/10.3390/ai4010015

Academic Editor: Tim Hulsen

Received: 6 January 2023
Revised: 14 February 2023
Accepted: 28 February 2023
Published: 2 March 2023

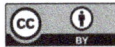

Copyright: © 2023 by the authors. Licensee MDPI, Basel, Switzerland. This article is an open access article distributed under the terms and conditions of the Creative Commons Attribution (CC BY) license (https://creativecommons.org/licenses/by/4.0/).

1. Introduction

User interfaces in computer applications can be in different forms such as graphical user interfaces, command lines, menu driven, form based and natural language [1,2]. Recent development of computer technology, Internet of Things (IoT) and artificial intelligence (AI) generated more advanced interfaces such as chatbots and virtual reality [3–5]. A chatbot is a software application designed to replace humans to provide user communication through an on-line chat conversation. Our research team proposes that there is a need to make the chatbot humanlike, by simulating the ways a human would behave and respond in the user conversation, especially when covering emotional and sensitive topics [6–8]. The chatbot is talking to real human beings, often worried and in distress. A chatbot should not just be vocalizing the written content available on a website. It should be constructed like a fictional character in literature, to whom the user can feel connected, who can be a reassuring voice in times of need. We named our chatbot the RT Bot.

Technically, the RT Bot has the necessary features, complete with routine testing, turning and updates necessary to pass the standard of the Turing test [9,10]. Nowadays, a chatbot in any domain is very popular as a virtual assistant to answer questions from users in business, industry and healthcare [11–13].

First, the RT Bot must be loaded with the necessary information. It is not just reading out information regarding cancer health that can be found in cancer centre or hospital websites. Such websites usually provide a list of topics which are neither interactive nor offer any personal touches, in attempting to understand the concerns of the users. Cancer patients, families and practitioners, on the other hand, are in challenging, often stressful, situations, wanting to access accurate information as efficiently as possible. On top of this, there is seldom any information specifically on radiotherapy, despite the large number of cancer patients, especially those with advanced stage (metastatic) disease that have to go through this process. Having "someone" with professional knowledge who can "listen" to them, provide the medical information with good will and encouragement goes a long way to help patients and families struggling with death [14,15]. As it is quite impossible to have real medical professionals to stand by around the clock to answer questions especially during the pandemic period, an educational chatbot would be essential to disseminate health information to the users. For example, the radiation treatment process is often a black box for cancer patients and families. They may scramble for answers everywhere, from visits to libraries, to Google search, asking Siri, or posting their questions to WhatsApp groups. However, they may not be getting the sort of accurate information they need. Recent innovative computer technology and technique such as IoT and AI apps in mobile devices can be used to provide the information about radiotherapy needed by patients and their families [16,17]. However, these still need to be customized to be relevant to the user's query.

The performance of a chatbot can be enhanced by AI, which makes the chatbot more powerful than a conventional website and Google searches, because the machine learns from the user's request and improves its knowledge base with each interaction [11]. It is situational, providing answers specific to the situations and environment of the query [18]. Machine learning (ML) and natural language processing (NLP) are two branches of AI generating the chatbot. Machine learning can read text to discern the sentiment of the user through natural language understanding [19]. The NLP applications try to understand natural human communication and respond to the user using a similar and natural language [20]. Machine learning is used to understand vast nuances in human language and to learn to answer in a way that the user is likely to comprehend. The innovation in AI through powerful ML algorithms and NLP can enable the chatbot to hold conversations with the user without too much human intervention.

Medical chatbots can carry out different functionalities. In cancer treatment, Bibault et al. [21] have investigated and found that chatbots can create bi-directional information exchange with patients, which could be leveraged for the treatment process, screening and follow-up. This AI-assisted chatbot can be deployed over various modalities such as text messaging, mobile applications and chat rooms. In healthcare, Chung et al. [22] proposed a chatbot-based healthcare service with a knowledgebase for cloud computing. They proposed a mobile health service based on a chatbot in response to accidents or change of conditions of patients with chronic disease, which may occur in everyday life. Lokman et al. [23] designed a chatbot that can function as a virtual diabetes physician. The chatbot allows diabetic patients to have diabetes management advice without going to the hospital. Hajare et al. [24], on the other hand, proposed a chatbot that not only can answer each and every query asked by the end user, but also focuses on a local database as well as a web database for educational purposes. The chatbot is built making use of the most recent technologies such as ML, NLP, pattern matching, data processing algorithms to enhance the performance. Setiaji et al. [25] draws attention to a human-to-machine conversation model using knowledge in a database. This chatbot includes a core and an interface that accesses that core in relational database management systems. The database stores the knowledge, and the interpreter stores the programs of function and procedure sets for pattern-matching requirements. The above AI-assisted chatbots in medicine show that the main challenges are to train the chatbot to understand the context of the user, to learn how the chatbot handles open-ended or unstructured inputs from the user, especially about emotional or sensitive topics.

In this paper, we present the design of an educational chatbot for different kinds of users: cancer patients and their families, general public and radiation staff working in the cancer centre or hospital. We will cover the different stages of design, including defining the problem, creating conversational flow, chatbot training, testing and evaluation, maintaining and updating. We also discuss the programming and implementation issues we encountered when creating the educational chatbot in radiotherapy. The objective of the chatbot is to conduct a basic and comprehensive information transfer from the chatbot provider to the user regarding simple knowledge in radiotherapy, customized for different kinds of users. The chatbot is designed taking advantage of some AI features such as NLP and informed by communication strategies for the targeted audience.

2. Materials and Methods

2.1. Overview of the Workflow

2.1.1. Identification of User Group

First, the scope of the project has to be defined by identifying the types of potential users and their needs. Such information can be gathered through workshops, meetings and conferences. In radiotherapy, the user groups may include the radiation staff working in the cancer centre, cancer patients, and people from the general public including the patient's family members. After understanding their needs, a chatbot can be created to address the issues. The chatbot is designed to simulate conversation with different kinds of human users through the internet. Figure 1 shows an example of the basic workflow of the chatbot. In Figure 1, the chatbot begins with questions identifying the user. The user may be a radiation staff member such as a radiotherapist or medical physicist looking for specific radiation treatment information in their fields (e.g., radiation safety), or a patient or his/her family member looking for general information about a specific radiation treatment process (e.g., external beam radiotherapy). Both groups of users have their specific needs. For example, radiation staff may want to confirm some specific rules and policies in radiation safety [26], while patients may want to understand some basic terms in external beam radiotherapy [27]. Therefore, it is necessary to classify and direct the user into his or her groups linked to the related database.

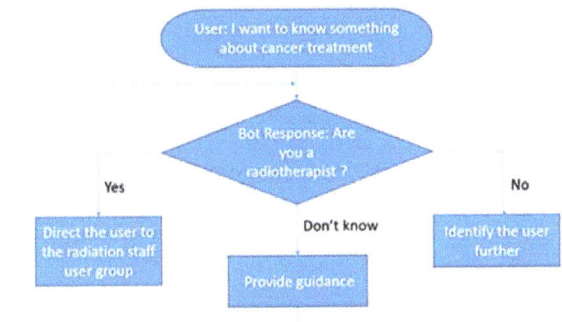

Figure 1. An example of the basic workflow of a chatbot.

The basic conversional flow for the chatbot is shown in Figure 1, when the user asks the chatbot what information about cancer treatment he wants to know. Then the chatbot will start to identify and categorize the user: e.g., a radiotherapist. If the answer is yes, the chatbot will direct the user to the staff user group. If the answer is no, further identification will follow. When the user finds it difficult to answer such a question, the chatbot will provide guidance or a choice. Such an initial communication approach through Q and A also builds the connection between the chatbot and the user. From the responses of the user, the chatbot tries to predict the type of information the user is looking for. This involves creating a set of intents, entities and actions that the chatbot will be able to recognize and respond to. In case the user cannot answer well or the chatbot cannot understand the response from the user, guidance will be provided by the chatbot to help the user to focus. The application of AI can help the chatbot to predict the response (intent) from the user accurately and provide more humanlike conversation.

2.1.2. Identification of Different Scenarios

The chatbot will put on a different persona with respect to the user's group. It first identifies the user's needs and then follows a suitable scenario tailored to the user based on the needs. To create an educational chatbot in radiotherapy, we use three user groups in the pilot, namely, patient and family, general public, and radiation staff or student. The approach and response of the chatbot as per each scenario to the user are different. For example, if the user is identified as a patient, the chatbot will act as a friend or mentor with friendly wording for the user. However, if the user is a radiation staff member, the chatbot will act professionally like an assistant trying to provide the requested information accurately, quickly and precisely. The scenarios can be a cancer patient looking for information about brain surgery, a user from the general public looking for information about breast cancer screening, or a medical physicist looking for dosimetric data on radiation beams. The chatbot needs to be trained with the data in the scenario of each user group, including both the input and expected output. Then the chatbot can understand and respond to different users appropriately. These scenarios can be identified by healthcare providers and clinical workers based on their experiences through interviews, meetings or workshops. If the chatbot cannot communicate to the user due to unexpected or unstructured wording, guidance will be provided by the chatbot to help the user. This guidance will be included in the script and workflow of the chatbot. Any unanswered questions will be added to a corpus of questions to be used to train the chatbot, so that it can become smarter with ML. This iterative approach is necessary, using what we learn from the former session to influence the inputs for the subsequent session. Improving the chatbot through iterations has the advantage of delivering the chatbot quickly, and while it is undergoing continuous improvement.

2.1.3. Communication Framework with Dialogue Tree and Layered Approach

The chatbot is designed using two phases of a communication framework. The first phase considers structured questions and answers based on the scenarios for patients and family, the general public and radiation staff. This means proceeding with a set of questions and answers like multiple choices, but with tips and feedback from the chatbot. This minimizes human monitoring and maximizes usage. In the second phase, after identifying the popular scenarios for each of the three user groups, the chatbot is added with the ability to answer open-ended questions asked by the users. This phase allows AI to learn from the Q and A through ML. We need to do this in Phase 2 after identifying the most needed scenarios in Phase 1 and build sufficiently substantial big data to train the chatbot in Phase 2 [26,27].

In the interaction logic of Phase 1, the user can select related items step by step as per his or her needs and finally acquire the information. For example, the chatbot first identifies the user's background as shown in Figure 2a. When the user selects the user group, a list of items will be provided. The list is based on the scenarios previously identified for the user group. For example, the general public likely wants to know information about cancer statistics, healthy life style and cancer screening, while radiation staff may want to know information about the radiotherapy process, radiation safety and so on. If the user is a patient and selects "Cancer sites", then a further breakdown of the item will be followed as shown in Figure 2b. The chatbot will ask the user which cancer sites he or she is interested in. A list of cancer sites such as brain, head-and-neck, breast and so on is shown to the user for selection. In this case, if the user selects "Brain", then further breakdown of such an item will be shown in Figure 2c. In the list, the user can select which category regarding brain cancer he or she wants to know about. If "Brain Radiotherapy" is selected, the chatbot will provide information related to such a topic. This is different from websites as this works through Q and A with the chatbot.

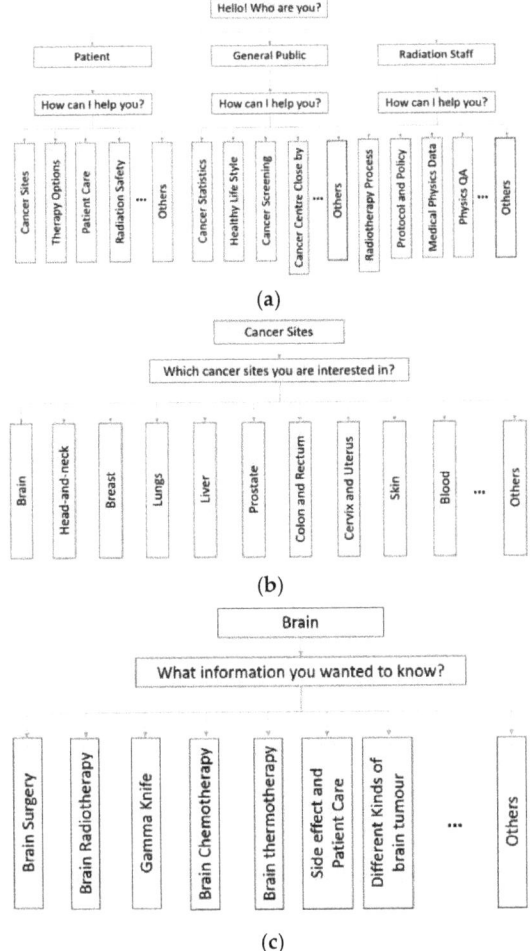

Figure 2. The interaction logic of the chatbot when the user (**a**) is identified in the "Patient" group and (**b**) selects to know information in "Cancer Sites" and then (**c**) wants to know information regarding the "Brain" site. The box in blue represents the enquiry from the chatbot and the box in green represents the selection of the user.

In Phase 1, for example, the interaction logic of the chatbot starts with a brief introduction and asks what it can help the user with (e.g., Figure 3: "Hello! I am RT Bot. How can I help you?"). The chatbot can answer most direct questions regarding radiotherapy such as "What is radiotherapy?" typed in by the user as shown in Figure 3. After answering, the chatbot follows if the user wants to know the definition of radiotherapy or how it works.

However, if the chatbot does not understand the user's text, a systematic guidance will be provided to the user as a structured Q and A set.

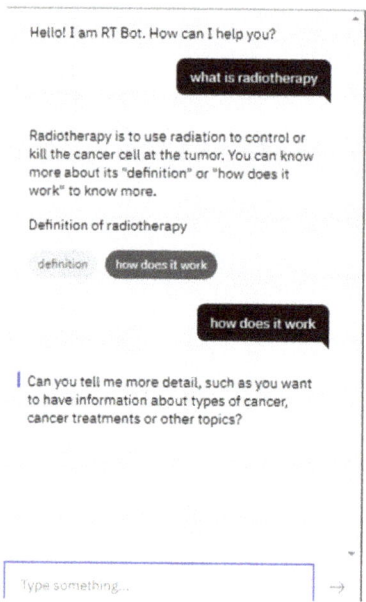

Figure 3. Chatbot in conversation to answer the question: "What is radiotherapy" from the user. In addition to the answer, the chatbot will provide further guidance, adding if the user would like to know more.

2.2. Artificial Intelligence used in Chatbot

The architectural diagram of the chatbot created on the IBM Watson Assistant platform can be seen in Figure 4. The chatbot is created by the Watson Assistant and can be integrated into social media or customized IoTs such as cell phones. The Watson Assistant provides AI features such as NLP and is linked to the IBM Cloud. The Cloud is further connected to other Watson services such as speech to text conversation and the backend systems.

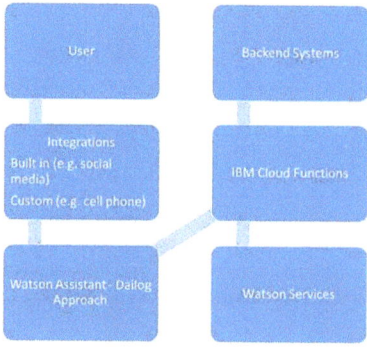

Figure 4. Architectural diagram showing how the chatbot is connected to the IBM Cloud platform.

The chatbot is powered by AI, which analyses the user's response, breaking down the text or speech to work out rules and recognize patterns. This means with the application of ML, the chatbot can convert the user's response into a structured format. One ML tool used in chatbots is the NLP technology which is included in various chatbot development platforms such as the IBM Watson Assistant [28,29]. The NLP includes pattern matching and linguistic analysis. For example, the IBM Watson Assistant can specifically recognize keywords from the user's response and weigh them to determine the intent of the sentence. This is then cross-referenced with the database of intents to evaluate the response that the chatbot can provide.

When the chatbot is communicating with the user using the Q and A approach, the questions are integrated individually into the dialogue nodes. While each node is self-contained, it also leads to the next question. The dialogue tool provides the user with the ability to access the dialogue tree. This allows the tree to control the dialogue nodes completely. The dialogue tree of the IBM Watson Assistant is shown in Figure 5. At a given node, such as the "Welcome" node in Figure 5, the user can give a variety of responses. In the Watson Assistant platform, for example, it is possible to set the response variation to either random, sequential, or multiline. To create a general flow of the dialogue tree, each node has an option button allowing the chatbot developer to add a new node either below or above it. Each node also has an option to have child nodes and this is important considering there are various ways that a user can answer a question.

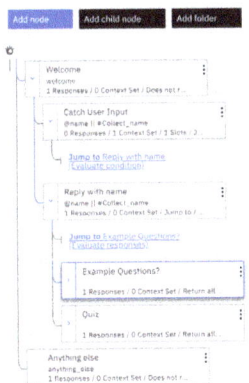

Figure 5. An example of the dialogue tree created by the IBM Watson Assistant.

A powerful tool provided by the IBM Watson Assistant to build the chatbot is the Intent, which allows the chatbot to process the user input and predict the intent of the user [30]. This tool is supported by the ML and NLP of the platform. As shown in Figure 5, for certain nodes of conversation to be accessed, the chatbot has to recognize the specific intents in the user's input. One example is the Hint node, which will pop up when the user does not understand the question from the chatbot and can only be accessed when the user asks for help. The node can be created by the Intent node to evaluate the possible user inputs as a response to that node. For example, if the user types "help" or "hint" as an answer for a question of the chatbot, an intent called "#Hint" is called. This and other intents are created by feeding the chatbot examples of the intent. The chatbot then runs these examples through ML and NLP and learns to recognize them from user input.

It should be noted that some intents require less than a few examples as the chatbot expects the user to answer only "Yes" or "No", as there are limited ways to write them. However, in some specific cases such as name collection when the chatbot asks the name of the user, the Intent works alongside Entities using the "Annotate Entities" function as shown in Figure 6. When the chatbot collects the user's name, the only part of the input that the chatbot is interested in is the name itself but it is not interested in other words. Therefore, the function of the "Annotate Entities" is to select the region of interest in the example sentences (i.e., the blue boxes in Figure 6). In this way, the chatbot may categorize any future names as entities, even the ones that it has not seen before. For the tool of Entities, the function can be considered a database that the chatbot has access to, can cross-reference and extract data. For example, a list of 6000 most common names in America can be used as a database [8]. The chatbot can extract names, when recognizing the related "#Collect_name" intent as shown in Figure 6.

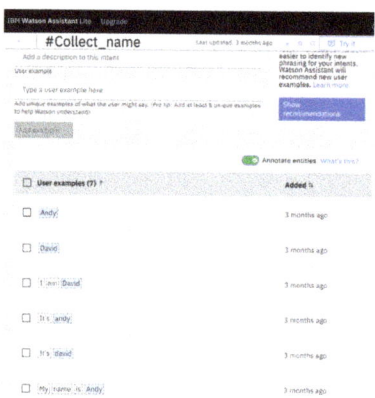

Figure 6. The Intent node named "#Collect_name" in the IBM Watson Assistant. The boxes in blue indicate the user's names that the chatbot is only interested in.

3. Results

To demonstrate the communication flow and running at the start, the chatbot created based on the architectural scheme in Figure 4 begins by introducing itself and asking the user questions to categorize the user into patient, radiation staff, from the general public or from the patient's family as shown in Figure 7.

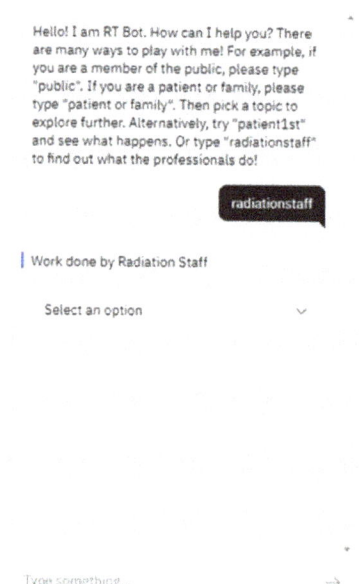

Figure 7. The chatbot introduced himself and tried to identify the user and whether he or she belonged to the group of radiation staff, general public or patient's family.

In this example, the user identified himself as radiation staff in the cancer centre. The chatbot then displayed a list of items showing a variety of information that the user might want to know (Figure 8).

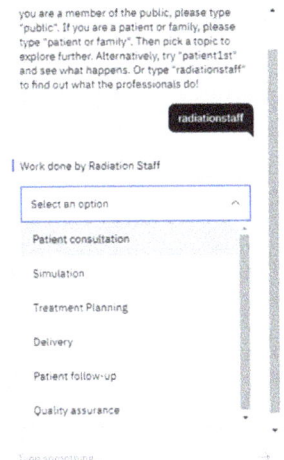

Figure 8. The chatbot displayed a list of items which the user might want to know.

The contents of the list included different categories of information such as patient consultation, simulation, treatment planning, treatment delivery, patient follow-up, quality assurance and so on. This list was designed specifically for the radiation staff. For patients and the general public, they had their own list of information. When the user (radiation staff) selected "Simulation" from the list, the chatbot further asked the user to clarify if he or she was interested in "CT-SIM" or "Conventional SIM". These are two common treatment simulation methods in radiotherapy. To answer that, the user only needed to click the icons to obtain the information as shown in Figure 9.

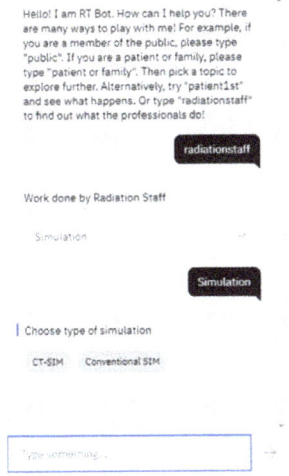

Figure 9. The chatbot noted the user wanted to know information regarding "Simulation" and further clarified which type of simulation, namely, "CT-SIM" or "Conventional SIM" the user wanted to know.

The workflow in Figures 7–9 can be found in Figure 10 for the group of radiation staff.

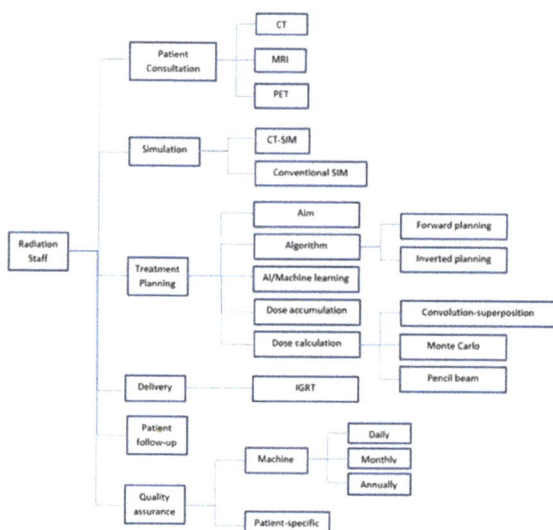

Figure 10. The workflow of the chatbot for the radiation staff regarding Figures 7–9.

Sometimes, the user may ask the chatbot a question directly. For example, the user asked the chatbot "What is clinical trial?" in radiotherapy as shown in Figure 11. In that case, the chatbot answered the question and asked the user if he or she wanted to know more, such as different phases of clinical trial. The user could then select a phase (Phase 1–4) from the chatbot. In Figure 11, the user picked up Phase 1. The chatbot would then explain further the Phase 1 trial in greater details.

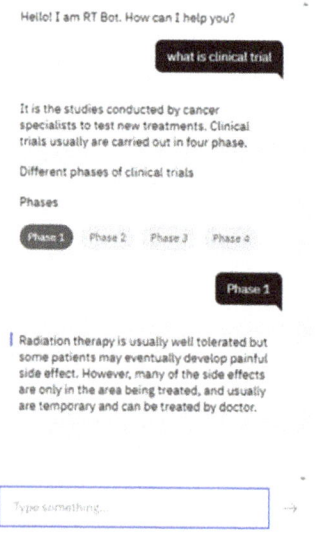

Figure 11. The user may ask the chatbot a question directly. In this example, the user asked the chatbot "What is clinical trial?". In addition to provide the answer to the user, the chatbot could further ask which phase of clinical trials (i.e., Phase 1–4) the user wanted, to refine the response.

4. Discussion

4.1. NLP and ML

George Bernard Shaw said: "Progress is impossible without change, and those who cannot change their minds cannot change anything." [31]. ML brought about sweeping changes in recent years and accounted for significant progress in medicine such as in creating medical chatbots. The Turing test is used to evaluate the intelligence of the machine, and the test is passed if a human being cannot distinguish the machine from another human being through conversation [32]. Since then, NPL was developed to enhance interactions between computer and human language. In the past, NLP depended on a set of hand-written rules coupled with dictionary look up to learn and understand the language from the user. It can be seen that such hand-written rules would only become more and more complex and unmanageable. ML, on the other hand, can simplify and enhance the learning process because the computer can automatically focus on some common cases selectively based on the ML algorithm. These automatic learning procedures supported by, for example, neural networks, can help to generate models to manipulate unfamiliar and erroneous user's input.

NLP includes a number of developed tasks in text and speech processing. These tasks include word segmentation, text-to-speech, stemming, sentence breaking, relationship extraction and so on [33]. Compared to other conversational and prescriptive medical chatbots, the goal of our educational chatbot is to provide information transfer to users who may be radiation staff, patients or people from the general public. Therefore, the main focus of the NPL in our design is to understand and classify the expression from user's with different backgrounds. In creating such a chatbot, some NLP tasks were used such as (1) *Name Entity Recognition*: this process helps to find out the entity of a person, location and organization from the user's input; (2) *Intent*: this process helps to execute an appropriate action to achieve the user's goal; (3) *Context*: this process differentiates the user's input to investigate if the message may have different meaning in the conversation; and (4) *Entity Linking*: this process helps to link any words which are referred to an entity such as a popular location, a well-known company or a famous person.

4.2. Programming and Implementation

In programming and running the educational chatbot, one issue found was the lack of global ability to restart the conversations freely by the user, as the chatbot is deposited on an IoT. For the IBM Watson Assistant, though the "Clear" function in the developer tools allows the conversation to reset back to the first node, when creating the chatbot in the platform, such a function is not available once the chatbot is published. Therefore, to implement this ability globally, every single node needs to be reworked manually. The solution is to add a new intent, linked to an exit node back to the first node. However, adding an exit node to some key parts of conversation would result in unforeseen error because the initial design of logic in programming did not foresee the need for this functionality.

Another programming issue in creating an educational chatbot for radiotherapy is the lack of ability to perform mathematical operations for the context variables. For example, when the chatbot offers a radiation safety test to the user (radiation staff) as training, it is desired that the chatbot could calculate the final mark of the test and provide a letter grade or percentage result to the user. In this case, the results can only be displayed in text format, where each question is either "Correct" or "Incorrect". When creating the chatbot, the development tool does not allow the developer to add up the context variables of the result of each question.

For the AI-assisted chatbot, NLP is used to understand and interpret user inputs. Sometimes, this is challenging and can be a difficult task due to the complexity and variability of human language. Moreover, the chatbot may have difficulty in understanding the context of a conversation. To avoid a poor understanding of open-ended or unstructured user inputs, and to address the difficulty in identifying intents and entities, the chatbot will first identify the user's background and classify the user into a user group (e.g., patient, radiation staff and general public). This can direct the chatbot to access the data related to the user's background. In addition, to further avoid confusion and inappropriate responses, the chatbot will include guidance with fixed options to help the user.

For integration and implementation, the chatbot can be included in a website. IBM Watson Assistant allows the developer to integrate the chatbot into different third-party media such as WhatsApp with Twilio, Slack, Facebook Messenger, SMS with Twilio and Intercom as shown in Figure 4. The chatbot can also be deposited into a website setting up through, for example, Weebly or WordPress. Since the educational chatbot in radiotherapy is quite specific, depositing it into a website allows the chatbot to be found by web crawlers. This ensured that if someone looks for a radiotherapy chatbot on a search engine, the chatbot can be found readily. This would not be the case if the chatbot was implemented through WhatsApp or Facebook.

For the privacy and security concerns, our educational chatbot only provides a single directional information flow from the chatbot to the user. Therefore, there is no storage and record of any user information such as personal data in the chatbot. Moreover, we do not find any significant time delay issue in the chatbot created using the IBM Watson platform.

4.3. Testing and Updating

Although the chatbot is powered by innovative computer technologies such as ML to provide humanlike communication to the user, various human user tests are necessary to find out any bugs in the chatbot and to evaluate its performance. This involves testing the chatbot with real users or simulated user input, and evaluating its performance based on accuracy and user satisfaction. The tests can be conducted by inviting different stakeholders to use the chatbot, including, people from the general public, patients and radiation staff, to test the chatbot for their respective databases. In the test, an evaluation template can be set up to measure different metrics regarding the user's experience in using the chatbot. For example, the test can ask the evaluators to score their experience on a scale in a range of grades, based on the metrics of information quality, user experience and navigability, or the test can be designed following the recent international standards for measuring the "quality in use" of medical chatbots [34]. The test can be carried out remotely through email invitation, or in person in a research meeting or conference, gathering a number of potential users such as radiation staff. To further evaluate and improve the chatbot, workshops for healthcare workers working with patients and families can be conducted to introduce the chatbot and ask them for feedback. These workshops are decent and essential in quality assurance to improve and fine-tune the chatbot.

When the educational chatbot is created and implemented, a continuous update of the contents and features are necessary. These include making adjustments to the conversational flow, adding new intents and entities or updating the training data. Although the chatbot has been validated before implementation, it may find it difficult to handle some edge cases which may not be covered by the training data, or the user may use an unexpected input. Moreover, some small errors which are missed in the validation process due to human variation may exist. These errors would be found occasionally by the users. Their feedbacks to the developer are important to further improve the chatbot. This process would take time but is worthwhile to continue in order to maintain the quality of the chatbot. Moreover, the content of the chatbot needs to be updated routinely to keep pace with new developments in radiotherapy, such as new cancer treatment techniques, new radiation safety policies or new statistical data in radiotherapy. The chatbot should be subject to continuous improvement, updated and modified frequently based on the feedback from the user, new features (e.g., new NLP algorithm) offered to the chatbot and new information in radiotherapy.

4.4. Chatbot Content Management

Building the content for the chatbot is a time-consuming process as the scope of information demanded by different groups of users can be extensive and under continuous update. Each item of information is subject to further breakdown of sub-items and so on. Since each item in the category is unique, the chatbot should provide information in a simple and comprehensive way as per different user classes. A careful selection and filtration of the content is necessary. For example, if the user asks for information about "Brain radiotherapy", a simple explanation should be displayed with a further question following a customized chatbot conversation stream. In this case, the chatbot can further ask the user if he or she wanted to know more about different options of brain radiotherapy such as gamma knife, cyber knife or stereotactic radiosurgery offered by a medical linear accelerator. In addition, plain English should be used for patient and user from the general public while technical terms should be used if the user group is radiation staff.

5. Conclusions

A chatbot integrated into the IoT can be designed using a layered structure and dialogue tree approach for educational purposes in radiotherapy. By taking advantage of some AI features such as NLP offered by some development platforms like the IBM Watson Assistant, the educational chatbot can be created with humanlike character. Using the Q and A approach, the chatbot can communicate with the user from different backgrounds and provide guidance to the user who is difficult to acquire information. It is concluded that the chatbot is not a one-off finished product, but needs to be updated and improved continuously to respond to the user's needs, and to keep pace with the advancements of computer technology and radiotherapy. Further work will include adding functional features in the chatbot and enabling the chatbot to handle multiple languages rather than English only.

Author Contributions: Conceptualization, J.C.L.C., L.S. and K.L.; methodology, J.C.L.C., L.S. and K.L.; software, J.C.L.C. and K.L.; validation, J.C.L.C., L.S. and K.L.; formal analysis, J.C.L.C. and K.L.; investigation, J.C.L.C. and K.L.; resources, J.C.L.C., L.S. and K.L.; data curation, J.C.L.C. and K.L.; writing—original draft preparation, J.C.L.C.; writing—review and editing, K.L.; visualization, J.C.L.C.; supervision, J.C.L.C., L.S. and K.L.; project administration, J.C.L.C., L.S. and K.L.; funding acquisition, J.C.L.C., L.S. and K.L. All authors have read and agreed to the published version of the manuscript.

Funding: This study was supported by a Canadian Institutes of Health Research Planning and Dissemination Grant—Institute Community Support (CIHR PCS–168296).

Institutional Review Board Statement: Not applicable.

Informed Consent Statement: Not applicable.

Data Availability Statement: No new data were created.

Acknowledgments: The authors would like to thank the support from David Kovacek and Nathanael Rebelo from the Toronto Metropolitan University, Toronto, Canada.

Conflicts of Interest: The authors declare no conflict of interest.

References

1. Darejeh, A.; Singh, D. A review on user interface design principles to increase software usability for users with less computer literacy. *J. Comput. Sci.* **2013**, *9*, 1443. [CrossRef]
2. Chow, J.C. Some computer graphical user interfaces in radiation therapy. *World J. Radiol.* **2016**, *8*, 255. [CrossRef] [PubMed]
3. Varitimiadis, S.; Kotis, K.; Pittou, D.; Konstantakis, G. Graph-Based Conversational AI: Towards a Distributed and Collaborative Multi-Chatbot Approach for Museums. *App. Sci.* **2021**, *11*, 9160. [CrossRef]
4. Siddique, S.; Chow, J.C.L. Artificial intelligence in radiotherapy. *Rep. Pract. Oncol. Radiother.* **2020**, *25*, 656–666. [CrossRef] [PubMed]
5. Chow, J.C.L. Internet-based computer technology on radiotherapy. *Rep. Pract. Oncol. Radiother.* **2017**, *22*, 455–462. [CrossRef] [PubMed]
6. Liebrecht, C.; van Hooijdonk, C. Creating humanlike chatbots: What chatbot developers could learn from webcare employees in adopting a conversational human voice. In *International Workshop on Chatbot Research and Design*; Springer: Cham, Switzerland, 2020; pp. 51–64.
7. Siddique, S.; Chow, J.C.L. Machine Learning in Healthcare Communication. *Encyclopedia* **2021**, *1*, 220–239. [CrossRef]

8. Kovacek, D.; Chow, J.C.L. An AI-assisted Chatbot for Radiation Safety Education in Radiotherapy. *IOP SciNotes* **2021**, *2*, 034002. [CrossRef]
9. Rebelo, N.; Sanders, L.; Li, K.; Chow, J.C.L. Learning the Treatment Process in Radiotherapy Using an Artificial Intelligence–Assisted Chatbot: Development Study. *JMIR Form. Res.* **2022**, *6*, e39443. [CrossRef]
10. Turing, A.M. Computing machinery and intelligence. In *Parsing the Turing Test: Philosophical and Methodological Issues in the Quest for the Thinking Computer*; Epstein, R., Roberts, G., Beber, G., Eds.; Springer: Dordrecht, The Netherlands, 2009; pp. 23–65.
11. Xu, L.; Sanders, L.; Li, K.; Chow, J.C. Chatbot for health care and oncology applications using artificial intelligence and machine learning: Systematic review. *JMIR Cancer* **2021**, *7*, e27850. [CrossRef]
12. Okuda, T.; Shoda, S. AI-based chatbot service for financial industry. *Fujitsu Sci. Tech. J.* **2018**, *54*, 4–8.
13. Heo, M.; Lee, K.J. Chatbot as a new business communication tool: The case of naver talktalk. *Bus. Commun. Res. Pract.* **2018**, *1*, 41–45. [CrossRef]
14. Bates, M. Health care chatbots are here to help. *IEEE Pulse* **2019**, *10*, 12–14. [CrossRef] [PubMed]
15. Denecke, K.; Tschanz, M.; Dorner, T.L.; May, R. Intelligent conversational agents in healthcare: Hype or hope. *Stud. Health Technol. Inform.* **2019**, *259*, 77–84. [PubMed]
16. Pearse, J.; Chow, J.C.L. An Internet of Things App for Monitor Unit Calculation in Superficial and Orthovoltage Skin Therapy. *IOP SciNotes* **2020**, *1*, 014002. [CrossRef]
17. Sheth, A.; Yip, H.Y.; Shekarpour, S. Extending patient-chatbot experience with internet-of-things and background knowledge: Case studies with healthcare applications. *IEEE Intell. Syst.* **2019**, *34*, 24–30. [CrossRef]
18. Chow, J.C. Artificial intelligence in radiotherapy and patient care. In *Artificial Intelligence in Medicine*; Springer International Publishing: Cham, Switzerland, 2021; pp. 1–13.
19. Ayanouz, S.; Abdelhakim, B.A.; Benhmed, M. A smart chatbot architecture based NLP and machine learning for health care assistance. In Proceedings of the 3rd International Conference on Networking, Information Systems & Security, Marrakech, Morocco, 31 March 2020; pp. 1–6.
20. Hirschberg, J.; Manning, C.D. Advances in natural language processing. *Science* **2015**, *349*, 261–266. [CrossRef]
21. Bibault, J.E.; Chaix, B.; Guillemassé, A.; Cousin, S.; Escande, A.; Perrin, M.; Pienkowski, A.; Delamon, G.; Nectoux, P.; Brouard, B. A chatbot versus physicians to provide information for patients with breast cancer: Blind, randomized controlled noninferiority trial. *J. Med. Internet Res.* **2019**, *21*, e15787. [CrossRef]
22. Chung, K.; Park, R.C. Chatbot-based heathcare service with a knowledge base for cloud computing. *Clust. Comput.* **2019**, *22*, 1925–1937. [CrossRef]
23. Lokman, A.S.; Zain, J.M.; Komputer, F.S.; Perisian, K. Designing a Chatbot for diabetic patients. In Proceedings of the International Conference on Software Engineering & Computer Systems (ICSECS'09), Penang, Malaysia, 19–21 October 2009; pp. 19–21.
24. Hajare, A.; Bhosale, P.; Nanaware, R.; Hiremath, G. Chatbot for Education System. *Int. J. Comput. Sci.* **2018**, *3*, 52–57.
25. Setiaji, B.; Wibowo, F.W. Chatbot using a knowledge in database: Human-to-machine conversation modeling. In Proceedings of the 2016 7th international conference on intelligent systems, modelling and simulation (ISMS), Bangkok, Thailand, 25 January 2016; IEEE: New York, NY, USA, 2016; pp. 72–77.
26. Li, K.; Chow, J.C.L. A Chatbot for the Staff in Radiotherapy Using Artificial Intelligence and Machine Learning. *Med. Phys.* **2021**, *48*, e426.
27. Chow, J.C.L.; Sanders, L.; Li, K. A radiotherapy chatbot for patients and the general public using machine learning. *Med. Phys.* **2021**, *48*, 4693–4694.
28. Nadkarni, P.M.; Ohno-Machado, L.; Chapman, W.W. Natural language processing: An introduction. *J. Am. Med. Inform. Assoc.* **2011**, *18*, 544–551. [CrossRef] [PubMed]
29. Lally, A.; Fodor, P. Natural language processing with prolog in the IBM Watson System. *Assoc. Log. Program. Newsl.* **2011**, *9*. Available online: http://www.cs.nmsu.edu/ALP/2011/03/natural-language-processing-with-prolog-in-the-ibm-watson-system/ (accessed on 1 March 2023).
30. Srivastava, S.; Prabhakar, T.V. Intent sets: Architectural choices for building practical chatbots. In Proceedings of the 2020 12th International Conference on Computer and Automation Engineering, Sydney, Australia, 14 February 2020; pp. 194–199.
31. George Bernard Shaw. *Everybody's Political What's What*; Dodd Mead: New York, NY, USA, 1945; p. 330.
32. Machinery, C. Computing machinery and intelligence-AM Turing. *Mind* **1950**, *59*, 433.
33. Shah, R.; Lahoti, S.; Lavanya, K. An intelligent chat-bot using natural language processing. *Int. J. Eng. Res.* **2017**, *6*, 281–286. [CrossRef]
34. Santa Barletta, V.; Caivano, D.; Colizzi, L.; Dimauro, G.; Piattini, M. Clinical-chatbot AHP evaluation based on "quality in use" of ISO/IEC 25010. *Int. J. Med. Inform.* **2023**, *170*, 104951. [CrossRef] [PubMed]

Disclaimer/Publisher's Note: The statements, opinions and data contained in all publications are solely those of the individual author(s) and contributor(s) and not of MDPI and/or the editor(s). MDPI and/or the editor(s) disclaim responsibility for any injury to people or property resulting from any ideas, methods, instructions or products referred to in the content.

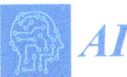

Review

Machine-Learning-Based Prediction Modelling in Primary Care: State-of-the-Art Review

Adham H. El-Sherbini [1], Hafeez Ul Hassan Virk [2], Zhen Wang [3,4], Benjamin S. Glicksberg [5] and Chayakrit Krittanawong [6,*]

1. Faculty of Health Sciences, Queen's University, Kingston, ON K7L 3N6, Canada
2. Harrington Heart & Vascular Institute, Case Western Reserve University, University Hospitals Cleveland Medical Center, Cleveland, OH 44115, USA
3. Robert D. and Patricia E. Kern Center for the Science of Health Care Delivery, Mayo Clinic, Rochester, MN 55901, USA
4. Division of Health Care Policy and Research, Department of Health Sciences Research, Mayo Clinic, Rochester, MN 55901, USA
5. The Hasso Plattner Institute for Digital Health at the Mount Sinai, Icahn School of Medicine at Mount Sinai, New York, NY 10029, USA
6. Cardiology Division, NYU School of Medicine and NYU Langone Health, New York, NY 10016, USA
* Correspondence: chayakrit.krittanawong@nyulangone.org

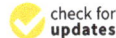

Citation: El-Sherbini, A.H.; Hassan Virk, H.U.; Wang, Z.; Glicksberg, B.S.; Krittanawong, C. Machine-Learning-Based Prediction Modelling in Primary Care: State-of-the-Art Review. *AI* 2023, 4, 437–460. https://doi.org/10.3390/ai4020024

Academic Editors: Tim Hulsen and Demos T. Tsahalis

Received: 14 March 2023
Revised: 8 May 2023
Accepted: 16 May 2023
Published: 23 May 2023

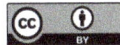

Copyright: © 2023 by the authors. Licensee MDPI, Basel, Switzerland. This article is an open access article distributed under the terms and conditions of the Creative Commons Attribution (CC BY) license (https://creativecommons.org/licenses/by/4.0/).

Abstract: Primary care has the potential to be transformed by artificial intelligence (AI) and, in particular, machine learning (ML). This review summarizes the potential of ML and its subsets in influencing two domains of primary care: pre-operative care and screening. ML can be utilized in preoperative treatment to forecast postoperative results and assist physicians in selecting surgical interventions. Clinicians can modify their strategy to reduce risk and enhance outcomes using ML algorithms to examine patient data and discover factors that increase the risk of worsened health outcomes. ML can also enhance the precision and effectiveness of screening tests. Healthcare professionals can identify diseases at an early and curable stage by using ML models to examine medical pictures, diagnostic modalities, and spot patterns that may suggest disease or anomalies. Before the onset of symptoms, ML can be used to identify people at an increased risk of developing specific disorders or diseases. ML algorithms can assess patient data such as medical history, genetics, and lifestyle factors to identify those at higher risk. This enables targeted interventions such as lifestyle adjustments or early screening. In general, using ML in primary care offers the potential to enhance patient outcomes, reduce healthcare costs, and boost productivity.

Keywords: artificial intelligence; machine learning; deep learning; primary care

1. Introduction

Artificial intelligence (AI) is a field of study that attempts to replicate natural human intelligence in machines [1]. The machines can then independently perform activities that would otherwise require human intelligence. AI can be broken down into several subsets, such as machine learning (ML) and deep learning (DL) [2]. ML makes a software application more accurate in predicting outcomes by feeding it with data rather than explicit programming. Comparatively, DL, a subset of ML, builds a hierarchy of knowledge based on learning from examples. These fundamental ideas of AI are utilized to develop analytic models to turn this productive technology into practice. Since its introduction in the 1950s, AI has made significant strides in manufacturing; sports analytics; autonomous vehicle; and more recently, primary care and preventive medicine [3].

Primary care and preventive medicine, otherwise expressed as day-to-day healthcare practices including outpatient settings, are a growing sector in the realms of AI and computer science. Although AI has endless applications in healthcare, particular sectors of primary care have been more progressive and accepting of AI and its potential. For instance, the Forward clinic is a primary care service incorporating standard doctor-led programs with technology to provide a more inclusive and long-term care [3]. The addition of the technology allows for 24/7 monitoring, skin cancer screening, testing of genes, and biometric monitoring. As with all AI interventions, the Forward clinic endures multiple challenges, such as additional physician training and fees. Although the Forward clinic is just a singular example of how AI can be integrated into primary care, AI's implementation into primary care can be further broken down into sections of healthcare, such as pre-operative care and screening. This review summarizes AI's, specifically ML's, short yet productive impact on primary care and preventive medicine and aims to inform primary care physicians about the potential integration of ML (Figure 1 and Table 1).

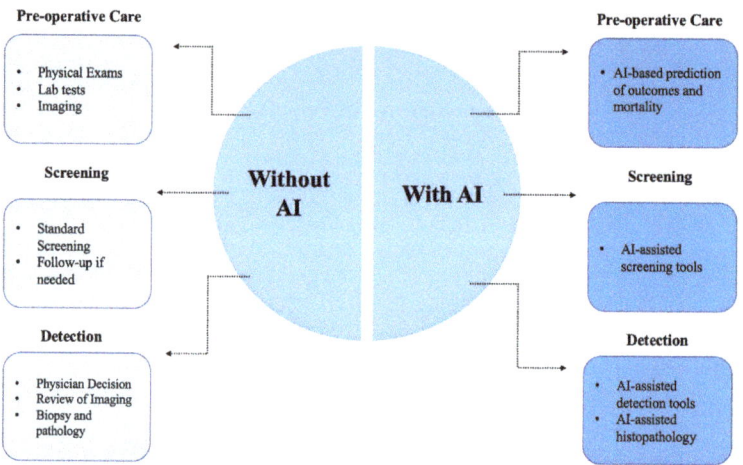

Figure 1. Current methods vs. AI-assisted methods in primary care. Figure Description: AI has the potential to assist current primary care methods in three domains: pre-operative care, screening, and detection. In pre-operative care, this includes using AI for predictions of outcomes and mortality. For screening, AI serves a prominent role in screening tools for numerous diseases. Similarly, AI can be used for real-time detection tools and AI-assisted histopathology tools.

Table 1. Abbreviations.

Name	Abbreviation
Acute kidney injury	AKI
Adaptive boosting	ADA
Age-related macular degeneration	AMD
Artificial intelligence	AI
Atherosclerotic cardiovascular disease	ACSVD
Atrial fibrillation	AF
Blood pressure	BP
Chronic kidney disease	CKD
Chronic obstructive pulmonary disease	COPD
Convolutional neural network	CNN
Coronary artery calcium score	CACS
Coronary artery disease	CAD
Decision tree	DT
Deep learning	DL
Deep neural network	DNN
Deep vein thrombus	DVT
Diabetes mellitus	DM
Electronic health records	EHR
Extreme gradient boosting	XGB

Table 1. Cont.

Name	Abbreviation
Familial hypercholesterolemia	FH
Generative adversarial network	GAN
Gradient boosting	GB
Gradient boosting tree	GBT
Heart failure	HF
Human immunodeficiency virus	HIV
K-nearest neighbors	KNN
Logistic regression	LR
Low-density lipoprotein	LDL
Machine learning	ML
Neural network	NN
Obstructive sleep apnea syndrome	OSAS
Photoplethysmogram	PPG
Potential pre-exposure prophylaxis	PrEP
Pulmonary embolism	PE
Pulmonary hypertension	PH
Random forest	RF
Support vector machine	SVM
Urinary tract infection	UTI

2. Pre-Operative Care

Pre-operative risk prediction and management have been promising areas of AI research and its application. PubMed and Google Scholar were searched using keywords for English literature published from inception to December 2022 (Figure 2). Studies were included if they reported outcomes regarding the effectiveness of ML models in pre-operative care or similar domains. Studies have utilized AI to predict mortality and postoperative complications. Such applications are necessary for clinical decision-making, forethought of healthcare resources such as ICU beds, the cost of the patient, and the possible need for transition of care [4]. Typically, researchers utilize a designated number of electronic health records (EHR) to train the analytic model and the remainder to test it. For instance, Chiew et al. utilized EHRs to predict post-surgical mortality in a tertiary academic hospital in Singapore [5]. The study compared five candidate models (Random Forest (RF), Adaptive Boosting (ADA), Gradient Boosting (GB), and Support Vector Machine (SVM)) and found that all GB was the greatest performing model (specificity (0.98), sensitivity (0.50), PPV (0.20), F1 score (0.28), and AUROC (0.96)). Five other studies by Fernandes et al., Jalai et al., COVIDSurg Collaborative, Sahara et al., and Pfitzner et al. have also evaluated how differing types of analytic models (Logistic Regression (LR), RF, Neural Network (NN), SVM, Extreme GB (XGB), Decision Tree (DT), GB, Deep Neural Network (DNN), GRU, and classification tree) can predict postoperative mortality [6–10]. The patient population included those undergoing cardiac surgery, pancreatic surgery, or hepatopancreatic surgery or those infected with SARS-CoV-2. Of the studies undergoing cardiac surgery, the selected ML models were good predictors of mortality and prolonged length of stay. In Fernandes et al., when utilizing pre-operative and intra-operative risk factors alongside intraoperative hypotension, XGB was the best performing model (AUROC (0.87), PPV (0.10), specificity (0.85), and sensitivity (0.71) [6]. In the other study by Jalai et al., deep neural network (DNN) was the best performing of the five models (accuracy (89%), F-score (0.89), and AUROC (0.95)) [7]. Neither study compared its models with established pre-operative risk scores, such as the Revised Cardiac Risk Index or Gupta score. Similarly, Pfitzner et al. used pre-, intra-, and short-term post-operative data on a number of models to assess its ability to predict pre-operative risk for those undergoing pancreatic surgery [8]. The study found maximum AUPRCs of 0.53 for postoperative complications and 0.51 for postoperative mortality, with LR as the best model. As for those undergoing hepatopancreatic surgery, Sahara et al. found that the classification tree model better predicted 30-day unpredicted deaths than the traditional American College of Surgeons National Surgery Quality Improvement Program surgical risk calculator [9]. Finally, a COVIDSurg Collaborative study that generated 78 AI models found that when combining an LR model with four features (ASA grade, RCRI, age, and pre-op respiratory support), an AUC of 0.80 in the testing dataset was achieved. This generated model was the best performing in predicting postoperative mortality among those infected with SARS-CoV-2 [10]. Ultimately, ML models present great promise in its integration into pre-operative care, particularly for simplifying pre-operative evaluations, as observed in Figure 3.

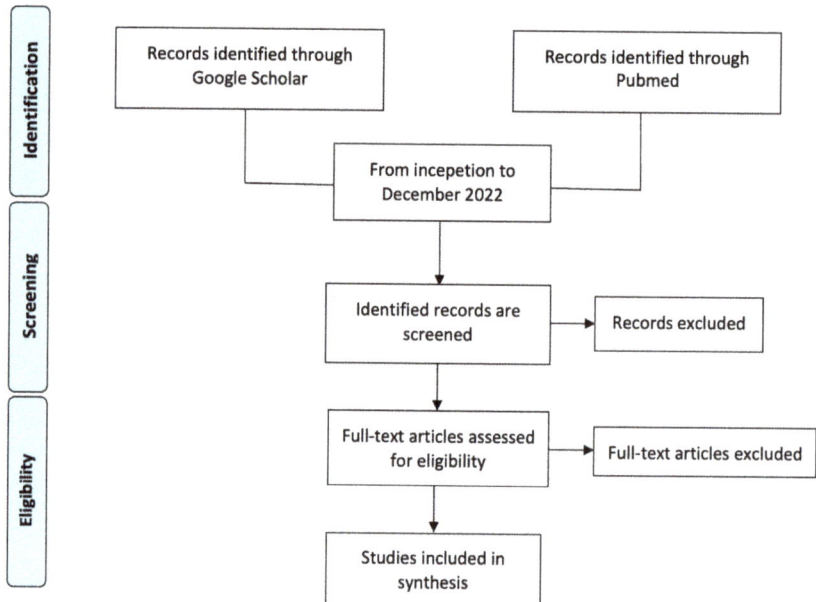

Figure 2. Literature Search Method. Figure Description: PubMed and Google Scholar were searched using keywords for English literature published from inception to December 2022. Observational studies, case–control studies, cohort studies, clinical trials, meta-analyses, reviews, and guidelines were reviewed.

Post-Operative Complications

Other pre-operative risk prediction objectives include assessing models on postoperative complications [11–13]. These studies have evaluated how varying ML models (SVM, LR, RF, GBT, DNN, GBT, and XGB) can predict a number of post-operative complications. One study utilized electronic anesthesia records (pre-operative and intra-operative data) to predict deep vein thrombus (DVT), delirium, pulmonary embolism, acute kidney injury (AKI), and pneumonia [11]. GBT was the most promising model, with AUROC scores of 0.905 (pneumonia), 0.848 (AKI), 0.881 (DVT), 0.831 (pulmonary embolism), and 0.762 (delirium). Similarly, Corey et al. utilized EHR data, including 194 clinical features, to train ML models on 14 postoperative complications [12]. Amongst the models, AUC scores ranged from 0.747 to 0.924, with the Lasso penalized regression being the best performing (sensitivity (0.775), specificity (0.749), and PPV (0.362)). Comparably, Bonde et al. trained three multi-labels DNNs to compete against traditional surgical risk prediction systems on post-operative complications [13]. The mean AUCs for the test dataset on models 1, 2, and 3 were 0.858, 0.863, and 0.874, all of which outperformed the ACS-SRC predictors. Ultimately, ML methods appear to be high-performing for predicting post-operative complications, but additional studies comparing models are required to validate the findings.

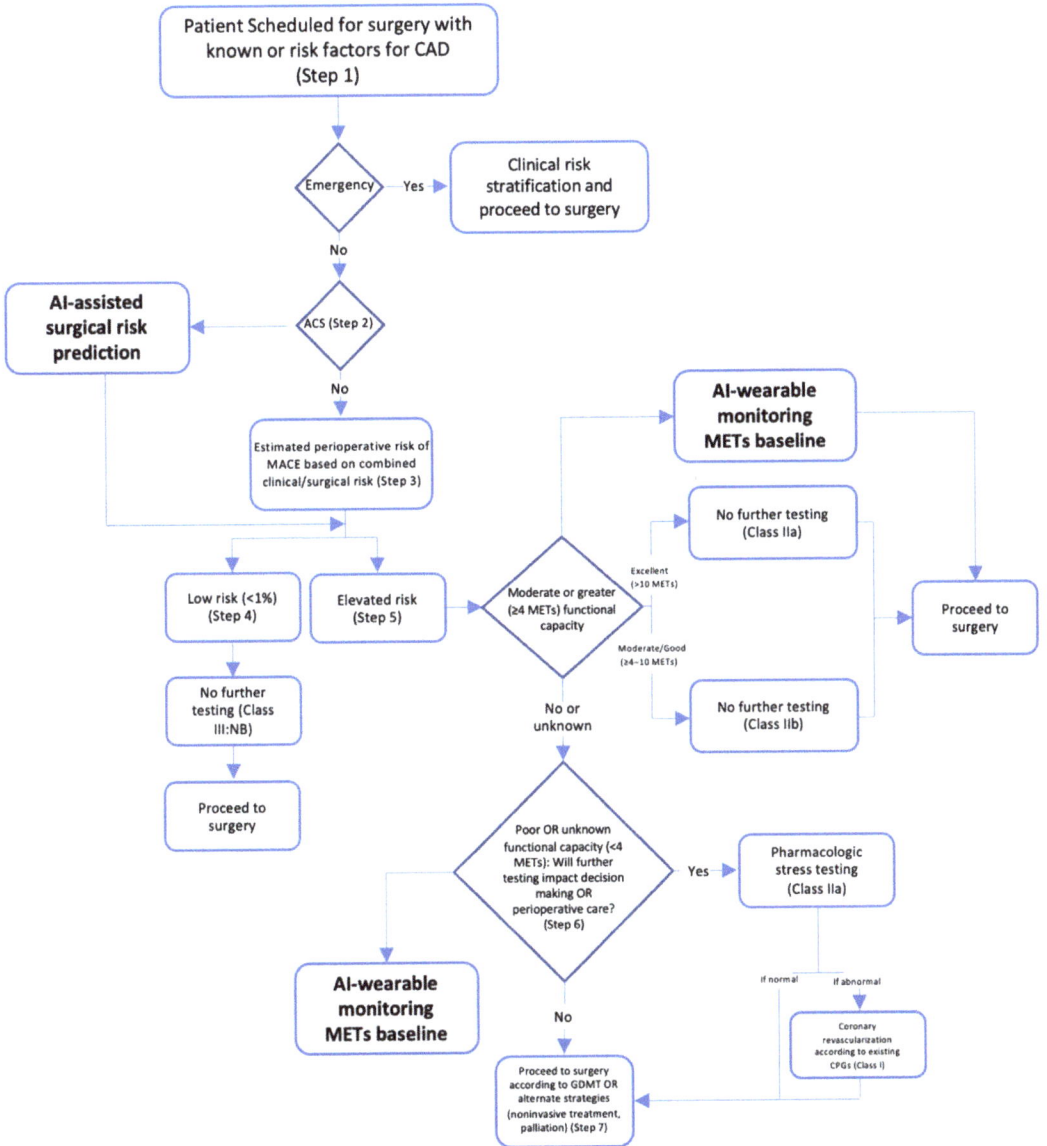

Figure 3. Example of AI in pre-operative evaluation. Figure Description: The integration of AI into pre-operative care allows for the refinement of more effective guidelines. For instance, in Figure 2, current guidelines recommend a seven-step pre-operative evaluation before surgery for patients with CAD risk factors. In this process, AI could be utilized to provide risk prediction and MET monitoring through wearable technology, ultimately cultivating a more straightforward process.

3. Screening

The applications of AI in screening are by far the most precedented. PubMed and Google Scholar were searched from inception to December 2022, and the databases were searched for studies investigating the role of ML in screening for several diseases and disorders.

3.1. Hypertension

One of these leading domains is hypertension, where studies have assessed the risk of hypertension and predicted resistant hypertension while concurrently estimating blood pressure (BP). Zhao et al. compared four analytical models (RF, CatBoost, MLP neural network, and LR) in predicting the risk of hypertension based on data from physical examinations [14]. RF was the best-performing model with an AUC of 0.92, an accuracy of 0.82, a sensitivity of 0.83, and a specificity of 0.81. In addition, no clinical or genetic data was utilized for training the models. Similarly, Alkaabi et al. utilized ML models (DT, RF, and LR) to assess the risk of developing hypertension in a more effective manner [15]. RF was the best-performing model (accuracy (82.1%), PPV (81.4%), sensitivity (82.1%), and AUC (86.9)). Clinical factors, such as education level, tobacco use, abdominal obesity, age, gender, history of diabetes, consumption of fruits and vegetables, employment, physical activity, mother's history of high BP, and history of high cholesterol, were all significant predictors of hypertension. Ye et al. investigated an XGBoost model that had AUC scores of 0.917 (retrospective) and 0.870 (prospective) in predicting hypertension. Similarly, LaFreniere et al. investigated an NN model which had 82% accuracy in predicting hypertension given the chosen risk factors [16,17]. Regarding BP, Khalid et al. compared three ML models (regression tree, SVM, and MLR) in estimating BPs from pulse waveforms derived from photoplethysmogram (PPG) signals [18]. The regression tree achieved the best systolic and diastolic BP accuracy, -0.1 ± 6.5 mmHg and -0.6 ± 5.2 mmHg, respectively. In summary, ML appears to be an effective tool for predicting hypertension and BP, though its clinical utility remains to be delineated, since hypertension can be diagnosed through non-invasive procedures.

3.2. Hypercholesterolemia

AI applications on hypercholesterolemia have outputted similar findings, as seen in Myers et al. [19]. Using data on diagnostic and procedures codes, prescriptions, and laboratory findings, the FIND FH model was trained on large healthcare databases to diagnose familial hypercholesterolemia (FH). The model achieved a PPV of 0.85, a sensitivity of 0.45, an AURPC of 0.55, and an AUROC score of 0.89. This model effectively identified those with FH for individuals at high risk of early heart attack and stroke. Comparatively, Pina et al. evaluated the accuracy of three ML models (CT, GBM, and NN) when trained on genetic tests to detect FH-causative genetic mutations [20]. All three models outperformed the clinical standard Dutch Lipid score in both cohorts. Similar findings have been produced for hyperlipidemia, where Liu et al. trained an LTSM network on 500 EHR samples [21]. The model achieved an ACC score of 0.94, an AUC score of 0.974, a sensitivity of 0.96, and a specificity of 0.92. Regarding low-density lipoproteins (LDLs), Tsigalou et al. and Cubukcu et al. concluded that ML models were productive alternatives to direct determination and equations [22,23]. In both studies, ML models (MLR, DNN, ANN, LR, and GB trees) outperformed the traditional equations: the Friedewald and Martin–Hopkins formulas. Although the researched algorithms show great potential, additional studies are warranted to validate these conclusions.

3.3. Cardiovascular Disease

Arguably, the largest field of primary care in which AI has made significant strides is predicting and assessing cardiovascular risk. As cardiovascular diseases are the leading cause of death globally, any advancements in risk prediction and early diagnosis are of substance. In 2017, Weng et al. compared four ML models (RF, LR, GB, and NN) in predicting cardiovascular risk through EHR [24]. The AUC scores of RF, LR, GB, and NN were 0.745, 0.760, 0.761, and 0.764, respectively. The study concluded that the applications of ML in cardiovascular risk prediction significantly improved the accuracy. Zhao et al. reproduced a similar study with LR, RF, GBT, CNN, and LSTM trained on longitudinal EHR and genetic data [25]. The event prediction was far better using the longitudinal feature for a 10-year CVD prediction. Kusunose et al. applied a CNN to identify those at risk of heart failure (HF) from a cohort of pulmonary hypertension

(PH) patients using chest x-rays [26]. The AUC scores of AI, chest x-rays, and human observers were 0.71, 0.60, and 0.63, respectively. In a unique perspective, Moradi et al. employed generative adversarial networks (GANs) for data augmentation on chest x-rays to assess its accuracy in detecting cardiovascular abnormalities when a CNN model was trained on it [27]. The GAN data augmentation outperformed traditional and no data augmentation scenarios on normal and abnormal chest X-ray images with accuracies of 0.8419, 0.8312, and 0.8193, respectively. Studies have also compared ML models relative to traditional risk scores, such as a study by Ambale-Venkatesh et al. [28]. A random survival forest model was assessed in its prediction of six cardiovascular outcomes compared with the Concordance index and Brier score. The model outperformed traditional risk scores (decreased Brier score by 10–25%), and age was the most significant predictor. Similarly, Alaa et al. compared an AutoPrognosis ML model with an established risk score (Framingham score), a Cox PH model with conventional risk factors, and a Cox PH model with all 473 variables (UK Biobank) [29]. The AUROC scores were 0.774, 0.724, 0.734, and 0.758, respectively. Pfohl et al. developed a "fair" atherosclerotic cardiovascular disease (ACSVD) risk prediction tool through EHR data [30]. The experiment ran through four experiments (standard, EQ_{race}, EQ_{gender}, and EQ_{age}) and achieved AUROC scores of 0.773, 0.742, 0.743, and 0.694, respectively. The tool has reduced discrepancies across races, genders, and ages in the prediction of ACSVD. Generally, AI can aid in mitigating gaps in ACSVD risk prevention guidelines, as observed in Figure 4. In the United States alone, one in every three patients undergoing elective cardiac catheterization is diagnosed with obstructive coronary artery disease (CAD). This begs the question of new methodologies to better diagnose the population. Al'Afref et al. assessed how applying an XGBoost model on Coronary Computed Tomography Angiography can predict obstructive CAD using clinical factors [31]. The ML model achieved an AUC score of 0.773, but more notably, when combined with the coronary artery calcium score (CACS), the AUC score was 0.881. Therefore, an ML model and CACS may accurately predict the presence of obstructive CAD. Based on the present literature, AI models screen effectively and predict cardiovascular risks while predominantly outperforming established risk scores.

3.4. Eye Disorders and Diseases

Another area of primary care that has used ML is vision-centric diseases, such as diabetic retinopathy, glaucoma, and age-related macular degeneration (AMD). Ting et al. assessed AI's metrics in this sector by training a DL system on retinal images (76,370 images of diabetic retinopathy, 125,189 images of possible glaucoma, and 72,610 images of AMD) [32]. For referable diabetic retinopathy, the model achieved an AUC of 0.936, a sensitivity of 0.905, and a specificity of 0.916. As for vision-threatening retinopathy, the AUC was 0.958, sensitivity was 1.00, and specificity was 0.911. For possible glaucoma images, the model achieved an AUC of 0.942, a sensitivity of 0.964, and a specificity of 0.872. Finally, the model on AMD testing retinal images achieved an AUC of 0.931, a sensitivity of 0.923, and a specificity of 0.887. Retinal fundus images can also be used by AI models to extract further information, such as predicting cardiovascular risk factors in the case of the study by Poplin et al. [33]. After training the model on 284,445 and validating it on two datasets, the model could predict age (mean absolute error (MAE) within 3.26 years), gender (AUC 0.97), smoking status (AUC 0.71), systolic blood pressure (MAE within 11.23 mmHG), and major adverse cardiac events (AUC 0.70). In another study, Kim et al. utilized retinal fundus images for training a CNN model to predict age and sex [34]. The MAE for patients, those with hypertension, those with diabetes mellitus (DM), and smokers were 3.06 years, 3.46 years, 3.55 years, and 2.65 years, respectively. Ultimately, well-trained ML models appear to be effective in predicting eye diseases.

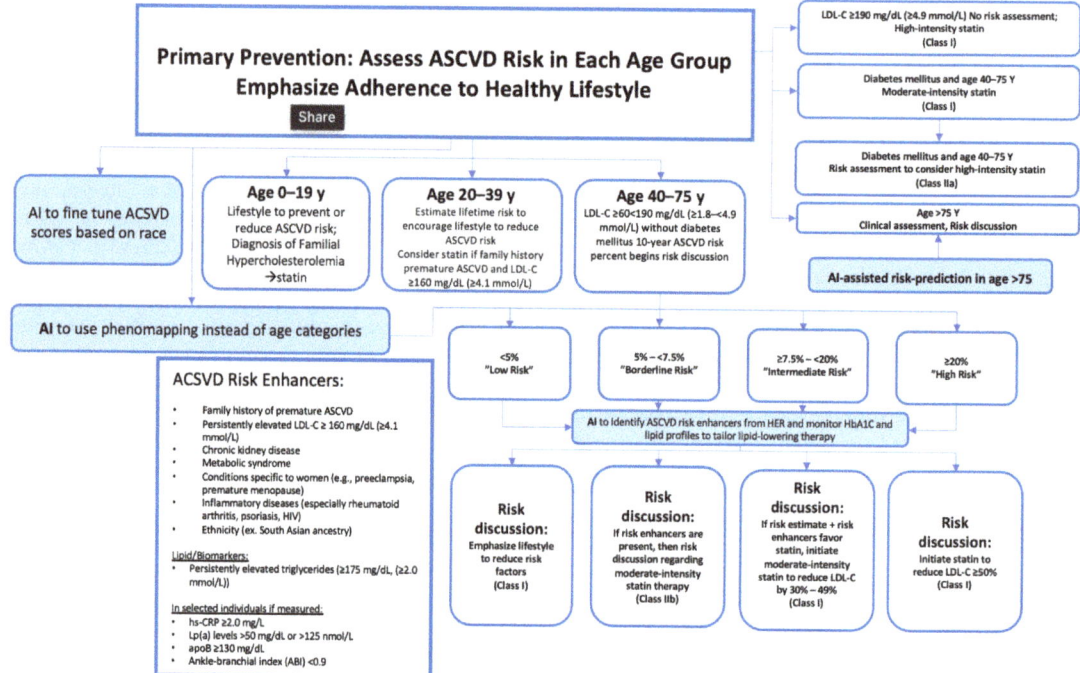

Figure 4. Example of AI in ASCVD assessment. Figure Description: ASCVD risk assessment is exceptionally extensive and varies significantly based on age groups. Although the guidelines are thorough, AI has the potential to address potential gaps in the evaluation. For instance, AI can provide risk prediction for individuals > 75 and it could fine-tune ACSVD scores based on race. AI could also detect risk enhancers of ASCVD based on HbA1C monitoring, EHR, and lipid profiles. This may allow for appropriate adjustments to lipid-lowering therapy. AI also has the potential to use phenomapping instead of age categories, allowing for stronger classification.

3.5. Diabetes

More than 400 million individuals globally are diagnosed with DM. AI's implementation into primary care has been shown to be effective when targeting this widespread disease's risk prediction. In one study, Alghamdi et al. used medical records of cardiorespiratory fitness to train and compare five models (DT, naïve bayes, LR, logistic model tree, and RF) in predicting DM. When RF, logistic model tree, and naïve bayes were ensembled with the developed predictive model classifier, a maximum AUC (0.92) was achieved. Similarly, through administrative data, Ravaut et al. trained a GB decision tree on 1,657,395 patients to predict T2DM 5 years prior to onset [35]. While validating the model on 243,442 patients and testing it on 236,506 patients, an AUC score of 0.8026 was achieved. In another study, Ravaut et al. also assessed if a GB decision tree can predict adverse complications of diabetes, including retinopathy, tissue infection, hyper/hypoglycemia, amputation, and cardiovascular events [36]. After being trained (1,029,366 patients), validated (272,864 patients), and tested (265,406 patients) on administrative data, the model achieved an AUC score of 0.777. To support the conclusion on DM, Debernah et al. found reasonably good accuracies in a Korean population, with DT (77.87%), LR (76.13%), and ANN having the lowest accuracy (73.23%) [37]. In Alhassan et al., when predicting T2DM, the LTSM and gated-recurrent unit outperformed MLP models with a 97.3% accuracy [38]. In India, Boutilier et al. attempted to find the best ML algorithm for predicting DM and hypertension in limited resource settings [39]. RF models had a higher prediction accuracy than established UK and US scores, with an improved AUC score from 0.671 to 0.910 for diabetes and from 0.698 to 0.792 for hypertension. With the current evidence, ML methods appear to be exceptionally effective in predicting diabetes; however, there lacks discussion on the benefits of using ML over a simple blood draw.

3.6. Cancer

In 2020, cancer was responsible for nearly 10 million deaths globally, making it a hotspot for ML implementations and strategies in primary care [40]. Fortunately, ML models have been proven to have potential in the early diagnosis and screening of lung, cervical, colorectal, breast, and prostate cancer [41]. Regarding lung cancer, Ardilla et al. trained a DL algorithm on CT images to predict the risk of lung cancer in 6716 national trial cases [42]. The model achieved an AUC score of 0.944. Similarly, Gould et al. compared an ML model in predicting a future lung cancer diagnosis with the 2012 Prostate, Lung, Colorectal and Ovarian Cancer Screening Trial risk model (mPLCOm2012) [43]. The novel algorithm outperformed the mPLCOm2012 in AUC scores (0.86 vs. 0.79) and sensitivity (0.401 vs. 0.279). Using NNs, Yeh et al. developed a model to screen patients at risk of lung cancer on EHR data [44]. For the overall population, the algorithm achieved an AUC score of 0.90 and 0.87 for patients over the age of 55 years. Guo et al. trained ML models on low-dose CT and found an accuracy of 0.6778, a F1 score of 0.6575, a sensitivity of 0.6252, and a specificity of 0.7357 [45]. More notably, the interactive pathways were BMI, DM, first smoke age, average drinks per month, years of smoking, year(s) since quitting smoking, sex, last dental visit, general health, insurance, education, last PAP test, and last sigmoidoscopy or colonoscopy. Concerning cervical cancer, CervDetect, a number of ML models that evaluate the risk of cervical cancer elements forming, has been a leader in this subject. In 2021, Mehmood et al. used cervical images to evaluate CervDetect and found a false negative rate of 100%, a false positive rate of 6.4%, an MSE error of 0.07111, and an accuracy of 0.936 [46]. Similarly, DeepCervix is another DL model that attempts to combat the high false-positive results in pap smear tests due to human error. Rahaman et al. trained DeepCervix, a hybrid deep fusion feature technique, on pap smear tests [47]. The DL-based model achieved accuracies of 0.9985, 0.9938, and 0.9914 for 2-class, 3-class, and 5-class classifications, respectively. Considering that 90% of cervical cancer is found in low-middle income settings, Bae et al. set out to implement an ML model onto endoscopic visual inspection following an application of acetic acid images [48]. Although resource-limited, the KNN model was the best performing, with an accuracy of 0.783, an AUC of 0.807, a specificity of 0.803, and a sensitivity of 0.75. In parallel, Wentzensen et al. developed a DL classifier with a cloud-based whole-slide imaging platform and trained it on P16/Ki-67 dual-stained (DS) slides for cervical cancer screening [48]. The model achieved a better specificity and equal sensitivity to manual DS and pap, resulting in lower positivity than manual DS and cytology. With respect to breast cancer screening, multiple studies have been conducted to achieve better accuracy in its diagnosis. Using screening mammograms, Shen et al. trained a DL algorithm on 1903 images and achieved an AUC of 0.88, and the four-model averaging improved the AUC score to 0.91 [49]. Similarly, using digital breast tomosynthesis images, Buda et al. achieved a sensitivity of 65% with a DL model for breast cancer screening [50]. Similarly, Haji Maghsoudi et al. developed Deep-LIBRA, an AI model trained on 15661 digital mammograms to estimate breast density and achieved an AUC of 0.612 [51]. The model had a strong agreement with the current gold standard. Another study by Ming et al. compared three ML models (MCMC GLMM, ADA, and RF) to the established BOADICEA model by training them on biennial mammograms [52]. When screening for lifetime risk of breast cancer, all models ($0.843 \leq$ AUROC ≤ 0.889) outperformed BOADICEA (AUROC = 0.639. Similar findings have been concluded in prostate cancer, where three studies (Perera et al., Chiu et al., and Bienecke et al.) compared numerous ML models (DNN, XGBoost, LightGBM, CatBoost, SVM, LR, RF, and multiplayer perceptron) [53–55]. Although all studies trained their respective models differently (PSA levels, prostate biopsy, or EHRs), all concluded that the ML algorithms were efficacious in predicting prostate cancer. Ultimately, there appears to be a substantial body of literature supporting the effectiveness of ML methods in predicting different types of cancer.

3.7. Human Immunodeficiency Virus and Sexually Transmitted Diseases

Another sector of primary care requiring additional applications to assist in its diagnosis and screening is the human immunodeficiency virus (HIV) and sexually transmitted diseases (STDs). In 2021, Turbe et al. trained a DL model on the rapid diagnostic test to classify rapid HIV in rural South Africa [56]. Relative to traditional reports of accuracy varying between 80 and 97%, this model achieved an accuracy of 98.9%. Similarly, Bao et al. compared 5 mL models predicting HIV and STIs [57]. GBM was the best performing, with AUROC scores of 0.763, 0.858, 0.755, and 0.68 for HIV, syphilis, gonorrhea, and chlamydia, respectively. Another study, Marcus et al., developed and assessed an HIV prediction model to find potential pre-exposure prophylaxis (PrEP) patients [58]. Using EHR data to train the model, the study reported an AUC score of 0.84. In terms of future predictions, Elder et al. compared 6 mL algorithms when determining patients at risk of additional STIs within the next 24–48 months through previous EHR data [59]. The Bayesian Additive RT was the best-performing model with an AUROC score of 0.75 and a sensitivity of 0.915. A number of studies have also reported plausible applications of AI on urinary tract infections (UTIs). Gadalla et al. have assessed how AI models can identify predictors for a UTI diagnosis through training on potential biomarkers and clinical data from urine [60]. The study concluded that clinical information was the strongest predictor, with an AUC score of 0.72, a PPV of 0.65, an NPV of 0.79, and an F1 score of 0.69. Comparatively, in Taylor et al., vitals, lab results, medication, chief complaints, physical exam findings, and demographics were all utilized for training, validating, and testing a number of ML algorithms to predict UTIs in ED patients [61]. The AUC scores ranged from 0.826 to 0.904, with XGBoost being the best-performing algorithm. Therefore, the benefits of using ML models to predict and screen for HIV and STDs are evident.

3.8. Obstructive Sleep Apnea Syndrome

There are a number of studies that have reported the use of ML for detecting obstructive sleep apnea syndrome (OSAS). For OSAS, findings have generally been positive, as in the case of a study by Tsai et al. [62]. LR, k-nearest neighbor, CNN, naïve Bayes, RF, and SVM were all compared for screening moderate-to-severe OSAS by being trained on demographic and information-based questionnaires. The study found that BMI was the most influential parameter, and RF achieved the highest accuracy in screening for both types. In another study, Alvarez et al. trained and tested a regression SVM on polysomnography and found that the dual-channel approach was a better performer than oximetry and airflow [63]. Mencar et al. used demographic and information questionaries again to predict OSAS severity [64]. SVM and RF were the best in classification, with the strongest average in classification being 44.7%. This study demonstrates some variability in studies attempting to define a conclusion between AI and OSAS. Overall, there is lack of literature to make a comprehensive conclusion regarding the use of ML for OSAS.

3.9. Osteoporosis

Regarding osteoporosis and related diseases, four studies have compared a number of AI models (XGBoost, LR, multiplayer perceptron, SVM, RF, ANN, extreme GB, stacking with five classifiers, and SVM with radial basis function kernel) [65–68]. Models were trained on EHR, CT and clinical data, or abdomen-pelvic CT. All studies concluded that ML methods were valid and presented great potential in screening for osteoporosis. An additional study trained ML models (RF, GB, NN, and LR) on genomic data for fracture prediction [69]. The study found that GB was the best-performing model, with an AUC score of 0.71 and an accuracy of 0.88. Ultimately, more studies are required to confirm the effectiveness of ML for predicting osteoporosis.

3.10. Chronic Conditions

Chronic obstructive pulmonary disease (COPD) is characterized by permanent lung damage and airway blockage. To enhance life quality and lower mortality rates, COPD must be diagnosed and treated early. The early identification, diagnosis, and prognosis of COPD can be aided by ML methods [70]. The likelihood of hospitalization, mortality, and COPD exacerbations have all been predicted using ML algorithms. These algorithms create predictive models using a variety of data sources, including patient demographics, clinical symptoms, and imaging data. For instance, Zeng et al. developed an ML algorithm trained on 278 candidate features [71]. The model achieved an AUROC of 0.866. Another chronic condition, chronic kidney disease (CKD), is characterized by a progressive decline in kidney function over time. Kidney failure can be prevented, and patient outcomes can be enhanced by early detection and care of CKD. The early detection, diagnosis, and management of CKD can be helped by ML algorithms. For instance, Nishat et al. developed an ML system to predict the probability of CKD. Eight supervised algorithms were developed, and RF was the best-performing mode reporting an accuracy of 99.75% [72]. At the final stage of CKD, known as ESKD, patients require dialysis or a kidney transplant. The early detection, diagnosis, and management of ESKD can be facilitated by ML algorithms. ML algorithms have been used to forecast mortality and the risk of ESKD in CKD patients. These algorithms create predictive models using a variety of data sources, including medical records, test results, and demographic information. For instance, Bai et al. trained five ML models on a longitudinal CKD cohort to predict ESKD [73]. LR, naive Bayes, and RF achieved similar predictability and sensitivity and outperformed the Kidney Failure Risk Equation. Since chronic conditions are a critical aspect of primary care, more studies involving a variety of ML models are needed to confirm MLs' potential.

3.11. Detecting COVID-19 and Influenza

ML has shown great promise in detecting and differentiating between common conditions, propagating more effective recommendations and guidelines (Figure 5). Specifically, detection research has rocketed with the rise and timeline of the COVID-19 virus [74]. Zhou et al. developed an XGBoost algorithm to distinguish between influenza and COVID-19 in case there are no laboratory results of pathogens [75]. The model used EHR data to achieve AUC scores of 0.94, 0.93, and 0.85 in the training, testing, and external validation datasets. Similarly, in Zan et al., a DL model, titled *DeepFlu*, was utilized to predict individuals at risk of symptomatic flu based on gene expression data of influenza A viruses (IAV) or the infection subtypes H1N1 or H3N2 [76]. The DeepFlu achieved an accuracy score of 0.70 and an AUROC of 0.787. In another study, Nadda et al. combined LSTM with an NN model to interpret patients' symptoms for disease detection [77]. For dengue and cold patients, the combination of models achieved AUCs of 0.829 and 0.776 for flu, dengue, and cold, and 0.662 for flu and cold. For influenza, Hogan et al. and Choo et al. trained multiple ML models on nasopharyngeal swab samples and the mHealth app, respectively, for influenza diagnosis and screening [78,79]. Both studies concluded that ML methods are capable of being utilized for infectious disease testing. Similar findings were presented for chronic coughs in Luo et al., where a DL model, BERT, could accurately detect chronic coughs through diagnosis and medication data [79]. Additionally, in Yoo et al., severe pharyngitis could be detected through the training of smartphone-based DL algorithms on self-taken throat images (AUROC 0.988) [80]. In summary, ML appears to be effective in screening and distinguishing between COVID-19, influenza, and related illnesses.

3.12. Detecting Atrial Fibrillation

Another large center for AI detection is atrial fibrillation (AF). Six studies have evaluated unique ways to detect AF through ML models [80–84]. Through wearable devices, countless algorithms (SVM, DNN, CNN, ENN, naïve Bayesian, LR, RF, GB, and W-PPG algorithm combined with W-ECG algorithm) have been trained on primary care data, RR intervals, W-PPG and W-ECG, electrocardiogram and pulse oximetry data, or waveform data. All studies concluded that ML is capable and has the potential to detect AF through wearable devices and through a number of different information. However, more studies to confirm these findings are required.

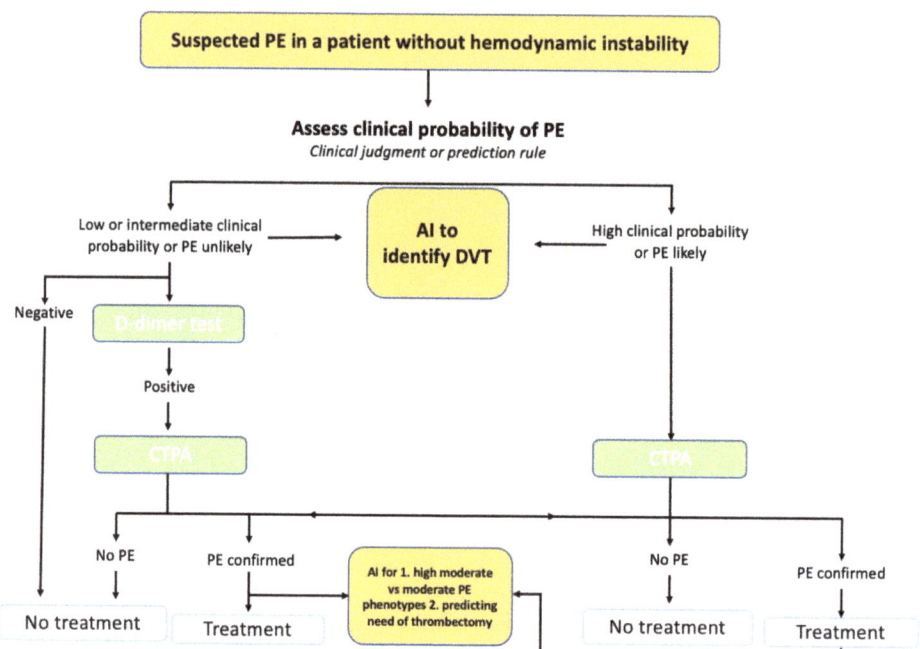

Figure 5. Example of AI in Pulmonary Embolism Evaluation. Figure Description: Current guidelines for a suspected pulmonary embolism (PE) in a patient without hemodynamic instability requires a clinical probability assessment of the PE. Based on the clinical judgment and a potential D-dimer test, a CT pulmonary angiogram is conducted to determine whether treatment or no treatment will occur. AI has the potential to be integrated into this process by potentially detecting deep vein thrombosis, detecting high moderate vs. moderate PE phenotypes, and predicting the risk of thrombectomy.

4. Limitations

While AI's applications have been relatively positive, several limitations have set back its implementation. For one, the introduction of AI into healthcare practices raises a number of concerns, such as a lack of trust, ethical issues, and the absence of accountability [85]. Certain human traits, such as empathy, comfort, and trust, are essential to a doctor–patient relationship, and the use of AI makes these components an issue. To add on, traditionally, physicians and healthcare workers are held accountable for their practice [86]. There is no law to keep ML models intact, and there is no defined ownership to take responsibility when an AI algorithm is at fault. This drawback raises several legal and ethical concerns yet to be answered. The common novelty in ML applications across primary care requires additional clinical trials to support the potential advantages. Table 2 presents all ongoing or completed clinical trials registered in ClinicalTrials.gov and found through the keywords "Artificial Intelligence" and "Primary Care", which were searched for ongoing or completed clinical trials investigating the role of AI in primary care. In addition, there remains mixed findings regarding the potential benefits of ML-based prediction models. For instance, in one systematic review of 71 studies, there was no evidence of a better performance from ML models compared with LR [87]. An additional drawback is that the implementation of ML is costly and would require additional education for incoming medical practitioners [88]. Regarding AI research, many studies suffer from a number of drawbacks that limit the quality of the results. These include a small sample, retrospective data, the inability to separate pre-operative and intra-operative data, missing data, the absence of external validation, data from a single institution, and several biases.

Table 2. Clinical Trials on Artificial Intelligence in Primary Care.

Trial or Registry	N	Aim	Inclusion Criteria	Exclusion Criteria	Status
NCT05166122	1600	Use AI to screen for diabetic retinopathy	>18 years, screened for diabetic retinopathy, with diabetes, can take retina pictures	Part of community hospital with ophthalmologist, previously diagnosed with some retinal conditions, laser retinal treatment, has other eye diseases	Recruiting
NCT05286034	4000	AI ChatBot to improve women participation in cervical cancer screening program	30–65, did not perform pap smear in last 4 years, living in deprived clusters	Outside age group, had pap smear in last 3 years, had hysterectomy including cervix, pregnant beyond 6 months, already scheduled screening appointment	Not yet recruiting
NCT04551287	16,164	Cervical cancer AI screening for cytopathological diagnosis	25–65 years old, availably of confirmed diagnosis results of cytological exam	Unsatisfactory samples of cytological exam, women diagnosed with other malignant tumors	Completed
NCT05435872	2000	AI for gastrointestinal endoscopy screening	Patients received gastroscopy and colonoscopy, endoscopic exam with AI can be accepted	Patients refusing to participate, patients with intolerance or contraindications to endoscopic exams	Recruiting
NCT05697601	2905	Finding predictors of ovarian and endometrial cancer for AI screening tool	Women with gynecological symptoms, women underwent routine gynecological exam	Unable to undergo serial gynecological exam	Recruiting
NCT04838756	100,000	AI for mammography screening	Women eligible for population-based mammography screening	None	Active, not recruiting
NCT05452993	330	AI screening for diabetic retinopathy	Adult patients with diabetes, ongoing diabetes treatment, regular pharmacy customer, informed consent	Unable to read, write, or give consent, refusing to share results with general practitioner	Not yet recruiting
NCT04778670	55,579	AI for large-scale breast screening	Participants in regular population-based breast cancer	Incomplete exam, breast implant, complete mastectomy, participant in surveillance program	Active, not recruiting
NCT05139797	300	AI-guided echo screening of rare diseases	Patients with high suspicion for cardiac amyloidosis by AI	Patients that decline to be seen at specialty clinic, patients that passed away	Recruiting
NCT05139940	2432	AI-enabled TB screening in Zambia	18 years or older with known HIV status	Individuals that do not meet inclusion criteria	Recruiting

Table 2. Cont.

Trial or Registry	N	Aim	Inclusion Criteria	Exclusion Criteria	Status
NCT04743479	5000	AI screening of pancreatic cancer	Subject can provide informed consent, detailed questionnaire filled, and subject has one of several listed conditions	Subject has been diagnosed with pancreatic cancer or other malignant tumors in past 5 years, subject contraindicates MRI or CT, subjects is in another clinical trial	Recruiting
NCT04949776	27,000	AI for breast cancer screening	50–69 years old, women studied in the program in the set period and for the first time	Unable to give consent, breast prostheses, symptoms or signs of suspected breast cancer	Recruiting
NCT05587452	950	AI screening for colorectal cancer	Informed consent, provide blood samples, diagnosed with colorectal cancer or colorectal adenoma	Pregnant or breastfeeding, diagnosed with another cancer, selective exclusions for colorectal cancer and healthy people	Recruiting
NCT05456126	125	AI for infant motor screening	Mothers older than 20, no history of recreational drugs, married or live with fathers. Specific criteria for term and preterm infants	None	Recruiting
NCT05024591	32,714	AI for breast cancer screening	Eligible for national screening, provides consent	History or current breast cancer, currently pregnant or plans to become pregnant, history of breast surgery, has mammography for diagnostic purposes	Recruiting
NCT04732208	410	AI screening of diabetic retinopathy using smartphone camera	Over 18 years, informed consent, established cases of DM, subjects dilated for ophthalmic evaluation	Acute vision loss, contraindicated for fundus imaging, treated for retinopathy, other retinal pathologies, at risk of acute angle closure glaucoma	Completed
NCT05311046	2400	AI screening for pediatric sepsis	3 months–17 years of age, diagnosed with sepsis, blood sample collection	Participating in outside interventions, parents or LARs that do not speak English or Spanish, pregnancy	Recruiting
NCT05391659	1200	AI screening for diabetic retinopathy	Diagnosed with DM, >18 years old, informed consent, fluent in written and oral Dutch	History of diabetic retinopathy or diabetic macular edema treatment, contraindicated for imaging by fundus imaging	Recruiting
NCT04307030	5000	AI screening for congenital heart disease by heart sounds	0–18 years of age, children with or without congenital heart disease, informed consent	>18 years of age, unable to undergo echo, not able to provide informed consent	Not yet recruiting
NCT04000087	358	ECG AI-guided screening for low ejection fraction	Primary care clinicians who are part of a participating care team	Primary care clinicians working in pediatrics, acute care, nursing homes, and resident care teams	Completed

Table 2. *Cont.*

Trial or Registry	N	Aim	Inclusion Criteria	Exclusion Criteria	Status
NCT04156880	1000	AI in mammography-based breast cancer screening	Women had undergone standard mammography, histopathology-proven diagnosis	Concurring lesions on mammograms, no available pathologic diagnosis or long term follow up exams, undergone breast surgery, diagnosed with other kinds of malignancy	Recruiting
NCT05645341	400	AI screening of malignant pigmented tumors on ocular surface	Dark-brown lesions on ocular surface	Non-pigmented ocular surface tumors and image quality does not meet clinical requirements	Recruiting
NCT05048095	15,500	AI in breast cancer screening	Women participating in regular breast cancer screening program	Women with breast implants or other foreign implants in mammogram and women with symptoms or signs of suspected breast cancer	Completed
NCT04894708	1572	AI for polyp detection in colonoscopy	>35 years, planned diagnostic colonoscopy's screening colonoscopy for men >50 or women >55	Colon bleeding, colon carcinoma, known polyps for removal, IBD, colonic stenosis, other suspected colon disease, follow-up care after colon cancer surgery, anticoagulant drugs, poor general condition, incomplete colonoscopy planned	Recruiting
NCT04160988	703	AI for screening diabetic retinopathy	>20 years, DM, image taken by color fundus, include includes macula and optic nerve	Color fundus image previously use, macula, optic nerve or other part is unclear	Completed
NCT04213183	1789	DL screening for hepatobiliary diseases	Quality of fundus and slit-lamp images is acceptable, more than 90% of fundus image area includes four main regions, more than 90% of slit-lamp image area includes three main regions	Images with light leakage (>10% of the area)	Completed
NCT04832594	2500	AI screening for breast cancer for supplemental MRI	Four-view screening mammography exam	Women in surveillance program, breast implants, prior breast cancer, breast feeding, MRI contraindication	Recruiting
NCT05704491	100	AI screening for diabetic retinopathy	DM diagnosis, diabetes duration >5 years, >18 years old, informed consent, fluent in writing and speaking German	History of laser treatment, contraindication to fundus imaging systems	Not yet recruiting
NCT04699864	630	AI for screening diabetic retinopathy	>18 years and older, informed consent, diagnostic for diabetes, diabetic patient followed and referred by physician	Patients less than 18 years old, no informed consent, patient already had treatment for retinal condition	Not yet recruiting

Table 2. Cont.

Trial or Registry	N	Aim	Inclusion Criteria	Exclusion Criteria	Status
NCT04859634	2000	AI for detecting multiple ocular fundus lesions	Participants who agree to take ultra-widefield fundus images	Patients that cannot cooperate with photographer, no informed consent	Recruiting
NCT05734820	312	AI screening colonoscopy	>45 years old, referred for screening colonoscopy, adequate bowel preparation, authorized for endoscopic approach	Pregnancy, clinical condition making endoscopy inviable, history of colorectal carcinoma, IBD, no informed consent	Recruiting
NCT04859530	5886	AI smartphone for cervical cancer screening	Informed consent	No initiation of sexual intercourse, pregnancy, condition altering cervix visualization, previous hysterectomy, health not sufficient	Recruiting
NCT03773458	500	AI for large-scale screening of scoliosis	Pretreatment back photos and whole spine standing X-ray or ultrasound images	Patients considered as non-idiopathic scoliosis	Completed
NCT05704920	2722	AI for lung cancer screening	50–80 years old, active or ex-smoker, smoking history of at least 20 pack-years, informed consent, affiliated with French social security	Clinical signs of cancer, recent chest scan, health problems affecting life expectancy or limiting ability to undergo lung surgery, vulnerable people	Not yet recruiting
NCT05236855	200	AI and spectroscopy for cervical cancer screening	Women undergoing standard HPV screening	NA	Not yet recruiting
NCT05527535	34,500	AI for diabetic retinopathy screening	T1DM or T2DM, no full-time ophthalmologist, >18 years old, eligible for fundus photo imaging	T1DM or T2DM with an ophthalmologist, previous diagnosed with macular edema, history of retinal laser, other ocular disease, not eligible for fundus imaging	Not yet recruiting
NCT05745480	2	NLP for screening opioid misuse	Adults hospitalized at UW health	NA	Recruiting
NCT05490823	1000	AI smartphone for anemia screening	Informed consent	Ophthalmic or fingernail surgery in past 30 days	Recruiting
NCT04896827	244	DL and AI for DNIC	18–70 years old, chronic or no chronic pain, informed consent	CVD, Raynaud syndrome, severe psychiatric disease, injuries or loss sensitivity, pregnant women	Recruiting
NCT05752045	1389	AI for screening eye diseases	>18 years, T1DM or T2DM, presenting screening for diabetic retinopathy, benefits of social security scheme, informed consent	Patient with known DR, any condition affecting study, presenting social or psychological factors, participates in another clinical research study	Not yet recruiting

Table 2. Cont.

Trial or Registry	N	Aim	Inclusion Criteria	Exclusion Criteria	Status
NCT05243121	5000	AI for MRI in screening breast cancer	Patients with clinical symptoms, undergoing full sequence BMRI exam, at least 6 months of follow-up results	Received therapy, contraindications of breast-enhanced MRI exams, prosthesis is implanted in affected breast, patients during lactation or pregnancy	Recruiting
NCT04996615	924	AI for identifying diabetic retinopathy and diabetic macular edema	Routine exams, routine laser treatment, diagnosed with T1DM or T2DM, presents visual acuity	Currently using AI system integrated into clinical care, inability to provide informed consent	Recruiting
NCT03975504	6000	AI for lung cancer screening	Eligible participants aged 45–75 years with one of several risk factors	Had CT scan of chest in past 12 months, history of any cancer within 5 years	Recruiting
NCT05626517	2000	Developing risk stratification tools using AI	21 years or older, sufficient English or Chinese language skills, informed consent	<21 years old, cardiac event, no informed consent	Not yet recruiting
NCT04994899	800	AI screening for mental health	13–79 years old, English-speaking	Previous participant, unable to verbally respond to standard questions, cannot participate in virtual visit, no informed consent	Recruiting
NCT05195385	2400	Lung cancer screening with low-dose CT scans	50–74 years, smoked at least 20 pack years, quit less than 15 years ago, gives consent, affiliated with social security system	Presence of clinical symptoms suggesting malignancy, evolving cancer, history of lung cancer, 2-year follow-up not possible, chest CT scan performed	Recruiting
NCT04240652	500,000	AI for diabetic retinopathy screening	T2DM or T1DM, subjects from other medical institutes are diabetes, non-diabetic patients and healthy participants	History of drug abuse, STDs, any condition not suitable for study	Recruiting
NCT04126239	1610	AI for food addiction screening test	BMI >30, able to give informed consent	Non-French speaker, unable to use internet tools	Recruiting
NCT04603404	430	Multimodality imaging in screening, diagnosis, and risk stratification of HFpEF	LVEF > 50%, NT-proBNP > 220pg/mL or BNP > pg/mL, symptoms and syndromes of HF, at least one criteria of cardiac structure	Special types of cardiomyopathies, infarction, myocardial fibrosis, severe arrhythmia, severe primary cardiac valvular disease, restrictive pericardial disease, refuses to participate in study	Recruiting
NCT05159661	1000	AI for screening brain connectivity and dementia risk estimation	Male and female 60–75 years, MCI diagnosis with MMSE > 25, MCI diagnosis with MoCa > 17	Confirmed dementia, history of cerebrovascular disease, AUD identification test, severe medical disorders associated with cognitive impairment, severe head trauma, severe mental disorders	Recruiting

Table 2. *Cont.*

Trial or Registry	N	Aim	Inclusion Criteria	Exclusion Criteria	Status
NCT05650086	700	AI for breast screening	Understands the study, informed consent, complies with schedule, >21 years, fits cohort specific criteria	Does not fit cohort specific criteria, unable to complete study procedures	Recruiting
NCT05426135	3000	AI for tumor risk assessment	Participants with suspected cancer, informed consent, detailed EHR data, healthy participants	Participants with primary clinical and pathological missing data, lost to follow-up, poor medical image quality	Recruiting
NCT05639348	650	AI for risk assessment of postoperative delirium	Surgical patients, >60 years old, planned postoperative hospital stay >2 days, informed consent	Preoperative delirium, insufficient knowledge in German or French, intracranial surgery, cardiac surgery, surgery within two previous weeks, unable to provide informed consent	Recruiting
NCT05466864	120	Screening of OSA using BSP	Hospitalized with acute ischemic stroke, 18–80, informed consent	History of AF, LVEF < 45%, aphasia, unstable cardiopulmonary status, recent surgery including tracheotomy in 30 days, narcotics, on O2, PAP device, ventilator, unable to understand instructions	Recruiting
NCT05655117	440	AI for detecting eye complications in diabetics	Diabetic patients aged 18–90	Severely ill patient or patient with cancer	Not yet recruiting
NCT03688906	3275	AI colorectal cancer screening test	Differs across three cohorts	Differs across three cohorts	Completed
NCT05246163	1500	AI smartphone for skin cancer detection	Patients with one or two lesions meeting one of several criteria, informed consent	Lack of informed consent	Recruiting
NCT05730192	950	AI for detection of gastrointestinal lesions in endoscopy	Screening or surveillance colonoscopy, age 40 or older, informed consent	Emergency colonoscopies, IBD, CRC, previous colonic resection, returning for elective colonoscopy, polyposis syndromes, contraindications	Not yet recruiting
NCT05566002	2000	AI evaluation of pulmonary hypertension	>18 years, previous received diagnostic imaging	Patients without RHC, quality of exams cannot meet requirement, severe loss of results	Recruiting

5. Implementing AI in Primary Care

Choosing the correct ML model for a primary care task depends on several factors, including the nature of the task, the available data, and the desired outcome (Table 3). First, a definition of the problem and the necessary data must be identified to select the appropriate model [89]. Subsequently, a suitable AI technique, such as supervised, unsupervised, or reinforcement learning, must be chosen. Following the selection of the model, evaluation of the model's performance using validation data and fine-tuning is necessary [89]. Several factors must be considered to evaluate the benefits and risks of implementing a specific AI model into a primary care routine. Accuracy and reliability must be assessed by testing the ML model's performance on validation data [89]. Clinical relevance must be determined by evaluating whether the model is based on relevant risk factors and whether the predictions are helpful for clinical decision-making. Potential benefits such as improving patient outcomes, reducing medical errors, increasing efficiency and productivity, and enhancing the quality of care must also be assessed. Ethical implications of using the AI model in primary care, such as the responsibility of healthcare providers to explain how the AI model works and how decisions are made, and potential issues related to patient autonomy and informed consent, must be considered. Finally, the cost-effectiveness of implementing the AI model, considering the costs of development, implementation, maintenance, and training, as well as potential cost savings and benefits, must be evaluated [90]. Finally, we can anticipate a number of ML technologies, such as sophisticated chatbots and virtual assistants, decision support tools, predictive analytics, wearable technology, and population health management, to become commonplace in primary care during the next two years. These tools could aid primary care providers in making better judgements, delivering more individualized care, and spotting high-risk patients or those needing more intense interventions. However, regulatory approval, patient and healthcare provider acceptance, and integration into current clinical workflows will all be necessary before ML can be deployed. Despite these obstacles, there will likely be major advancements in integrating AI into primary care in the upcoming years, given the rate of technological advancement and the growing desire for more individualized and effective healthcare.

Table 3. Machine learning models.

ML Model	Advantages	Limitations	Clinical Applications in Primary Care
Logistic Regression	Easy to implement and interpret, handles binary and multi-class classification	Does not perform well with outliers, assumes linear relationship	Diagnostic tests, selection of treatment, prognostic modeling, predicting disease risk
Convolutional Neural Network	Excels in video and image recognition, learns hierarchical features	Needs a lot of data and resource, interpretation is limited	Image classification, diagnosing from medical imaging
Support Vector Machine	Handles non-linear decision boundaries, great generalization	Precise kernel function and hyperparameters selection, difficult with noisy data	Diagnosing disease, risk stratification, classifying clinical data
K-Nearest Neighbors	Easy, simple, handles non-linear decision boundaries	Needs a lot of memory and time, sensitivities to certain features	Assisting in disease progression through forecasting
Random Forest	Performs well with high-dimensional data, handles non-linear effects	Hard to interpret, overfits noisy data	Identifying risk factors, predicting outcomes,
Adaptive Boosting	Handles regression and classification problems, combines weak learners	Overfits with weak learners, sensitive to noisy data	Predicting risk of disease, and detecting high risk
Gradient Boosting	Performs with large datasets, handles regression and classification	Overfits with weak learners, sensitive to noisy data	Forecasting outcomes and diagnosing disease
Neural Network	Handles large datasets, performs well on speech and image recognition	Needs a lot of computational resources and data, overfits if complex	Diagnosing disease, selecting treatment, predicting risk of disease
Extreme Gradient Boosting	Fast with large datasets, handles regression and classification	Needs tuning of hyperparameters, overfits with complex weak learners	Predicting outcomes, detecting high-risk patients, diagnosing disease

Table 3. *Cont.*

ML Model	Advantages	Limitations	Clinical Applications in Primary Care
Decision Tree	Simple, easy, handles categorical and numerical data	Overfits with noisy data, sensitivity to variations in training	Identifying risk factors, diagnosing disease, predicting risk of disease
Deep Neural Network	Good performer with large datasets, automatically learns hierarchical features	Requires a lot of data, overfits with complex network	Diagnosing disease, detecting high-risk patients, predicting the risk of disease
Gated Recurrent Unit	Great performer with time-series data, handles variable-length sequences	Sensitivity to some conditions and parameters, poor generalization to new data	Predicting risk of disease, diagnosing diseases, and determining outcomes
XGBoost	Fast, accurate, handles regressions and classification problems	Needs tuning of hyperparameters, overfits with noisy data	Predicting outcomes, identifying risk factors
CatBoost	Handles categorical data, handles regression and classification problems	Needs resources and data, needs tuning of hyperparameters	Identifying risk factors, forecasting outcomes
Naïve Bayes	Simple, efficient, handles high-dimensional data	Independent between features, poor performer with correlated features	Diagnosing diseases, forecasting risk of disease
Logistic Model Tree	Combination of DT and LR to get non-linear effects	Overfits with noisy data, needs tuning of hyperparameters	Determining risk factors, predicting risk of disease
Long Short-Term Memory	Good performer with time-series data, handles variable-length sequence	Computational complexity, difficult interpretation, overfitting, difficult to handle long sequences	Forecasting outcomes, diagnosing diseases, forecasting risk of disease

6. Conclusions

AI in primary care and preventive medicine is a relatively new field of study that has developed endless possibilities. The applications are widespread, as seen through a number of studies on all facets of primary care. Although there is some variability within the findings of studies in specific fields, the general development and implementation of ML algorithms are successful and constructive. The models are usually more effective than previously established models or scores. Future research should focus on tackling the aforementioned limitations and furthering the research on promising sectors of primary care.

Author Contributions: Conceptualization, C.K.; methodology, C.K.; software, H.U.H.V.; validation, C.K., Z.W. and H.U.H.V.; investigation, A.H.E.-S. and C.K.; resources, C.K.; data curation, A.H.E.-S.; writing—original draft preparation, A.H.E.-S.; writing—review and editing, A.H.E.-S., H.U.H.V., Z.W., C.K. and B.S.G.; visualization, H.U.H.V.; supervision, C.K.; project administration. All authors have read and agreed to the published version of the manuscript.

Funding: This research received no external funding.

Institutional Review Board Statement: Not applicable.

Informed Consent Statement: Not applicable.

Data Availability Statement: No new data were created in this study.

Conflicts of Interest: The authors declare no conflict of interest.

References

1. Collins, C.; Dennehy, D.; Conboy, K.; Mikalef, P. Artificial intelligence in information systems research: A systematic literature review and research agenda. *Int. J. Inf. Manag.* **2021**, *60*, 102383. [CrossRef]
2. Kersting, K. Machine Learning and Artificial Intelligence: Two Fellow Travelers on the Quest for Intelligent Behavior in Machines. *Front. Big Data* **2018**, *1*, 6. [CrossRef] [PubMed]
3. Ghuwalewala, S.; Kulkarni, V.; Pant, R.; Kharat, A. Levels of Autonomous Radiology. *Interact. J. Med. Res.* **2022**, *11*, e38655. [CrossRef]
4. Bignami, E.G.; Cozzani, F.; Del Rio, P.; Bellini, V. Artificial intelligence and perioperative medicine. *Minerva Anestesiol.* **2020**, *87*, 755–756. [CrossRef] [PubMed]
5. Chiew, C.J.; Liu, N.; Wong, T.H.; Sim, Y.E.; Abdullah, H.R. Utilizing Machine Learning Methods for Preoperative Prediction of Postsurgical Mortality and Intensive Care Unit Admission. *Ann. Surg.* **2020**, *272*, 1133–1139. [CrossRef]
6. Fernandes, M.P.B.; de la Hoz, M.A.; Rangasamy, V.; Subramaniam, B. Machine Learning Models with Preoperative Risk Factors and Intraoperative Hypotension Parameters Predict Mortality After Cardiac Surgery. *J. Cardiothorac. Vasc. Anesth.* **2021**, *35*, 857–865. [CrossRef] [PubMed]
7. Jalali, A.; Lonsdale, H.; Do, N.; Peck, J.; Gupta, M.; Kutty, S.; Ghazarian, S.R.; Jacobs, J.P.; Rehman, M.; Ahumada, L.M. Deep Learning for Improved Risk Prediction in Surgical Outcomes. *Sci. Rep.* **2020**, *10*, 9289. [CrossRef]
8. Pfitzner, B.; Chromik, J.; Brabender, R.; Fischer, E.; Kromer, A.; Winter, A.; Moosburner, S.; Sauer, I.M.; Malinka, T.; Pratschke, J.; et al. Perioperative Risk Assessment in Pancreatic Surgery Using Machine Learning. In Proceedings of the 2021 43rd Annual International Conference of the IEEE Engineering in Medicine & Biology Society (EMBC), Scotland, UK, 1–5 November 2021; IEEE: Piscataway, NJ, USA, 2021; pp. 2211–2214. [CrossRef]
9. Sahara, K.; Paredes, A.Z.; Tsilimigras, D.I.; Sasaki, K.; Moro, A.; Hyer, J.M.; Mehta, R.; Farooq, S.A.; Wu, L.; Endo, I.; et al. Machine learning predicts unpredicted deaths with high accuracy following hepatopancreatic surgery. *HepatoBiliary Surg. Nutr.* **2021**, *10*, 20–30. [CrossRef]
10. COVIDSurg Collaborativ; Dajti, I.; Valenzuela, J.I.; Boccalatte, L.A.; Gemelli, N.A.; Smith, D.E.; Dudi-Venkata, N.N.; Kroon, H.M.; Sammour, T.; Roberts, M.; et al. Machine learning risk prediction of mortality for patients undergoing surgery with perioperative SARS-CoV-2: The COVIDSurg mortality score. *Br. J. Surg.* **2021**, *108*, 1274–1292. [CrossRef]
11. Xue, B.; Li, D.; Lu, C.; King, C.R.; Wildes, T.; Avidan, M.S.; Kannampallil, T.; Abraham, J. Use of Machine Learning to Develop and Evaluate Models Using Preoperative and Intraoperative Data to Identify Risks of Postoperative Complications. *JAMA Netw. Open* **2021**, *4*, e212240. [CrossRef]
12. Corey, K.M.; Kashyap, S.; Lorenzi, E.; Lagoo-Deenadayalan, S.A.; Heller, K.; Whalen, K.; Balu, S.; Heflin, M.T.; McDonald, S.R.; Swaminathan, M.; et al. Development and validation of machine learning models to identify high-risk surgical patients using automatically curated electronic health record data (Pythia): A retrospective, single-site study. *PLOS Med.* **2018**, *15*, e1002701. [CrossRef]
13. Bonde, A.; Varadarajan, K.M.; Bonde, N.; Troelsen, A.; Muratoglu, O.K.; Malchau, H.; Yang, A.D.; Alam, H.; Sillesen, M. Assessing the utility of deep neural networks in predicting postoperative surgical complications: A retrospective study. *Lancet Digit. Health* **2021**, *3*, e471–e485. [CrossRef]
14. Zhao, H.; Zhang, X.; Xu, Y.; Gao, L.; Ma, Z.; Sun, Y.; Wang, W. Predicting the Risk of Hypertension Based on Several Easy-to-Collect Risk Factors: A Machine Learning Method. *Front. Public Health* **2021**, *9*, 619429. [CrossRef]
15. Alkaabi, L.A.; Ahmed, L.S.; Al Attiyah, M.F.; Abdel-Rahman, M.E. Predicting hypertension using machine learning: Findings from Qatar Biobank Study. *PLoS ONE* **2020**, *15*, e0240370. [CrossRef]
16. Ye, C.; Fu, T.; Hao, S.; Zhang, Y.; Wang, O.; Jin, B.; Xia, M.; Liu, M.; Zhou, X.; Wu, Q.; et al. Prediction of Incident Hypertension Within the Next Year: Prospective Study Using Statewide Electronic Health Records and Machine Learning. *J. Med. Internet Res.* **2018**, *20*, e22. [CrossRef]
17. LaFreniere, D.; Zulkernine, F.; Barber, D.; Martin, K. Using machine learning to predict hypertension from a clinical dataset. In Proceedings of the 2016 IEEE Symposium Series on Computational Intelligence (SSCI), Athens, Greece, 6–9 December 2016; IEEE: Piscataway, NJ, USA, 2016; pp. 1–7. [CrossRef]
18. Khalid, S.G.; Zhang, J.; Chen, F.; Zheng, D. Blood Pressure Estimation Using Photoplethysmography Only: Comparison between Different Machine Learning Approaches. *J. Healthc. Eng.* **2018**, *2018*, 1548647. [CrossRef]
19. Myers, K.D.; Knowles, J.W.; Staszak, D.; Shapiro, M.D.; Howard, W.; Yadava, M.; Zuzick, D.; Williamson, L.; Shah, N.H.; Banda, J.; et al. Precision screening for familial hypercholesterolaemia: A machine learning study applied to electronic health encounter data. *Lancet Digit. Health* **2019**, *1*, e393–e402. [CrossRef]
20. Pina, A.; Helgadottir, S.; Mancina, R.M.; Pavanello, C.; Pirazzi, C.; Montalcini, T.; Henriques, R.; Calabresi, L.; Wiklund, O.; Macedo, M.P.; et al. Virtual genetic diagnosis for familial hypercholesterolemia powered by machine learning. *Eur. J. Prev. Cardiol.* **2020**, *27*, 1639–1646. [CrossRef]
21. Liu, Y.; Zhang, Q.; Zhao, G.; Liu, G.; Liu, Z. Deep Learning-Based Method of Diagnosing Hyperlipidemia and Providing Diagnostic Markers Automatically. *Diabetes Metab. Syndr. Obes. Targets Ther.* **2020**, *13*, 679–691. [CrossRef]
22. Tsigalou, C.; Panopoulou, M.; Papadopoulos, C.; Karvelas, A.; Tsairidis, D.; Anagnostopoulos, K. Estimation of low-density lipoprotein cholesterol by machine learning methods. *Clin. Chim. Acta* **2021**, *517*, 108–116. [CrossRef]

23. Çubukçu, H.C.; Topcu, D.I. Estimation of Low-Density Lipoprotein Cholesterol Concentration Using Machine Learning. *Lab. Med.* **2022**, *53*, 161–171. [CrossRef] [PubMed]
24. Weng, S.F.; Reps, J.; Kai, J.; Garibaldi, J.M.; Qureshi, N. Can machine-learning improve cardiovascular risk prediction using routine clinical data? *PLoS ONE* **2017**, *12*, e0174944. [CrossRef] [PubMed]
25. Zhao, J.; Feng, Q.; Wu, P.; Lupu, R.A.; Wilke, R.A.; Wells, Q.S.; Denny, J.C.; Wei, W.-Q. Learning from Longitudinal Data in Electronic Health Record and Genetic Data to Improve Cardiovascular Event Prediction. *Sci. Rep.* **2019**, *9*, 717. [CrossRef] [PubMed]
26. Kusunose, K.; Hirata, Y.; Tsuji, T.; Kotoku, J.; Sata, M. Deep learning to predict elevated pulmonary artery pressure in patients with suspected pulmonary hypertension using standard chest X-ray. *Sci. Rep.* **2020**, *10*, 19311. [CrossRef]
27. Madani, A.; Moradi, M.; Karargyris, A.; Syeda-Mahmood, T. Chest X-ray generation and data augmentation for cardiovascular abnormality classification. In *Medical Imaging 2018: Image Processing*; Angelini, E.D., Landman, B.A., Eds.; SPIE: Houston, TX, USA, 2018; p. 57. [CrossRef]
28. Ambale-Venkatesh, B.; Yang, X.; Wu, C.O.; Liu, K.; Hundley, W.G.; McClelland, R.; Gomes, A.S.; Folsom, A.R.; Shea, S.; Guallar, E.; et al. Cardiovascular Event Prediction by Machine Learning: The Multi-Ethnic Study of Atherosclerosis. *Circ. Res.* **2017**, *121*, 1092–1101. [CrossRef]
29. Alaa, A.M.; Bolton, T.; Di Angelantonio, E.; Rudd, J.H.F.; van der Schaar, M. Cardiovascular disease risk prediction using automated machine learning: A prospective study of 423,604 UK Biobank participants. *PLoS ONE* **2019**, *14*, e0213653. [CrossRef]
30. Pfohl, S.; Marafino, B.; Coulet, A.; Rodriguez, F.; Palaniappan, L.; Shah, N.H. Creating Fair Models of Atherosclerotic Cardiovascular Disease Risk. In Proceedings of the 2019 AAAI/ACM Conference on AI, Ethics, and Society, Honolulu, HI, USA, 27–28 January 2019. [CrossRef]
31. Al'aref, S.J.; Maliakal, G.; Singh, G.; van Rosendael, A.R.; Ma, X.; Xu, Z.; Alawamlh, O.A.H.; Lee, B.; Pandey, M.; Achenbach, S.; et al. Machine learning of clinical variables and coronary artery calcium scoring for the prediction of obstructive coronary artery disease on coronary computed tomography angiography: Analysis from the CONFIRM registry. *Eur. Heart J.* **2020**, *41*, 359–367. [CrossRef]
32. Ting, D.S.W.; Cheung, C.Y.-L.; Lim, G.; Tan, G.S.W.; Quang, N.D.; Gan, A.; Hamzah, H.; Garcia-Franco, R.; Yeo, I.Y.S.; Lee, S.Y.; et al. Development and Validation of a Deep Learning System for Diabetic Retinopathy and Related Eye Diseases Using Retinal Images From Multiethnic Populations With Diabetes. *JAMA* **2017**, *318*, 2211–2223. [CrossRef]
33. Poplin, R.; Varadarajan, A.V.; Blumer, K.; Liu, Y.; McConnell, M.V.; Corrado, G.S.; Peng, L.; Webster, D.R. Prediction of cardiovascular risk factors from retinal fundus photographs via deep learning. *Nat. Biomed. Eng.* **2018**, *2*, 158–164. [CrossRef]
34. Kim, Y.D.; Noh, K.J.; Byun, S.J.; Lee, S.; Kim, T.; Sunwoo, L.; Lee, K.J.; Kang, S.-H.; Park, K.H.; Park, S.J. Effects of Hypertension, Diabetes, and Smoking on Age and Sex Prediction from Retinal Fundus Images. *Sci. Rep.* **2020**, *10*, 4623. [CrossRef]
35. Ravaut, M.; Harish, V.; Sadeghi, H.; Leung, K.K.; Volkovs, M.; Kornas, K.; Watson, T.; Poutanen, T.; Rosella, L.C. Development and Validation of a Machine Learning Model Using Administrative Health Data to Predict Onset of Type 2 Diabetes. *JAMA Netw. Open* **2021**, *4*, e2111315. [CrossRef]
36. Ravaut, M.; Sadeghi, H.; Leung, K.K.; Volkovs, M.; Kornas, K.; Harish, V.; Watson, T.; Lewis, G.F.; Weisman, A.; Poutanen, T.; et al. Predicting adverse outcomes due to diabetes complications with machine learning using administrative health data. *Npj Digit. Med.* **2021**, *4*, 24. [CrossRef]
37. Deberneh, H.M.; Kim, I. Prediction of Type 2 Diabetes Based on Machine Learning Algorithm. *Int. J. Environ. Res. Public Health* **2021**, *18*, 3317. [CrossRef]
38. Alhassan, Z.; McGough, A.S.; Alshammari, R.; Daghstani, T.; Budgen, D.; Al Moubayed, N. Type-2 Diabetes Mellitus Diagnosis from Time Series Clinical Data Using Deep Learning Models. In *Artificial Neural Networks and Machine Learning—ICANN 2018*; Kůrková, V., Manolopoulos, Y., Hammer, B., Iliadis, L., Maglogiannis, I., Eds.; Lecture Notes in Computer Science; Springer International Publishing: Cham, Switzerland, 2018; Volume 11141, pp. 468–478. [CrossRef]
39. Boutilier, J.J.; Chan, T.C.Y.; Ranjan, M.; Deo, S. Risk Stratification for Early Detection of Diabetes and Hypertension in Resource-Limited Settings: Machine Learning Analysis. *J. Med. Internet Res.* **2021**, *23*, e20123. [CrossRef]
40. Sung, H.; Ferlay, J.; Siegel, R.L.; Laversanne, M.; Soerjomataram, I.; Jemal, A.; Bray, F. Global Cancer Statistics 2020: GLOBOCAN Estimates of Incidence and Mortality Worldwide for 36 Cancers in 185 Countries. *CA Cancer J. Clin.* **2021**, *71*, 209–249. [CrossRef]
41. Alharbi, F.; Vakanski, A. Machine Learning Methods for Cancer Classification Using Gene Expression Data: A Review. *Bioengineering* **2023**, *10*, 173. [CrossRef]
42. Ardila, D.; Kiraly, A.P.; Bharadwaj, S.; Choi, B.; Reicher, J.J.; Peng, L.; Tse, D.; Etemadi, M.; Ye, W.; Corrado, G.; et al. End-to-end lung cancer screening with three-dimensional deep learning on low-dose chest computed tomography. *Nat. Med.* **2019**, *25*, 954–961. [CrossRef]
43. Gould, M.K.; Huang, B.Z.; Tammemagi, M.C.; Kinar, Y.; Shiff, R. Machine Learning for Early Lung Cancer Identification Using Routine Clinical and Laboratory Data. *Am. J. Respir. Crit. Care Med.* **2021**, *204*, 445–453. [CrossRef]
44. Yeh, M.C.-H.; Wang, Y.-H.; Yang, H.-C.; Bai, K.-J.; Wang, H.-H.; Li, Y.-C.J. Artificial Intelligence–Based Prediction of Lung Cancer Risk Using Nonimaging Electronic Medical Records: Deep Learning Approach. *J. Med. Internet Res.* **2021**, *23*, e26256. [CrossRef]
45. Guo, Y.; Yin, S.; Chen, S.; Ge, Y. Predictors of underutilization of lung cancer screening: A machine learning approach. *Eur. J. Cancer Prev.* **2022**, *31*, 523–529. [CrossRef]

46. Mehmood, M.; Rizwan, M.; Ml, M.G.; Abbas, S. Machine Learning Assisted Cervical Cancer Detection. *Front. Public Health* **2021**, *9*, 788376. [CrossRef] [PubMed]
47. Rahaman, M.; Li, C.; Yao, Y.; Kulwa, F.; Wu, X.; Li, X.; Wang, Q. DeepCervix: A deep learning-based framework for the classification of cervical cells using hybrid deep feature fusion techniques. *Comput. Biol. Med.* **2021**, *136*, 104649. [CrossRef] [PubMed]
48. Wentzensen, N.; Lahrmann, B.; Clarke, M.A.; Kinney, W.; Tokugawa, D.; Poitras, N.; Locke, A.; Bartels, L.; Krauthoff, A.; Walker, J.; et al. Accuracy and Efficiency of Deep-Learning–Based Automation of Dual Stain Cytology in Cervical Cancer Screening. *JNCI J. Natl. Cancer Inst.* **2020**, *113*, 72–79. [CrossRef] [PubMed]
49. Shen, L.; Margolies, L.R.; Rothstein, J.H.; Fluder, E.; McBride, R.; Sieh, W. Deep Learning to Improve Breast Cancer Detection on Screening Mammography. *Sci. Rep.* **2019**, *9*, 12495. [CrossRef]
50. Buda, M.; Saha, A.; Walsh, R.; Ghate, S.; Li, N.; Swiecicki, A.; Lo, J.Y.; Mazurowski, M.A. A Data Set and Deep Learning Algorithm for the Detection of Masses and Architectural Distortions in Digital Breast Tomosynthesis Images. *JAMA Netw. Open* **2021**, *4*, e2119100. [CrossRef]
51. Maghsoudi, O.H.; Gastounioti, A.; Scott, C.; Pantalone, L.; Wu, F.-F.; Cohen, E.A.; Winham, S.; Conant, E.F.; Vachon, C.; Kontos, D. Deep-LIBRA: An artificial-intelligence method for robust quantification of breast density with independent validation in breast cancer risk assessment. *Med. Image Anal.* **2021**, *73*, 102138. [CrossRef]
52. Ming, C.; Viassolo, V.; Probst-Hensch, N.; Dinov, I.D.; Chappuis, P.O.; Katapodi, M.C. Machine learning-based lifetime breast cancer risk reclassification compared with the BOADICEA model: Impact on screening recommendations. *Br. J. Cancer* **2020**, *123*, 860–867. [CrossRef]
53. Perera, M.; Mirchandani, R.; Papa, N.; Breemer, G.; Effeindzourou, A.; Smith, L.; Swindle, P.; Smith, E. PSA-based machine learning model improves prostate cancer risk stratification in a screening population. *World J. Urol.* **2021**, *39*, 1897–1902. [CrossRef]
54. Chiu, P.K.-F.; Shen, X.; Wang, G.; Ho, C.-L.; Leung, C.-H.; Ng, C.-F.; Choi, K.-S.; Teoh, J.Y.-C. Enhancement of prostate cancer diagnosis by machine learning techniques: An algorithm development and validation study. *Prostate Cancer Prostatic Dis.* **2021**, *25*, 672–676. [CrossRef]
55. Beinecke, J.M.; Anders, P.; Schurrat, T.; Heider, D.; Luster, M.; Librizzi, D.; Hauschild, A.-C. Evaluation of machine learning strategies for imaging confirmed prostate cancer recurrence prediction on electronic health records. *Comput. Biol. Med.* **2022**, *143*, 105263. [CrossRef]
56. Turbé, V.; Herbst, C.; Mngomezulu, T.; Meshkinfamfard, S.; Dlamini, N.; Mhlongo, T.; Smit, T.; Cherepanova, V.; Shimada, K.; Budd, J.; et al. Deep learning of HIV field-based rapid tests. *Nat. Med.* **2021**, *27*, 1165–1170. [CrossRef]
57. Bao, Y.; Medland, N.A.; Fairley, C.K.; Wu, J.; Shang, X.; Chow, E.P.; Xu, X.; Ge, Z.; Zhuang, X.; Zhang, L. Predicting the diagnosis of HIV and sexually transmitted infections among men who have sex with men using machine learning approaches. *J. Infect.* **2020**, *82*, 48–59. [CrossRef]
58. Marcus, J.L.; Hurley, L.B.; Krakower, D.S.; Alexeeff, S.; Silverberg, M.J.; Volk, J.E. Use of electronic health record data and machine learning to identify candidates for HIV pre-exposure prophylaxis: A modelling study. *Lancet HIV* **2019**, *6*, e688–e695. [CrossRef]
59. Elder, H.R.; Gruber, S.; Willis, S.J.; Cocoros, N.; Callahan, M.; Flagg, E.W.; Klompas, M.; Hsu, K.K. Can Machine Learning Help Identify Patients at Risk for Recurrent Sexually Transmitted Infections? *Sex. Transm. Dis.* **2020**, *48*, 56–62. [CrossRef]
60. Gadalla, A.A.H.; Friberg, I.M.; Kift-Morgan, A.; Zhang, J.; Eberl, M.; Topley, N.; Weeks, I.; Cuff, S.; Wootton, M.; Gal, M.; et al. Identification of clinical and urine biomarkers for uncomplicated urinary tract infection using machine learning algorithms. *Sci. Rep.* **2019**, *9*, 19694. [CrossRef]
61. Taylor, R.A.; Moore, C.L.; Cheung, K.-H.; Brandt, C. Predicting urinary tract infections in the emergency department with machine learning. *PLoS ONE* **2018**, *13*, e0194085. [CrossRef]
62. Tsai, C.-Y.; Liu, W.-T.; Lin, Y.-T.; Lin, S.-Y.; Houghton, R.; Hsu, W.-H.; Wu, D.; Lee, H.-C.; Wu, C.-J.; Li, L.Y.J.; et al. Machine learning approaches for screening the risk of obstructive sleep apnea in the Taiwan population based on body profile. *Inform. Health Soc. Care* **2021**, *47*, 373–388. [CrossRef]
63. Álvarez, D.; Cerezo-Hernández, A.; Crespo, A.; Gutiérrez-Tobal, G.C.; Vaquerizo-Villar, F.; Barroso-García, V.; Moreno, F.; Arroyo, C.A.; Ruiz, T.; Hornero, R.; et al. A machine learning-based test for adult sleep apnoea screening at home using oximetry and airflow. *Sci. Rep.* **2020**, *10*, 5332. [CrossRef]
64. Mencar, C.; Gallo, C.; Mantero, M.; Tarsia, P.; Carpagnano, G.E.; Barbaro, M.P.F.; Lacedonia, D. Application of machine learning to predict obstructive sleep apnea syndrome severity. *Health Inform. J.* **2020**, *26*, 298–317. [CrossRef]
65. Park, H.W.; Jung, H.; Back, K.Y.; Choi, H.J.; Ryu, K.S.; Cha, H.S.; Lee, E.K.; Hong, A.R.; Hwangbo, Y. Application of Machine Learning to Identify Clinically Meaningful Risk Group for Osteoporosis in Individuals Under the Recommended Age for Dual-Energy X-Ray Absorptiometry. *Calcif. Tissue Int.* **2021**, *109*, 645–655. [CrossRef]
66. Kim, S.K.; Yoo, T.K.; Oh, E.; Kim, D.W. Osteoporosis risk prediction using machine learning and conventional methods. In Proceedings of the 2013 35th Annual International Conference of the IEEE Engineering in Medicine and Biology Society (EMBC), Osaka, Japan, 3–7 July 2013; IEEE: Piscataway, NJ, USA, 2013; pp. 188–191. [CrossRef]
67. Liu, L.; Si, M.; Ma, H.; Cong, M.; Xu, Q.; Sun, Q.; Wu, W.; Wang, C.; Fagan, M.J.; Mur, L.A.J.; et al. A hierarchical opportunistic screening model for osteoporosis using machine learning applied to clinical data and CT images. *BMC Bioinform.* **2022**, *23*, 63. [CrossRef] [PubMed]

68. Lim, H.K.; Ha, H.I.; Park, S.-Y.; Han, J. Prediction of femoral osteoporosis using machine-learning analysis with radiomics features and abdomen-pelvic CT: A retrospective single center preliminary study. *PLoS ONE* **2021**, *16*, e0247330. [CrossRef] [PubMed]
69. Wu, Q.; Nasoz, F.; Jung, J.; Bhattarai, B.; Han, M.V. Machine Learning Approaches for Fracture Risk Assessment: A Comparative Analysis of Genomic and Phenotypic Data in 5130 Older Men. *Calcif. Tissue Int.* **2020**, *107*, 353–361. [CrossRef] [PubMed]
70. Moslemi, A.; Kontogianni, K.; Brock, J.; Wood, S.; Herth, F.; Kirby, M. Differentiating COPD and asthma using quantitative CT imaging and machine learning. *Eur. Respir. J.* **2022**, *60*, 2103078. [CrossRef] [PubMed]
71. Zeng, S.; Arjomandi, M.; Tong, Y.; Liao, Z.C.; Luo, G. Developing a Machine Learning Model to Predict Severe Chronic Obstructive Pulmonary Disease Exacerbations: Retrospective Cohort Study. *J. Med. Internet Res.* **2022**, *24*, e28953. [CrossRef]
72. Nishat, M.; Faisal, F.; Dip, R.; Nasrullah, S.; Ahsan, R.; Shikder, F.; Asif, M.A. Hoque A Comprehensive Analysis on Detecting Chronic Kidney Disease by Employing Machine Learning Algorithms. *EAI Endorsed Trans. Pervasive Health Technol.* **2018**, *7*, 170671. [CrossRef]
73. Bai, Q.; Su, C.; Tang, W.; Li, Y. Machine learning to predict end stage kidney disease in chronic kidney disease. *Sci. Rep.* **2022**, *12*, 8377. [CrossRef]
74. Heidari, A.; Navimipour, N.J.; Unal, M.; Toumaj, S. Machine learning applications for COVID-19 outbreak management. *Neural Comput. Appl.* **2022**, *34*, 15313–15348. [CrossRef]
75. Zhou, X.; Wang, Z.; Li, S.; Liu, T.; Wang, X.; Xia, J.; Zhao, Y. Machine Learning-Based Decision Model to Distinguish Between COVID-19 and Influenza: A Retrospective, Two-Centered, Diagnostic Study. *Risk Manag. Healthc. Policy* **2021**, *14*, 595–604. [CrossRef]
76. Zan, A.; Xie, Z.-R.; Hsu, Y.-C.; Chen, Y.-H.; Lin, T.-H.; Chang, Y.-S.; Chang, K.Y. DeepFlu: A deep learning approach for forecasting symptomatic influenza A infection based on pre-exposure gene expression. *Comput. Methods Programs Biomed.* **2021**, *213*, 106495. [CrossRef]
77. Nadda, W.; Boonchieng, W.; Boonchieng, E. Influenza, dengue and common cold detection using LSTM with fully connected neural network and keywords selection. *BioData Min.* **2022**, *15*, 5. [CrossRef]
78. Hogan, C.A.; Rajpurkar, P.; Sowrirajan, H.; Phillips, N.A.; Le, A.T.; Wu, M.; Garamani, N.; Sahoo, M.K.; Wood, M.L.; Huang, C.; et al. Nasopharyngeal metabolomics and machine learning approach for the diagnosis of influenza. *EbioMedicine* **2021**, *71*, 103546. [CrossRef]
79. Choo, H.; Kim, M.; Choi, J.; Shin, J.; Shin, S.-Y. Influenza Screening via Deep Learning Using a Combination of Epidemiological and Patient-Generated Health Data: Development and Validation Study. *J. Med. Internet Res.* **2020**, *22*, e21369. [CrossRef]
80. Lown, M.; Brown, M.; Brown, C.; Yue, A.M.; Shah, B.N.; Corbett, S.J.; Lewith, G.; Stuart, B.; Moore, M.; Little, P. Machine learning detection of Atrial Fibrillation using wearable technology. *PLoS ONE* **2020**, *15*, e0227401. [CrossRef]
81. Ali, F.; Hasan, B.; Ahmad, H.; Hoodbhoy, Z.; Bhuriwala, Z.; Hanif, M.; Ansari, S.U.; Chowdhury, D. Detection of subclinical rheumatic heart disease in children using a deep learning algorithm on digital stethoscope: A study protocol. *BMJ Open* **2021**, *11*, e044070. [CrossRef]
82. Kwon, S.; Hong, J.; Choi, E.-K.; Lee, E.; Hostallero, D.E.; Kang, W.J.; Lee, B.; Jeong, E.-R.; Koo, B.-K.; Oh, S.; et al. Deep Learning Approaches to Detect Atrial Fibrillation Using Photoplethysmographic Signals: Algorithms Development Study. *JMIR mHealth uHealth* **2019**, *7*, e12770. [CrossRef]
83. Tiwari, P.; Colborn, K.L.; Smith, D.E.; Xing, F.; Ghosh, D.; Rosenberg, M.A. Assessment of a Machine Learning Model Applied to Harmonized Electronic Health Record Data for the Prediction of Incident Atrial Fibrillation. *JAMA Netw. Open* **2020**, *3*, e1919396. [CrossRef]
84. Sekelj, S.; Sandler, B.; Johnston, E.; Pollock, K.G.; Hill, N.R.; Gordon, J.; Tsang, C.; Khan, S.; Ng, F.S.; Farooqui, U. Detecting undiagnosed atrial fibrillation in UK primary care: Validation of a machine learning prediction algorithm in a retrospective cohort study. *Eur. J. Prev. Cardiol.* **2021**, *28*, 598–605. [CrossRef]
85. Kelly, C.J.; Karthikesalingam, A.; Suleyman, M.; Corrado, G.; King, D. Key challenges for delivering clinical impact with artificial intelligence. *BMC Med.* **2019**, *17*, 195. [CrossRef]
86. Sunarti, S.; Rahman, F.F.; Naufal, M.; Risky, M.; Febriyanto, K.; Masnina, R. Artificial intelligence in healthcare: Opportunities and risk for future. *Gac. Sanit.* **2021**, *35*, S67–S70. [CrossRef]
87. Christodoulou, E.; Ma, J.; Collins, G.S.; Steyerberg, E.W.; Verbakel, J.Y.; Van Calster, B. A systematic review shows no performance benefit of machine learning over logistic regression for clinical prediction models. *J. Clin. Epidemiol.* **2019**, *110*, 12–22. [CrossRef]
88. Ahuja, A.S. The impact of artificial intelligence in medicine on the future role of the physician. *PeerJ* **2019**, *7*, e7702. [CrossRef] [PubMed]
89. Raschka, S. Model Evaluation, Model Selection, and Algorithm Selection in Machine Learning. *arXiv* **2018**, arXiv:1811.12808. [CrossRef]
90. de Vos, J.; Visser, L.A.; de Beer, A.A.; Fornasa, M.; Thoral, P.J.; Elbers, P.W.; Cinà, G. The Potential Cost-Effectiveness of a Machine Learning Tool That Can Prevent Untimely Intensive Care Unit Discharge. *Value Health* **2021**, *25*, 359–367. [CrossRef] [PubMed]

Disclaimer/Publisher's Note: The statements, opinions and data contained in all publications are solely those of the individual author(s) and contributor(s) and not of MDPI and/or the editor(s). MDPI and/or the editor(s) disclaim responsibility for any injury to people or property resulting from any ideas, methods, instructions or products referred to in the content.

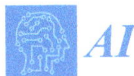

Commentary

Predictive Analytics with a Transdisciplinary Framework in Promoting Patient-Centric Care of Polychronic Conditions: Trends, Challenges, and Solutions

Thomas T. H. Wan [1,*] and Hunter S. Wan [2]

1 School of Global Health Management and Informatics, University of Central Florida, 500 W Livingston Street, Orlando, FL 32801, USA
2 Department of Biology, Grove City College, 100 Campus Drive, Grove City, PA 16127, USA; wanhs20@gcc.edu
* Correspondence: thomas.wan@ucf.edu

Abstract: Context. This commentary is based on an innovative approach to the development of predictive analytics. It is centered on the development of predictive models for varying stages of chronic disease through integrating all types of datasets, adds various new features to a theoretically driven data warehousing, creates purpose-specific prediction models, and integrates multi-criteria predictions of chronic disease progression based on a biomedical evolutionary learning platform. After merging across-center databases based on the risk factors identified from modeling the predictors of chronic disease progression, the collaborative investigators could conduct multi-center verification of the predictive model and further develop a clinical decision support system coupled with visualization of a shared decision-making feature for patient care. The Study Problem. The success of health services management research is dependent upon the stability of pattern detection and the usefulness of nosological classification formulated from big-data-to-knowledge research on chronic conditions. However, longitudinal observations with multiple waves of predictors and outcomes are needed to capture the evolution of polychronic conditions. Motivation. The transitional probabilities could be estimated from big-data analysis with further verification. Simulation or predictive models could then generate a useful explanatory pathogenesis of the end-stage-disorder or outcomes. Hence, the clinical decision support system for patient-centered interventions could be systematically designed and executed. Methodology. A customized algorithm for polychronic conditions coupled with constraints-oriented reasoning approaches is suggested. Based on theoretical specifications of causal inquiries, we could mitigate the effects of multiple confounding factors in conducting evaluation research on the determinants of patient care outcomes. This is what we consider as the mechanism for avoiding the black-box expression in the formulation of predictive analytics. The remaining task is to gather new data to verify the practical utility of the proposed and validated predictive equation(s). More specifically, this includes two approaches guiding future research on chronic disease and care management: (1) To develop a biomedical evolutionary learning platform to predict the risk of polychronic conditions at various stages, especially for predicting the micro- and macro-cardiovascular complications experienced by patients with Type 2 diabetes for multidisciplinary care; and (2) to formulate appropriate prescriptive intervention services, such as patient-centered care management interventions for a high-risk group of patients with polychronic conditions. Conclusions. The commentary has identified trends, challenges, and solutions in conducting innovative AI-based healthcare research that can improve understandings of disease-state transitions from diabetes to other chronic polychronic conditions. Hence, better predictive models could be further formulated to expand from inductive (problem solving) to deductive (theory based and hypothesis testing) inquiries in care management research.

Keywords: polychronic conditions; predictive analytics; care management interventions; patient care outcomes and modeling; decision support system design and evaluation

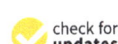

Citation: Wan, T.T.H.; Wan, H.S. Predictive Analytics with a Transdisciplinary Framework in Promoting Patient-Centric Care of Polychronic Conditions: Trends, Challenges, and Solutions. *AI* **2023**, *4*, 482–490. https://doi.org/10.3390/ai4030026

Academic Editor: Tim Hulsen

Received: 20 May 2023
Revised: 8 July 2023
Accepted: 11 July 2023
Published: 13 July 2023

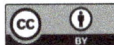

Copyright: © 2023 by the authors. Licensee MDPI, Basel, Switzerland. This article is an open access article distributed under the terms and conditions of the Creative Commons Attribution (CC BY) license (https:// creativecommons.org/licenses/by/ 4.0/).

1. Introduction

A transdisciplinary framework for chronic disease research has been established by health services researchers [1,2] in the selection of relevant variables for the prediction of disease transition during a life course, as particularly related to Type 2 diabetes [3–5], heart failure [6,7], and chronic kidney disease [8]. The Centers for Medicare and Medicaid Services (CMS) has strongly advocated for the use of practical selfcare management strategies to tackle chronic disease management under severe resource constraints [9,10]. It offers a detailed analytical plan with problem-solving steps for delivering high-quality research results.

The concomitant development of the theoretical framework and methodological rigor required for verifying predictive analytics is germane to the formulation of artificial intelligence applications in healthcare. This care management approach may generate pertinent information for implementing and evaluating effective multidisciplinary care for chronic diseases. The present research and review paper offers a novel approach to the design and implementation of Support Vector Machine (SVM), a simple supervised machine learning algorithm used for classification and/or regression. The SVM-based predictive models enhance the prescriptive clinical care for polychronic conditions [11,12]. The transdisciplinary and collaborative nature of confirmatory research may generate useful care management and policy-relevant information to guide the improvement of chronic disease care for a targeted group of high-risk patient population members [13].

The central research inquiry is to address what and how AI healthcare research on the management of chronic diseases can be solidified and guided by the development of theoretically sound and methodologically rigorous approaches to selfcare management research. The purpose of this commentary is twofold: (1) To develop a biomedical evolutionary learning platform for predicting the micro- and macro-cardiovascular complications experienced by patients with chronic conditions for multidisciplinary care; and (2) to formulate appropriate prescriptive intervention services, such as patient-centered care management interventions, for a high-risk group of patients with polychronic conditions.

2. Critical Issues for Chronic Disease and Care Management Research

This paper addresses four critical issues pertaining to the application of artificial intelligence technologies: (1) global trends in chronic care and outcomes evaluation, (2) critical needs for assessing patient-centered care interventions, (3) challenges and solutions for chronic care in promoting coordinated or guided care, and (4) opportunities in transdisciplinary and collaborative care management research.

2.1. Global Trends in Chronic Care and Outcomes Evaluation

As the growth of an aging population is associated with an increase in demand for care, it is natural to pay special attention to the complex needs of frail elders. Four specific care management trends are presented below. First, the path to polychronic conditions reflects the need for covering both physical and mental health domains. The reciprocal relationship between them should be better investigated by health services researchers. Second, chronic care management has emerged as a highly specialized field in clinical medicine. Integrated care coupled with chronic care management requires the development of transdisciplinary orientation and teamwork in the phase of design, implementation, and evaluation of care plans. In the United States, the joint efforts of two governmental agencies such as the Agency for Health Research and Quality (AHRQ) and the CMS have led the ways in formulating chronic care management guidelines. Second, the growth of community-based care as an option or alternative to the institutionalization of the elderly facilitates the growth of post-acute care and long-term care in numerous countries. For instance, Taiwan has ventured into a long-term care (LTC) alternative movement in 2007. To date, Taiwan has ventured into an era of LTC 2.0. with strong financial support for the growth of community-based long term care alternatives. Third, patient engagement is essential for success in performing patient care outcomes assessment and evaluation. The use of logic models in program planning and evaluation has signified how the structure-process-performance-outcomes framework of chronic care management could help optimize global collaboration in chronic care management research. Fourth, assisted technology development has shaped how care is managed and delivered. Furthermore, embracing new applications of information technology and addressing the healthcare labor shortage are two important tasks for global collaboration. It is anticipated that social robotics and other AI-based communication applications may transfer the landscape of chronic care management from a low to a high technology platform.

2.2. Critical Needs for Assessing Patient-Centered Care Interventions

Patient-centered care is characterized by several important principles: (1) problem identification [14] before alleviating the problem, (2) targeting high-risk patients for care management interventions [15], (3) designing and implementing patient-centered care modalities [4,6], and (4) conducting a patient outcome-based evaluation guided by the logic model [9,16]. It is important to note that patient-centered care is characterized by important principles such as respect for a patient's preference or choice, the provision of coordinated and integrated care, encouragement in shared information and decision-making, presence of personal comfort and emotional support, family involvement and support groups, continuity of care, and equitable care provision.

2.3. Challenges and Solutions for Designing Chronic Care Modalities in Promoting Coordinated or Guided Care

Challenge One. The Lack of Theoretical Guidance in Selecting Predictor Variables

Longitudinal patient-care datasets could be used to generate predictive models in varying stages of chronic disease. This is an efficient approach for the investigation of the progressive nature of chronic disease. However, a lack of theoretical guidance in selecting predictor variables has seriously affected the predictability of empirical models.

Solutions: The retrospective approach could be replaced by the prospective study approach, using a small set of predictor variables in the evaluation of progressive paths of polychronic conditions. Two-level modeling of the determinants of health and healthcare enables the examination of joint and interaction effects of personal/behavioral factors at the micro-level analysis and ecological/contextual factors at the macro-level analysis. In addition, the exploration of interaction effects of micro- and macro-level variables is essential to the development of predictive models that can detect the influence of contextual and cultural factors on personal and public health. For instance, here are four research questions pertaining to the study for improving selfcare management of chronic conditions: (1) What are the dominant human factors involved in selfcare? (2) What are the contextual or ecological variables that may interact with personal or human factors in the design of selfcare management strategies? (3) How are patient care outcomes specified and measured? (4) What is the value-based appraisal and evaluation of an innovative chronic care modality? The Patient-Centered Outcomes Research Institute (PCORI) [17] has played a vital role in helping people make informed decisions and improving healthcare delivery and outcomes by producing and promoting high-integrity, evidence-based information that comes from research guided by patients, caregivers, and the broader healthcare community.

Challenge Two. Inadequate Validation of Multidisciplinary Care

The sensitivity and specificity of each predictive model derived from SVM have not been systematically examined to determine the validity of multidisciplinary patient care since stringent and pre-determined criteria, ranging from the proximal, intermediate, and distal outcomes, and measured at the patient- and population-level, have yet to be formulated in evaluation research. Furthermore, the development of "precision care" or personal care modalities should consider both the quality and efficiency of care plans simultaneously [17].

Solutions: The validation criteria of a predictive model should be decided and set in advance so that the predictive power of selfcare management strategies can be determined and enhanced. The prescriptive nature of patient-centered care strategies should consider individual choices or self-efficacy, rather than simply based on the relative cost of care options. The critical research question for validating the effectiveness of multidisciplinary care for polychronic conditions should include the follow inquiry: What is the dose-response relationship of the amount and type of innovative care services for patient care outcomes?

Challenge Three. The Need for Conducting Prospective or Experimental Studies

Under the pay-for-performance and other incentive policies for promoting selfcare management of polychronic conditions, only prospective studies have potential to generate useful information for designing, implementing, and evaluating chronic care models supplemented by the clinical decision support system. However, limited theoretical specifications for formulating polychronic care management are available to guide the design of interventions. Thus, the usefulness of patient-centered care components for the design of care plans is yet to be ascertained and standardized in empirical research.

Solutions: Clarification is needed to differentiate multidisciplinary care and integrated care in clinical practice. The use of a complex factorial design for outcomes evaluation is an efficient and powerful analytical strategy to generate practical solutions for chronic care problems. It is important to develop or select a theoretically guided framework, such as the logic model, in conducting the implementation of care interventions [16]. When multiple datasets are merged or pooled together for performing statistical analysis, it is important to delineate important confounding factors such as the contextual and provider variations in the establishment of predictive models. The study questions pertaining to the implementation research should address the consistency and integrity of patient adherence to the prescribed intervention. This refers to the identification of treatment integrity when a randomized controlled trial is being conducted.

Challenge Four. The Rationale for Establishing an Integrated or Guided Care Model

A clear rationale for formalizing an integrated or guided care model at the early stage of chronic disease is imperative and essential to the achievement of optimal health outcomes for a target group of high-risk patients who are likely to experience polychronic conditions later in life.

Solutions: Chronic disease progression or transition is an important concept for studying the chronicity of the disease. It is also important to consider both time-varying and time-constant predictors of the disease evolution or progression when predictive analytics are being formulated. A multivariate modeling approach is preferred since it could simultaneously investigate the main effects and interaction effects of personal, organizational, ecological, and contextual variables in the analysis. Furthermore, the temporal sequence of service utilization and outcome variables should be captured in the design of a multi-wave longitudinal study. Thus, the sequential or causal effects of the intervention on the proximal, intermediate, and distal outcomes could be delineated from the analysis.

2.4. Opportunities for Collaborative and Transdisciplinary Research on Chronic Care Management

Figure 1 portrays a variety of discipline-free analytical methods that could be used in the evaluation of the effectiveness of multilevel predictors of chronic care innovations such as selfcare management strategies. For instance, the prediction of disease transitions over time (e.g., the evolution of diabetes to cardiovascular disorders and chronic kidney disease in varying severity stages) requires having a panel study design capturing the longitudinal data observed from an early to advanced stage of the illness. Thus, the treatments or interventions could be better monitored and followed up by collaborative research teams. Furthermore, the longitudinal study design will require the collection of multi-waves of patient care data for performing parametric and non-parametric statistical modeling of predictors [17]. Moreover, the ultimate solution for developing disease-specific detection, AI-based diagnostics and prevention strategies, relies on the standardization of measurements and metrics used in the design, implementation, and evaluation of healthcare outcomes [18–20].

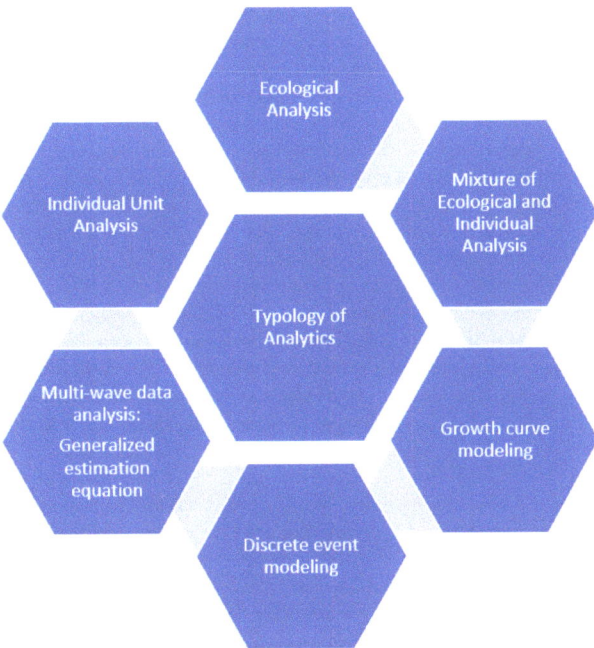

Figure 1. Disciplinary Free Methods or Modeling Approaches.

The risk identification approach to constructing predictive equations has been extensively used by epidemiologists [19,21]. The development of predictive analytics for enhancing the validity of clinical decision support tools is a logical step for improving the disease management program for diabetes and related complications and critical care events. However, this is not a breakthrough idea, but rather is just a practical step for optimizing diabetes care. The stability of the predictive equations and modeling approaches should be examined, using repeated measures of disease transition or progression. The interplay or the reciprocal relationship between the micro- and macro-vascular changes for diabetes should be determined if the causal links among multiple measures or events are to be established and validated [22,23].

3. Transdisciplinary Science in Search for Theoretically Relevant Predictors of Polychronic Conditions and Outcomes

The Society for Design and Process Science is leading the way to identify theoretically sound frameworks to guide the design and implementation of clinical and administrative decision support systems for promoting selfcare management of chronic conditions [1,21]. By employing advanced data science technologies, theory-based constructs, or domains identified by collaborative scientists in the formulation of the data warehouse, practitioners may facilitate the convergence and integration of personal and social determinants of health into health services and management research. The simultaneity in considering personal and societal (ecological and contextual) factors in explaining the variations in healthcare outcomes enables the detection of interplays among multiple predictors such as personal, behavioral, organizational, ecological, and information technological factors. This reliance on theoretical guidance of care technology and management will foster changes in the design, implementation, and evaluation of healthcare innovations. This theoretically guided approach enables researchers to establish a scientific core for the data system containing useful constructs or domains to be used for formulating predictive analytics. More specifically, as data science is maturing, AI technology, such as ChatGPT in healthcare, will shape the direction of selfcare management strategies and policy developments for promoting the physical and mental health of the population.

Three specific research agendas are suggested for furthering the scientific pursuit of chronic care management. First, the field of predictive analytics should develop a sociobiomedical evolutionary learning platform to predict the risk of polychronic conditions at various stages. The trajectories of chronic disease should be clearly delineated or estimated from transitional probabilities at the population level. The big-data approach to merging the micro- and macro-data generated from public and private health insurance databases, coupled with theoretical specifications of relevant predicators measured at both personal and ecological levels, could effectively validate the disease patterns. Thus, the integrity of care management designed for the high-risk patient population for polychronic conditions could be adequately evaluated. Second, disease management strategies or toolboxes should help maximize both efficiency and effectiveness in achieving the ultimate goals of advancing quality and human dignity [24]. Third, scientific methods for protecting privacy and confidentiality in the release of healthcare data should be employed, particularly in the design of perturbations of personal data containing individual or geographic identifiers.

4. Conclusions

This commentary is unique and original in three ways. First, it identifies the major gaps in care management research and articulates the important role of developing theoretical frameworks coupled with rigorous multivariate modeling approaches for the causal analysis of factors influencing the care process and outcomes of patients with polychronic conditions. Second, we advocate the need to conduct rigorous care management research that will improve the design, process, and patient care outcomes. Third, we also specify the directions for future AI-based healthcare research that will overcome some challenges in designing and performing high-quality and innovative research.

Chronic disease may evolve from a single disease state into polychronic conditions. For example, Type 2 diabetes could evolve with both micro- and macro-vascular complications and further develop into polychronic conditions such as heart failure and chronic kidney disease. Thus, clinical researchers must make boundary spinning efforts to suggest viable and effective interventions for multiple chronic conditions. This is why chronic care management must provide not only specialty care but also comprehensive preventive and maintenance care for treating each target patient as a whole person. In the realm of multidisciplinary and comprehensive care, clinicians should establish clear criteria or quantifiable metrics for assessing and achieving optimal healthcare outcomes. As clinical researchers, it is imperative to design and execute intervention studies that will capture both micro (personal) and macro (provider and ecological) variants or predictive variables. Thus, clinically meaningful results or outcomes could be scientifically gathered via predetermined criteria for clinical evaluation of the effectiveness and efficiency of polychronic care. Commentary on trends, challenges, and solutions in conducting AI healthcare research can improve understandings of disease-state transitions from diabetes to other polychronic conditions. Hence, better predictive models could be further formulated to expand from inductive (problem solving) to deductive (theory centering and hypothesis testing) inquiries in care management research.

As digital health becomes more mature, the big-data-to-knowledge approach may be supplemented by the advance of machine and deep learning methods and guided by a theoretically meaningful framework for developing parsimonious models for maximizing the power of predictive analytics for performing high-quality health services evaluation and care management research [25]. One important development in population health management is the need to identify high-risk and target groups for interventions and then formulating and implementing decision support systems coupled with visualizations of changes in clinical and health outcomes of patients with polychronic conditions [13].

Finally, patient-centered care needs to be accentuated by an emphasis on patient engagement [10,26]. When patients are more aware of the choices available to them, selfcare management could further motivate them to take necessary and sufficient actions for reducing the burden of chronic illness. For optimizing the predictive analytics, it is imperative that an empirical approach, such as using neural network analysis and SVM, should be supplemented by sound theoretical specifications of predictive variables that could identify the causal sequala associated with unstable or declined health outcomes such as the concomitant development of multiple conditions and complications [13], unplanned hospitalization [27,28], and the transition from metabolic syndromes to cardiovascular disorders [29–32], chronic kidney disease [33–36], and mortality [37–41].

Author Contributions: T.T.H.W.: design, implementation, and critique of the AI healthcare applications; H.S.W.: review of the literature, editing, and referencing the paper. All authors have read and agreed to the published version of the manuscript.

Funding: This research received no external funding.

Institutional Review Board Statement: Not applicable.

Informed Consent Statement: Not applicable.

Data Availability Statement: Not applicable.

Conflicts of Interest: The authors declare no conflict of interest.

References

1. Wan, T.T. Convergence of Artificial Intelligence Research in Healthcare: Trends and Approaches. *J. Integr. Des. Process Sci.* **2020**, 1–15, Preprint. [CrossRef]
2. Wan, T.T.H.; Terry, A.; McKee, B.; Kattan, W. KMAP-O framework for care management research of patients with type 2 diabetes. *World J. Diabetes* **2017**, *8*, 165–171. [CrossRef] [PubMed]
3. Wan, T.T.; Wang, B.L. An Integrated Social and Behavioral System Approach to Evaluation of Healthcare Information Technology for Polychronic Conditions. *J. Integr. Des. Process Sci.* **2021**, *25*, 148–160. [CrossRef]
4. Luh, S.; Lin, Y.M.; Wu, P.H. A single framework of precision performance of diabetes disease prognosis for better care with collaboration. *J. Integr. Des. Process Sci.* **2022**, Pre-press. [CrossRef]
5. Lin, M.-Y.; Liu, J.-S.; Huang, T.-Y.; Wu, P.-H.; Chiu, Y.-W.; Kang, Y.; Hsu, C.-C.; Hwang, S.-J.; Luh, H. Data Analysis of the Risks of Type 2 Diabetes Mellitus Complications before Death Using a Data-Driven Modelling Approach: Methodologies and Challenges in Prolonged Diseases. *Information* **2021**, *12*, 326. [CrossRef]
6. Liu, X.; Liu, L.; Li, Y.; Cao, X. The association between physical symptoms and self-care behaviours in heart failure patients with inadequate self-care behaviours: A cross-sectional study. *BMC Cardiovasc. Disord.* **2023**, *23*, 205. [CrossRef] [PubMed]
7. Wan, T.T.H.; Terry, A.; Cobb, E.; McKee, B.; Tregerman, R.; Barbaro, S.D.S. Strategies to modify the risk of heart failure read-mission: A systematic review and meta analysis. *Health Serv. Res.-Manag. Epidemiol.* **2017**, *4*, 2333392817701050.
8. Hsu, C.-C.; Hwang, S.-J.; Wen, C.-P.; Chang, H.-Y.; Chen, T.; Shiu, R.-S.; Horng, S.-S.; Chang, Y.-K.; Yang, W.-C. High Prevalence and Low Awareness of CKD in Taiwan: A Study on the Relationship Between Serum Creatinine and Awareness From a Nationally Representative Survey. *Am. J. Kidney Dis.* **2006**, *48*, 727–738. [CrossRef]
9. Centers for Medicare and Medicaid Services. *CMS Vendor Guidelines*; Centers for Medicare and Medicaid Services: Baltimore, MD, USA, 2022.
10. Nielsen, M.; Buelt, L.; Patel, K.; Nichols, L.M. The Patient-Centered Medical Home's Impact on Cost and Quality: Annual Review of Evidence, 2014–2015. Patient-Centered Primary Care Collaborative. 2016. Available online: https://www.pcpcc.org/sites/default/files/resources (accessed on 11 July 2023).
11. Xie, Z.; Nikolayeva, O.; Luo, J.; Li, D. Building Risk Prediction Models for Type 2 Diabetes Using Machine Learning Techniques. *Prev. Chronic Dis.* **2019**, *16*, E130. [CrossRef]
12. Agliata, A.; Giordano, D.; Bardozzo, F.; Bottiglieri, S.; Facchiano, A.; Tagliaferri, R. Machine Learning as a Support for the Diagnosis of Type 2 Diabetes. *Int. J. Mol. Sci.* **2023**, *24*, 6775. [CrossRef]
13. Wan, T.T.H. *Population Health Management for Polychronic Conditions: Evidence Based Research Approaches*; Springer: New York, NY, USA, 2018.
14. Nash, D.; Wohlforth, C. *How COVID Crashed the System: A Guide to Fixing American Health Care*; Rowan & Littlefield Publishers: New York, NY, USA, 2022.
15. Wan, T.T.H. Artificial intelligence research in primary care management. *Qual. Prim. Care* **2018**, *26*, 114–116.

16. Goff, Z.; House, A.; Guthrie, E.; Weston, H.; Mansbridge, L. Diabetes care in the acute psychiatric inpatient setting: A logic model for service delivery. *Gen. Hosp. Psychiatry* **2022**, *78*, 135–137. [CrossRef]
17. Wan, T.T.; Matthews, S.; Luh, H.; Zeng, Y.; Wang, Z.; Yang, L. A Proposed Multi-Criteria Optimization Approach to Enhance Clinical Outcomes Evaluation for Diabetes Care: A Commentary. *Health Serv. Res. Manag. Epidemiol.* **2022**, *9*, 23333928221089125. [CrossRef] [PubMed]
18. Cabral, B.P.; Braga, L.A.M.; Syed-Abdul, S.; Mota, F.B. Future of Artificial Intelligence Applications in Cancer Care: A Global Cross-Sectional Survey of Researchers. *Curr. Oncol.* **2023**, *30*, 3432–3446. [CrossRef]
19. Lai, H.; Huang, H.; Keshavjee, K.; Guergachi, A.; Gao, X. Predictive models for diabetes mellitus using machine learning techniques. *BMC Endocr. Disord.* **2019**, *19*, 101. [CrossRef] [PubMed]
20. Li, Q.; Xie, W.; Li, L.; Wang, L.; You, Q.; Chen, L.; Li, J.; Ke, Y.; Fang, J.; Liu, L.; et al. Development a validation of a pre-diction model for elevated arterial stiffness in Chinese patients with diabetes using machine learning. *Front. Physiol.* **2021**, *12*, 714195. [CrossRef]
21. Rav-Marathe, K.; Wan, T.T.; Marathe, S. The Effect of Health Education on Clinical and Self-Reported Outcomes of Diabetes in a Medical Practice. *J. Integr. Des. Process Sci.* **2016**, *20*, 45–63. [CrossRef]
22. Fowler, M.J. Microvascular and Macrovascular Complications of Diabetes. *Clin. Diabetes* **2011**, *29*, 116–122. [CrossRef]
23. Ismail-Beigi, F.; Craven, T.; Banerji, M.A.; Basile, J.; Calles, J.; Cohen, R.M.; Cuddihy, R.; Cushman, W.C.; Genuth, S.; Grimm, R.H., Jr.; et al. Effect of intensive treatment of hyperglycaemia on microvascular outcomes in type 2 diabetes: An analysis of the ACCORD randomized trial. *Lancet* **2010**, *376*, 419–430. [CrossRef]
24. Fiedler, B.A.; Wan, T.T.H. Disease management organization approach to chronic illness. *Int. J. Public Policy* **2010**, *6*, 260–277. [CrossRef]
25. Wan, T.T.H. *Evidence-Based Health Care Management: Multivariate Modeling Approaches*; Kluwer Academic Publishers: Boston, MA, USA, 2002.
26. Cianfrocco, H. Paving a Path for Better Polychronic Care: How Collaboration, Prioritization, and Engagement Can Improve Outcomes. Harvard Business Review Analytical Services. 2021. Available online: www.optum.com/content/dam/optum3 /optum/en/resources/white-papers/hbras_optum-white-paper-1-21-2021.pdf (accessed on 11 July 2023).
27. Yang, X.; Ma, R.C.; So, W.-Y.; Kong, A.P.; Ko, G.T.; Ho, C.-S.; Lam, C.W.; Cockram, C.S.; Tong, P.C.; Chan, J.C. Development and validation of a risk score for hospitalization for heart failure in patients with Type 2 Diabetes Mellitus. *Cardiovasc. Diabetol.* **2008**, *7*, 9. [CrossRef] [PubMed]
28. Chen, J.; Yi, Q.; Wang, Y.; Wang, J.; Yu, H.; Zhang, J.; Hu, M.; Xu, J.; Wu, Z.; Hou, L.; et al. Long-term glycemic variability and risk of adverse health outcomes in patients with diabetes: A systematic review and meta-analysis of cohort studies. *Diabetes Res. Clin. Pract.* **2022**, *192*, 110085. [CrossRef] [PubMed]
29. The ADVANCE Collaborative Group; Patel, A.; MacMahon, S.; Chalmers, J.; Neal, B.; Billot, L.; Woodward, M.; Marre, M.; Cooper, M.; Glasziou, P.; et al. Intensive Blood Glucose Control and Vascular Outcomes in Patients with Type 2 Diabetes. *N. Engl. J. Med.* **2008**, *358*, 2560–2572. [CrossRef] [PubMed]
30. Levey, A.S.; Stevens, L.A.; Schmid, C.H.; Zhang, Y.L.; Castro, A.F., 3rd; Feldman, H.I.; Kusek, J.W.; Eggers, P.; Van Lente, F.; Greene, T.; et al. A new equation to estimate glomerular filtration rate. *Ann. Intern. Med.* **2009**, *150*, 604–612. [CrossRef] [PubMed]
31. Xu, F.; Zhu, J.; Sun, N.; Wang, L.; Xie, C.; Tang, Q.; Mao, X.; Fu, X.; Brickell, A.; Hao, Y.; et al. Development and validation of prediction models for hypertension risks in rural Chinese populations. *J. Glob. Health* **2019**, *9*, 020601. [CrossRef] [PubMed]
32. Li, T.-C.; Wang, H.-C.; Li, C.-I.; Liu, C.-S.; Lin, W.-Y.; Lin, C.-H.; Yang, S.-Y.; Lin, C.-C. Establishment and validation of a prediction model for ischemic stroke risks in patients with type 2 diabetes. *Diabetes Res. Clin. Prac.* **2018**, *138*, 220–228. [CrossRef]
33. Garlo, K.G.; White, W.B.; Bakris, G.L.; Zannad, F.; Wilson, C.A.; Kupfer, S.; Vaduganathan, M.; Morrow, D.A.; Cannon, C.P.; Charytan, D.M. Kidney Biomarkers and Decline in eGFR in Patients with Type 2 Diabetes. *Clin. J. Am. Soc. Nephrol.* **2018**, *13*, 398–405. [CrossRef]
34. Lin, C.-C.; Niu, M.J.; Li, C.-I.; Liu, C.-S.; Lin, C.-H.; Yang, S.-Y.; Li, T.-C. Development and validation of a risk prediction model for chronic kidney disease among individuals with type 2 diabetes. *Sci. Rep.* **2022**, *12*, 4794. [CrossRef]
35. Nelson, R.G.; Grams, M.E.; Ballew, S.H.; Sang, Y.; Azizi, F.; Chadban, S.J.; Chaker, L.; Dunning, S.C.; Fox, C.; Hirakawa, Y.; et al. Development of Risk Prediction Equations for Incident Chronic Kidney Disease. *JAMA* **2019**, *322*, 2104–2114. [CrossRef]
36. Jardine, M.J.; Hata, J.; Woodward, M.; Perkovic, V.; Ninomiya, T.; Arima, H.; Zoungas, S.; Cass, A.; Patel, A.; Marre, M.; et al. Prediction of Kidney-Related Outcomes in Patients With Type 2 Diabetes. *Am. J. Kidney Dis.* **2012**, *60*, 770–778. [CrossRef]
37. Li, T.-C.; Li, C.-I.; Liu, C.-S.; Lin, W.-Y.; Lin, C.-H.; Yang, S.-Y.; Chiang, J.-H.; Lin, C.-C. Development and validation of prediction models for the risks of diabetes-related hospitalization and in-hospital mortality in patients with type 2 diabetes. *Metab. Clin. Exp.* **2018**, *85*, 38–47. [CrossRef] [PubMed]
38. Liu, C.; Li, C.; Wang, M.; Yang, S.; Li, T.; Lin, C. Building clinical risk score systems for predicting the all-cause and expanded cardiovascular-specific mortality of patients with type 2 diabetes. *Diabetes Obes. Metab.* **2021**, *23*, 467–479. [CrossRef]
39. De Cosmo, S.; Copetti, M.; Lamacchia, O.; Fontana, A.; Massa, M.; Morini, E.; Pacilli, A.; Fariello, S.; Palena, A.; Rauseo, A.; et al. Development and Validation of a Predicting Model of All-Cause Mortality in Patients With Type 2 Diabetes. *Diabetes Care* **2013**, *36*, 2830–2835. [CrossRef]

40. Robinson, T.E.; Elley, C.R.; Kenealy, T.; Drury, P.L. Development and validation of a predictive risk model for all-cause mortality in type 2 diabetes. *Diabetes Res. Clin. Pract.* **2015**, *108*, 482–488. [CrossRef] [PubMed]
41. Ramírez-Prado, D.; Palazón-Bru, A.; Rosa, D.M.F.-D.; Carbonell-Torregrosa, M.; Martínez-Díaz, A.M.; Gil-Guillén, V.F. Predictive models for all-cause and cardiovascular mortality in type 2 diabetic inpatients. A cohort study. *Int. J. Clin. Prac.* **2015**, *69*, 474–484. [CrossRef] [PubMed]

Disclaimer/Publisher's Note: The statements, opinions and data contained in all publications are solely those of the individual author(s) and contributor(s) and not of MDPI and/or the editor(s). MDPI and/or the editor(s) disclaim responsibility for any injury to people or property resulting from any ideas, methods, instructions or products referred to in the content.

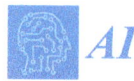

Article

Evaluating the Performance of Automated Machine Learning (AutoML) Tools for Heart Disease Diagnosis and Prediction

Lauren M. Paladino [1], Alexander Hughes [1], Alexander Perera [1], Oguzhan Topsakal [1] and Tahir Cetin Akinci [2,3,*]

1 Department of Computer Science, Florida Polytechnic University, Lakeland, FL 33805, USA; lpaladino7605@floridapoly.edu (L.M.P.); ahughes3300@floridapoly.edu (A.H.); aperera3727@floridapoly.edu (A.P.); otopsakal@floridapoly.edu (O.T.)
2 Winston Chung Global Energy Center (WCGEC), University of California at Riverside (UCR), Riverside, CA 92521, USA
3 Electrical Engineering Department, Istanbul Technical University (ITU), Istanbul 34469, Turkey
* Correspondence: tahircetin.akinci@ucr.edu

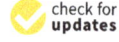

Citation: Paladino, L.M.; Hughes, A.; Perera, A.; Topsakal, O.; Akinci, T.C. Evaluating the Performance of Automated Machine Learning (AutoML) Tools for Heart Disease Diagnosis and Prediction. *AI* 2023, *4*, 1036–1058. https://doi.org/10.3390/ai4040053

Academic Editor: Tim Hulsen

Received: 13 September 2023
Revised: 24 November 2023
Accepted: 27 November 2023
Published: 1 December 2023

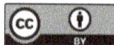

Copyright: © 2023 by the authors. Licensee MDPI, Basel, Switzerland. This article is an open access article distributed under the terms and conditions of the Creative Commons Attribution (CC BY) license (https://creativecommons.org/licenses/by/4.0/).

Abstract: Globally, over 17 million people annually die from cardiovascular diseases, with heart disease being the leading cause of mortality in the United States. The ever-increasing volume of data related to heart disease opens up possibilities for employing machine learning (ML) techniques in diagnosing and predicting heart conditions. While applying ML demands a certain level of computer science expertise—often a barrier for healthcare professionals—automated machine learning (AutoML) tools significantly lower this barrier. They enable users to construct the most effective ML models without in-depth technical knowledge. Despite their potential, there has been a lack of research comparing the performance of different AutoML tools on heart disease data. Addressing this gap, our study evaluates three AutoML tools—PyCaret, AutoGluon, and AutoKeras—against three datasets (Cleveland, Hungarian, and a combined dataset). To evaluate the efficacy of AutoML against conventional machine learning methodologies, we crafted ten machine learning models using the standard practices of exploratory data analysis (EDA), data cleansing, feature engineering, and others, utilizing the sklearn library. Our toolkit included an array of models—logistic regression, support vector machines, decision trees, random forest, and various ensemble models. Employing 5-fold cross-validation, these traditionally developed models demonstrated accuracy rates spanning from 55% to 60%. This performance is markedly inferior to that of AutoML tools, indicating the latter's superior capability in generating predictive models. Among AutoML tools, AutoGluon emerged as the superior tool, consistently achieving accuracy rates between 78% and 86% across the datasets. PyCaret's performance varied, with accuracy rates from 65% to 83%, indicating a dependency on the nature of the dataset. AutoKeras showed the most fluctuation in performance, with accuracies ranging from 54% to 83%. Our findings suggest that AutoML tools can simplify the generation of robust ML models that potentially surpass those crafted through traditional ML methodologies. However, we must also consider the limitations of AutoML tools and explore strategies to overcome them. The successful deployment of high-performance ML models designed via AutoML could revolutionize the treatment and prevention of heart disease globally, significantly impacting patient care.

Keywords: AutoML; machine learning; cardiovascular disease; coronary artery disease; diagnosis; heart disease; prediction; AutoGluon; AutoKeras; PyCaret

1. Introduction

The term "cardiovascular disease" (CVD) applies to any disorder affecting the cardiovascular system (heart and blood vessels) [1]. Over 17 million people die from CVD annually globally [2], and heart disease specifically is the leading cause of death in the United States, killing almost 700,000 people in 2020 [3]. Atherosclerosis, or the buildup of plaque within the arteries, leads to coronary artery disease (CAD), one of the most common types of heart disease [3]. Risk factors for CVD include obesity, hypertension, hyperglycemia, and "high alcohol intake" [4]. Doctors usually diagnose CAD through a combination of physical examination, family history, and diagnostic tests including angiography, a type of contrast X-ray that measures the extent of narrowing of the blood vessels [5–7]. Other diagnostic tools include electrocardiography, sonography, and blood testing [4]. The public health importance of addressing heart disease, along with the abundant and continuously growing data, means that machine learning (ML) techniques could be utilized to find meaningful patterns in clinical data and predict the presence of heart disease. Numerous researchers have explored applying ML to medical diagnosis using many different techniques and ensembles, as discussed in the Related Work section below. However, to apply ML, a certain level of computer science knowledge is required, which may be a barrier to widespread use by healthcare professionals [8]. Steps in a typical machine learning project include framing the problem, obtaining the data, conducting exploratory data analysis, preparing the data, exploring the different models, and fine-tuning the models. AutoML tools allow for the implementation of complex models, including feature engineering and hyperparameter optimization, requiring fewer lines of code and less technical knowledge than traditional ML methods. AutoML can automate the steps of data preparation, model selection, and the fine-tuning of models. By utilizing AutoML frameworks, it is possible to develop a cost-effective way to predict heart disease, providing health professionals with a powerful tool for heart disease prediction and diagnosis [4]. AutoML frameworks are machine learning tools that automate many of the more complex machine learning processes to allow non-experts access. This enables someone with less technical knowledge and with fewer lines to use powerful machine learning algorithms. AutoML tools provide access to a range of ML models that make implementing machine learning applications using various datasets much easier. Most AutoML tools are capable of data preprocessing, hyperparameter tuning, and model training automatically without extensive code or data manipulation [9–11].

This study aims to assess the efficacy of automated machine learning (AutoML) tools in the diagnosis of heart disease—a domain where, to our current knowledge, there is yet to be a comprehensive comparative analysis of various AutoML frameworks. We have conducted a thorough investigation of three widely used AutoML Python libraries—PyCaret, AutoGluon, and AutoKeras—across three distinct datasets: Cleveland, Hungarian, and a synthesized dataset amalgamating four separate databases.

Given the grave implications of cardiovascular diseases, and with heart disease at the forefront as a major global health concern, the need for advanced, accurate diagnostic methods is more pressing than ever. Our research delves into the potential of AutoML tools to meet this need, scrutinizing their capabilities in contrast to traditional machine learning techniques. For a robust comparison, we meticulously engineered ten machine learning models using conventional processes, such as exploratory data analysis (EDA), data cleansing, and feature engineering, applying the comprehensive tools provided by the sklearn library.

The ambition of our work is to illuminate the strengths and possible applications of AutoML in refining the diagnosis of heart disease, thereby contributing meaningfully to both the healthcare sector and the field of machine learning. Through this exploration, we intend to delineate the extent to which AutoML tools can not only streamline the diagnostic process but also potentially increase its precision, offering a significant step forward in combating this global health challenge.

In the following sections, we provide a synthesis of pertinent literature, laying the groundwork for the context of our research. Subsequently, we elucidate the methodology adopted in our study, detailing the selection and application of AutoML tools, as well as the datasets chosen for evaluation. Within our methodological exposition, we articulate the conventional techniques implemented to construct a high-performing model manually.

We then proceed to delineate the results obtained, paving the way for an in-depth discussion that interprets the findings within the broader scope of current knowledge and practice. Finally, we encapsulate the study by highlighting its key contributions and the significance of our findings, drawing attention to the implications of our work in the field of heart disease diagnosis through advanced machine learning technologies.

2. Related Works

Medical data analysis and prediction is a critical research area, and dozens of research groups have already applied non-automated ML techniques to heart disease specifically. Hazra et al., Khan et al., and Marimuthi et al. have reviewed and summarized some of the extant research and the accuracies achieved [12–14]. Applied techniques include artificial neural networks (ANN), decision trees, K-nearest neighbor, naïve Bayes, logistic regression, support vector machines (SVM), and association rules, with most researchers obtaining high accuracies [12–14]. Decision trees, ANN, and SVM are three of the most frequently used methods, and many groups had improved success using ensembles of multiple methods [12–14]. Nagavelli et al. compared several different machine learning algorithms in 2022 in their paper titled "Machine Learning Technology-Based Heart Disease Detection Models." The authors of the paper used SVM, the naïve Bayes weight approach, and XGBoost algorithms. The Cleveland dataset and the Statlog dataset, which is a smaller version of the Cleveland, were used for the machine learning algorithms. DBSCAN was used to remove outlier data, and Python library XGBoost V0.81 was used to implement the XGBoost portion of the algorithm. Their results showed that XGBoost had the highest accuracy, with lower accuracy for the SVM and naïve Bayes approaches [15].

In another paper, titled "Heart Disease Diagnosis and Prediction Using Machine Learning and Data Mining Techniques: A Review", the authors reviewed a list of relevant machine learning information [10]. The paper explained several different machine learning algorithms that have been used in heart disease datasets, including decision trees, K-means, SVM, naïve Bayes, artificial neural networks (ANN), Iterative Dichotomiser 3 (ID3), classification and regression trees (CART), random forest, a-priori, fuzzy logic, and association rules. During this review, several tools and environments for data learning were examined, including WEKA (Waikato Environment for Knowledge Learning), RapidMiner, TANAGRA, Apache Mahout, MATLAB, Java, C, and Orange. These machine learning algorithms and tools were extracted from a survey of 35 research papers and represent what has been used in non-automated machine-learning research for heart disease [12]. Various software systems (e.g., WEKA, RapidMiner, TANAGRA) and programming languages (e.g., Java, MATLAB, Python) are available for the implementation of ML models. WEKA, based on Java, was one of the more commonly referenced tools in the papers by Hazra et al., Khan et al., and Marimuthi et al. [12–14]. Singh et al. used WEKA for predicting heart disease, with a dataset of 303 records and a multilayer perceptron neural network (MLPNN) with backpropagation [6,16–19].

It is important to note that new technologies are emerging for disease diagnosis including heart disease diagnosis. For example, hyperspectral and multispectral imaging systems are non-invasive diagnostic tools that capture and analyze a wide spectrum of light to identify, assess, and map various biological materials. These systems are increasingly being applied in the field of medical diagnosis, including for the detection and analysis of diseases [16,17]. The data from these systems are also being utilized in machine/deep learning models for improved diagnosis [18,19].

Pol et al. used Python and the AutoML tool PyCaret to predict the presence or absence of heart disease [8]. Padmanabhan et al. used Python and Auto-Sklearn on the same Cleveland Heart Disease dataset as Pol et al. [20]. Valarmathi and Sheela used the AutoML tool TPOT with the Cleveland dataset, but only when tuning the hyperparameters of their random forest and XG boost classifier models [21]. With the growth of AutoML tools, there has been a concern regarding if AutoML is comparable to previous machine learning methods. A paper titled "Physician-Friendly Machine Learning: A Case Study with Cardiovascular Disease Risk Prediction" compared the performance of the AutoML tool Auto-Sklearn to that of more traditional manual machine learning techniques for accuracy [20]. In the paper, a graduate student who was experienced in creating machine learning models was allowed one month to develop models using manual techniques using the scikit-learn python library. Then, models were created using the Auto-Sklearn tool to automatically create the model, which took around 30 min to complete and only required four lines of Python code. The results showed comparable results of the models. The paper concluded that their research strongly suggests that AutoML is a useful approach that allows less experienced users to quickly create models that are competitive and comparable to models created by experienced machine learning users [20]. Pol et al. used another popular Python AutoML tool, PyCaret, in their paper titled "AutoML: Building A Classification Model with PyCaret." PyCaret was used with a heart disease dataset and trained on a 70/30 train/test split with normalization turned on. PyCaret was then used to train the dataset with all algorithms available in its library. The paper concluded the results were "favorable" for classification with logistic regression for their heart disease dataset [8].

Romero et al. benchmarked the performance of the AutoML tools AutoSklearn, H2O, and TPOT in disease prediction. They used medical claims data of more than 12 million people to predict six different diseases. These did not include heart disease. While the dataset used was large, the disease prevalence was very low, with the highest prevalence being for chronic kidney disease at 0.63%. They found that the performance of the different tools varied for different diseases, with prostate cancer prediction having some of the highest accuracies and type 2 diabetes some of the lowest. Performance between the tools themselves also varied. H2O produced some of the most accurate models across the diseases examined, though Romero et al. noted that the variation between the tools was not large [22].

In their 2021 paper, Ferreira et al. [9] compared the performance of eight open-source AutoML tools. Like us, they used default settings for the different tools when possible. Though they did not use the same datasets as we did, the tools they used included Auto-Gluon and AutoKeras, two of the three used in this paper. AutoGluon was significantly faster than the other tools. AutoKeras was one of the fastest deep learning/neural network tools that they used. While it was the slowest tool used here, it was the only deep learning tool used in this study. Ferreira et al. found that no single AutoML tool performed better than the others across all datasets [9].

3. Methodology

In the following sections, available AutoML tools are introduced first, followed by the ones included in this study and the inclusion criteria. Then, the existing datasets and the details of the selected datasets are given, and the selected performance criteria are also introduced in detail.

3.1. AutoML Tools

There are several open-source and proprietary AutoML tools available. The following well-known AutoML tools (listed in alphabetical order) were considered for our study. AutoGL is open source and was created at Tsinghua University for AutoML on graphs and contains four modules, including auto feature engineering, model training, hyperparameter optimization, and auto ensemble [23,24]. AutoGluon is an open-source tool created by Amazon that can automate machine learning and deep learning algorithms for text, images, and datasets [25–27]. AutoGluon evaluates and compares a variety of models and assists in selecting the best model to utilize and fine-tune. It is developed to support very specific problem types: regression and classification using tabular data, image classification, and object detection. AutoGluon provides a user-friendly interface and tools that allow for data to be trained effectively within a single line of code as it automatically balances efficiency and performance, allowing for less headaches with hyperparameter editing [28]. AutoKeras is an AutoML system based on Keras and TensorFlow and was developed at DATA Lab at the Texas AM campus [29–31]. AutoKeras allows for the building and training of deep neural networks and automates the process of hyperparameter tuning and model selection with an easy-to-use interface [29]. Auto-Sklearn was built around scikit-learn and automatically searches for the best machine learning algorithm for a dataset, along with hyperparameter optimization [32,33]. Auto-Sklearn provides efficient processes to learn the data and continue learning from similarly identified datasets through "meta-learning" and a Bayesian optimizer, which learns from the preprocessed data, features, and classifier to determine the best model approach [34]. While Auto-Sklearn can be an effective approach, reliance on the data being large enough is a necessity [34,35]. MLBox is a library for Python that offers powerful AutoML tools and predictive models for classification and regression. It can use deep learning, stacking, and LightGBM and offers interpretations of prediction models [36]. Neural Network Intelligence is an automated machine learning toolkit created by Microsoft that searches for the best hyperparameters and neural architecture by running trial jobs automatically [37]. PyCaret provides an ideal experience for productivity and low-effort ML solutions and designs and launches quick prototypes [38,39]. PyCaret quickly tests a variety of models, providing the data scientist with an effective understanding of what models work efficiently and accurately between classification and regression tasks [8]. TPOT (tree-based pipeline optimization tool) is another open-source automated machine learning tool for Python, built on top of scikit-learn, that optimizes machine learning pipelines [40]. TPOT is still in active development and can automate many steps of the machine learning process, such as feature selection, feature preprocessing, feature construction, model selection, and parameter optimization [40]. TPOT explores thousands of possible pipelines using genetic algorithms and returns the best one for a given dataset [40,41].

3.2. Details of the Selected AutoML Tools

Effective AutoML modeling choices for the various heart disease datasets were narrowed down to AutoGluon, AutoKeras, and PyCaret. AutoGluon was chosen due to its high performance and ease of use [38]. It evaluates several different machine learning algorithms to find the best model for the data. These algorithms include ExtraTreeEntr, RandomForestEntr, WeightedEnsemble-L2, ExtraTreesGini, RandomForestGini, XGBoost, KneighborsUnif, and KNeighborsDist. Random forest is a machine learning algorithm that uses multiple randomized decision trees (an algorithm based on splitting binary decision nodes) to make predictions. The extra trees algorithm is similar to random forest except that the split in the decision trees is randomly selected. The models with the Gini and Entr suffixes indicate the measures used to determine how a decision tree node splits. These measures are referred to as the Gini index and Entropy, which is a measure of the purity of the split [42]. XGBoost is an extreme gradient-boosted tree with an ensemble algorithm, with each tree boosting misclassified attributes of the previous tree [43]. K-nearest neighbor is a machine learning algorithm that uses classification based on data points that are close to each other. Weighted ensemble algorithms combine multiple model predictions, where each model's contribution is weighted based on how accurate the model is, creating a single model based on the combination [44].

AutoKeras trains deep neural networks and performs model selection and hyperparameter tuning, with little user input required [29]. Some of the highest accuracies achieved by previous research groups predicting heart disease using traditional methods were obtained using neural networks [12,13]. Due to AutoKeras's ease of use and other researchers' success using neural networks, AutoKeras was another tool that was selected. AutoKeras offers classification and regression tools for image, text, and structured data. It also offers a TimeSeriesForecaster and more advanced tools for multi-modal and multi-task analyses and customized model development [29]. Default settings were used for the AutoKeras StructuredDataClassifier, including max-trials = 100, epochs = 1000, and validation-split = 0.2.

PyCaret, being built from the sklearn groundwork, allows for more adaptability and model evaluation but relies more on the strength of the dataset and preprocessing preparation. PyCaret operates by applying multiple machine learning models and algorithms to either preprocessed or unprocessed data to determine which machine learning model best applies to the data given and grants the most accurate model to utilize [39]. A variety of models are used within PyCaret [45], which include logistic regression, quadratic discriminate analysis (QDA), light gradient boosting machine, linear discriminant analysis (LDA), SVM, naïve Bayes (NB), and several other classifiers. PyCaret functions with a user setup that establishes what the target variable for prediction is amongst all models that are given within the PyCaret utility. PyCaret has various performance metrics embedded that allowed the authors to compare the various algorithms, including a confusion matrix, class prediction error, and precision–recall curve [8]. Post-data preprocessing enables significantly better results within the model evaluation step and leads to model tuning, which further refines the best-selected model and prepares it for prediction analysis [46]. The prediction function best operates after the best-selected model undergoes tuning and then proceeds to test the given model with the test data that split after data preprocessing. PyCaret does not just focus on singularly labeled data but also works within multiclass data, which expands the capacity that it can operate with and provides further data analysis [47].

The selection criteria prioritized open-source tools that were compatible with the latest version of Python. Compatibility ensured that the selected tools were actively maintained and could be seamlessly used in Google Colab, our chosen analysis environment. To provide a diverse range of approaches, we aimed to include a variety of tools. Auto Gluon is predominantly based on decision tree methods, while Pycaret incorporates other machine learning algorithms such as QDA, LDA, SVM, and NB, along with ensembles. Given the limited availability of deep learning approaches for small datasets, only one neural network tool, AutoKeras, was included [9,35]. Although it is possible to use the tools collectively, in this study, we evaluated each tool as an independent solution.

3.3. Dataset

Multiple resources are available for datasets, such as Google [48], IEEE [49], Mendeley [48–50], Kaggle [50], and the University of California, Irvine (UCI) [51]. However, patient privacy is an important consideration when handling health data, with HIPAA requiring "IRB waiver or patient authorization for research" use of protected health information [52–55]. Some datasets are freely accessible, while others require a research request or an access fee. Two open-access heart disease datasets available from UCI are the Cleveland Heart Disease [54] and the Statlog (Heart) datasets [56]. Most of the previous studies utilizing ML to predict heart disease used the Cleveland Heart Disease dataset when training and testing their models, including Marimuthu et al. [14], Pol et al. [8], Valarmathi et al. [20], Padmanabhan et al. [20], six research groups reviewed by Hazra et al. [9], and three different research groups surveyed by Khan et al. [12]. Researchers Dangare et al. [5], El Bialy et al. [55], Nagavelli et al. [15], Sarra et al. [56], and Ahmed [57] used both the Cleveland and Statlog datasets in their analyses.

3.4. Details of the Selected Datasets

The Cleveland and Statlog datasets were both considered for use in this research due to them being easily accessible and having been used by other researchers, allowing for direct comparisons of results. However, when performing preliminary exploratory analysis, we observed very similar patterns in the histograms and attribute distributions. This suggested the possibility that the Statlog dataset is a subset of the Cleveland dataset, despite other researchers having used both datasets in their analyses. The source of the Statlog dataset is not clear in its documentation, so we compared the datasets and confirmed that Statlog is a subset of Cleveland, making it unsuitable and redundant for our use. The second dataset chosen was the Hungarian Heart Disease dataset, which is available from the same UCI repository location as Cleveland. The Cleveland and Hungarian datasets are of a similar size, with 303 and 294 observations, respectively, but Cleveland is more complete, with fewer missing values: 6 versus 781. Besides these two datasets, two additional datasets, UCI: Switzerland (123 samples) and Long Beach, CA (V.A. Medical Center) (200 samples) were utilized to form a larger third dataset containing 920 total samples. All datasets use the same 13 attributes and a label, as shown in Table 1. General statistics for the datasets are in Tables 2 and 3. Distributions for the different attributes for the combined dataset are shown in Figure 1, 2 and 3 and are separated by heart disease status: HD positive versus HD negative.

Table 1. Attribute descriptions of datasets.

Attribute	Description
Age	Age in years
Sex	Sex (1 = male; 0 = female)
Cp	Chest pain type
Trestbps	Resting blood pressure (in mm Hg on admission to hospital)
Chol	Serum cholesterol in mg/dL
Fbs	Fasting blood sugar > 120 mg/dL (1 = true; 0 = false)
Restecg	Resting electrocardiographic results
Thalach	Maximum heart rate achieved
Exang	Exercise-induced angina (1 = yes; 0 = no)
Oldpeak	ST depression induced by exercise relative to rest
Slope	The slope of the peak exercise ST segment
Ca	Number of major vessels (0–3) colored by fluoroscopy
Thal	3 = normal; 6 = fixed defect; 7 = reversible defect
Num	Diagnosis of heart disease (angiographic disease status)

Table 2. Number of missing values per attribute by dataset.

Attribute	Cleveland	Hungarian	Switzerland	VA
Trestbps	0	1	2	56
Chol	0	23	0	7
Fbs	0	8	75	7
ReThalach	0	1	1	53
Exang	0	1	1	53
Oldpeak	0	0	6	53
Slope	0	190	17	102
Ca	4	290	118	198
Thal	2	266	52	166

Attributes not shown were complete.

Table 3. Attribute correlations with label.

Attribute	Cleveland	Hungarian	Combined
Thalach	−0.417167	−0.331074	−0.385972
Fbs	0.025264	0.162869	dropped
Chol	0.085164	0.202372	-0.234679
Trestbps	0.150825	0.139582	0.103828
Restecg	0.169202	−0.031988	0.062304
Age	0.223120	0.159315	0.282700
Sex	0.276816	0.272781	0.307284
Slope	0.339213	dropped	dropped
Cp	0.414446	0.505864	0.471712
Oldpeak	0.424510	0.545700	0.373382
Exang	0.431894	0.584541	0.443433
Ca	0.460033	dropped	dropped
Thal	0.522057	dropped	dropped

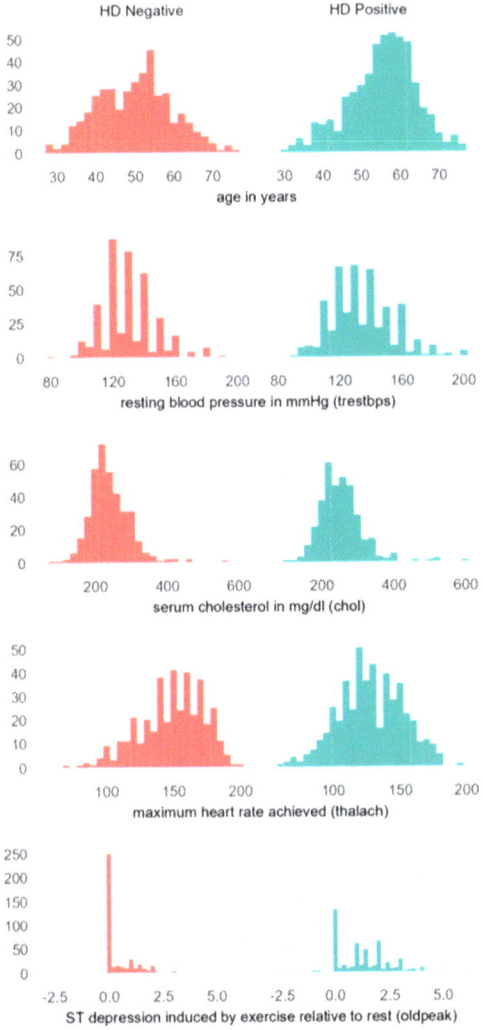

Figure 1. Histograms of five continuous attributes from the combined dataset, filtered for heart disease (+) positive and (−) negative patients.

Table 2 shows the number of missing values per attribute for each of the datasets used. Age and sex are omitted from the table as they were complete in all datasets. The number of missing values varied between datasets, with Cleveland being the most complete. Certain attributes, like ca, thal, and slope, were excluded from analyses using the Hungarian, Switzerland, or VA datasets due to very few observations being available. In addition to the number of major vessels colored by fluoroscopy (ca), thalassemia, and slope, fasting blood sugar (fbs) was also excluded from the combined dataset due to the large number of missing values in the Switzerland dataset.

Histograms of the continuous attributes are shown in Figure 1, with heart disease-positive patients on the right and negative on the left. The histograms clearly show the differences between heart disease-positive and -negative patients. First of all, when the age data were examined, it was seen that the age of positive patients was higher than that of negative patients. This situation reflects that positive patients' age distribution is skewed compared to negative patients. It was observed that trestbps (resting blood pressure) data were generally reported in ten-unit increments. While it is noteworthy that the trestbps values of negative patients were close to values such as 120, 130, and 140, an abnormal outlier value of 0 was observed in positive patients. In Chol (serum cholesterol) data, there were many outliers close to 0 in positive patients, while there were fewer outliers in negative patients. These outliers were not specified in the dataset documentation, with missing data denoted by "−9" or NaN. However, it is physically impossible for cholesterol or blood pressure to be 0. Considering these outliers, the trestbps and cholesterol data appeared to have similar skewness and kurtosis characteristics in positive patients compared to negative patients, with higher mean values in positive patients. While Thalach (maximum heart rate reached) data showed an approximately symmetrical distribution for positive patients, the distribution was negatively skewed in negative patients and had a higher mean value. Oldpeak (ST depression caused by exercise) data contained many 0 values. These 0 values appeared to be actual observations and not missing values, given the magnitude of the neighboring observations, but this was not noted in the data documentation or a quick literature search. Additionally, approximately twice as many 0 values were observed in positive patients than in negative patients. These data are presented in detail in Figure 1 and reveal significant differences in the datasets.

Figures 2 and 3 show the differences in different characteristics between heart disease-positive and negative patients. Female patients (0) constituted a significant proportion (about one-third) of the heart disease-negative group, while representing a smaller proportion (about one-tenth) of heart disease-positive cases. The "cp" feature indicated that patients with heart disease predominantly experience asymptomatic chest pain (4), while typical angina (1) was rarely seen in heart disease-negative cases. Compared with other individual features, the differences in "fbs" (fasting blood glucose) and "restecg" (resting electrocardiography results) between the two groups of patients were less pronounced. "Exang" (exercise-induced angina) was rare in heart disease-negative patients but common in more than half of heart disease-positive cases. By understanding these complex patterns between different characteristics, changes in factors affecting the diagnosis of heart disease could be clearly observed, as shown in Figures 2 and 3.

Discrete attributes are shown in Figures 2 and 3. Women (0) were found to make up less than a quarter of all patients but almost a third of heart disease-negative patients and only about a tenth of heart disease (+) positive patients. In analysis, this makes sex an important feature. Results obtained from analyses where data are not combined with sex may be very different. Cp describes chest pain. Heart disease patients were found to predominantly exhibit asymptomatic chest pain (4), while little typical angina (1) was seen among negative patients. The differences in fasting blood sugar (fbs) and resting electrocardiographic results (restecg) between heart disease (+) positive and (−) negative patients were not as large as those for other discrete attributes. Very few heart disease (−) negative patients were found to experience exercise-induced angina (exang), while more than half of positive patients did.

The slope was flat (2) for most positive patients and rarely downsloping (3) for negative patients. The number of major vessels colored by fluoroscopy, ca, was seen to be predominantly 0 for negative patients, but it is not known if this value is an observation or only represents a missing observation. It was observed most heart disease (−) negative patients were normal for thalassemia, and most heart disease-positive patients had a reversible defect. Num was the label, for which 0 indicated heart disease (−) negative and 1 through 4 indicated heart disease-positive. All prior research we found using the Cleveland dataset used a binary label. We chose to do the same for our analyses.

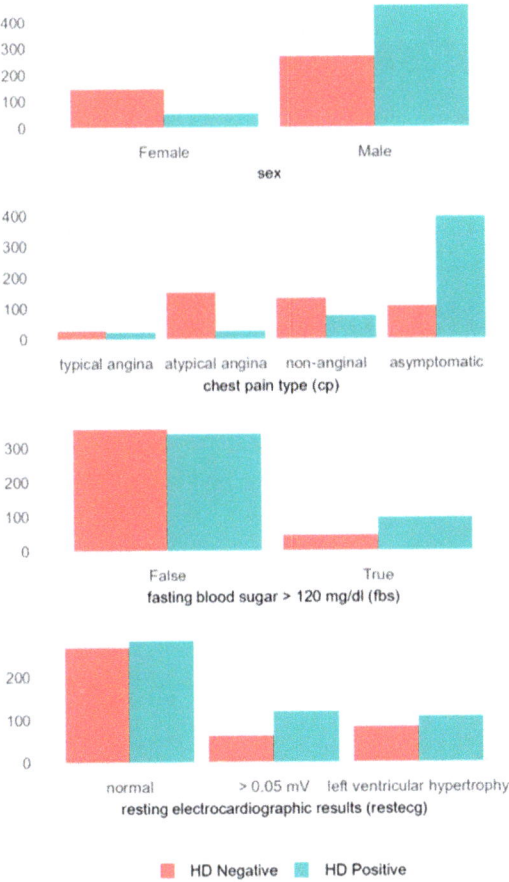

Figure 2. Distributions of the first four of the eight discrete attributes from the combined dataset, filtered for heart disease (+) positive and (−) negative patients, excluding the binary label.

Table 3 shows the correlations of the different attributes with the dependent variable, num. The attributes chosen for analysis for each of the datasets are shown with unused features marked as "dropped". The number of major vessels colored by fluoroscopy (ca) and thalassemia were both highly correlated with num in the Cleveland dataset, meaning their exclusion in the Hungarian and combined datasets may have negatively impacted prediction accuracy. Slope also had a correlation above 0.2 for the Cleveland dataset, though not as high as for the number of major vessels colored by fluoroscopy (ca) or thalassemia. The slope may be worthy of inclusion in future analyses with larger datasets, provided there is an adequate number of observations available, as it has been found to be a useful predictor in other applications [54]. The exclusion of fasting blood sugar (fbs) from the combined dataset was supported by the relatively low correlations in the Cleveland and Hungarian datasets.

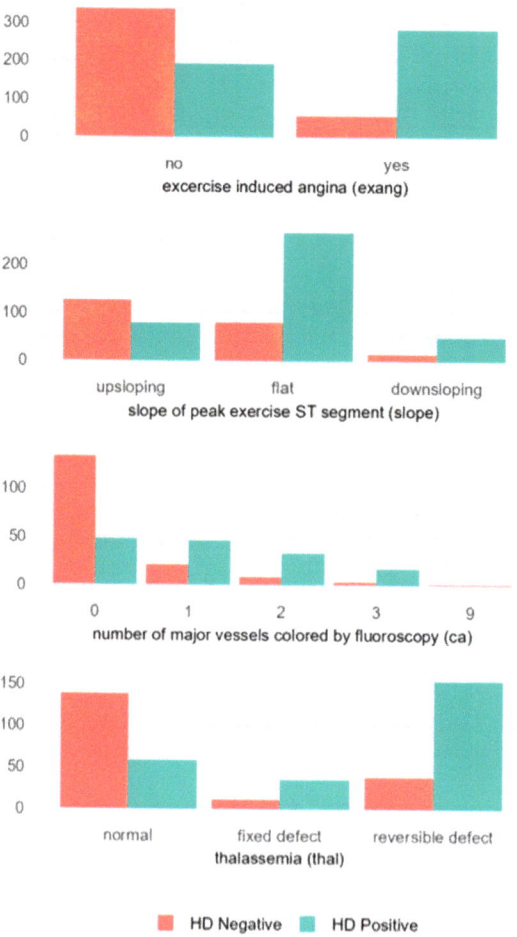

Figure 3. Distributions of the last four of the eight discrete attributes from the combined dataset, filtered for heart disease (+) positive and (−) negative patients, excluding the binary label.

3.5. Performance Metrics Used

Accuracy and F1 score metrics were used to evaluate the performance of the AutoML tools. Accuracy (ACC) is a measure of how well the model predicts the outcome. The formula for accuracy is the number of correct predictions divided by the total number of predictions (Equation (1)). This metric, however, can be biased due to data imbalances and thus lead to skewed results.

$$\text{Accuracy} = \frac{(TP + TN)}{(TP + TN + FP + FN)} \qquad (1)$$

One metric that takes this into account and is commonly used for machine learning is the F1 score. The F1 score is the harmonic mean between precision and recall (2 times the product of precision and recall divided by the total sum of precision and recall) (Equation (4)). Precision is defined as the number of true positives divided by the sum of true positives and false positives (Equation (2)). The recall metric is the number of true positives divided by the total number of true positives and false negatives (Equation (3)) [58].

$$\text{Precision} = \frac{TP}{(TP + FP)} \quad (2)$$

$$\text{Recall} = \frac{(TP)}{(TP + FN)} \quad (3)$$

$$\text{F1 score} = 2\frac{(precision \times recall)}{(precision + recall)} \quad (4)$$

3.6. Applying Traditional Steps of Manually Generating the Well-Performing Model

To benchmark the performance of AutoML-generated models against those produced by traditional manual techniques, we meticulously followed a series of steps to develop a classification model using sklearn libraries for heart disease using the Cleveland Heart Disease dataset:

(1). Data Cleaning: Rows with missing information in the "ca" and "thal" columns were removed to ensure data integrity.
(2). Data Type Conversion: All fields were converted to numeric data types to facilitate subsequent analysis and modeling.
(3). Correlation Analysis: The correlations between the fields and the target label were analyzed. Four fields ("chol", "fbs", "trestbps", "restecg") with correlations below 0.2 were identified and subsequently dropped from the dataset.
(4). Data Scaling: The remaining data were scaled to normalize the feature values and ensure comparability across different variables.
(5). Cross-validation: Cross-validation (k = 5) accuracy scores were calculated for 10 different machine learning algorithms. The algorithms used were stochastic gradient descent (SGD), logistic regression, support vector machine with a linear kernel, support vector machine with an RBF kernel, decision tree classifier, random forest classifier, extra trees classifier, AdaBoost classifier, gradient boosting classifier, and XGBoost.
(6). Hyperparameter Tuning: The top-performing algorithms (AdaBoost, rando forest, gradient boosting, XGBoost) were selected for further improvement through hyperparameter tuning. A grid search was performed using various combinations of hyperparameters, including n-estimators (100, 200, 300, 400, 500), learning-rate (0.3, 0.1, 0.05), max-features (1, 0.7, 0.5, 0.4, 0.3), subsample (1, 0.5, 0.3), max-samples (1, 0.5, 0.3, 0.2), and bootstrap (True, False).
(7). Ensemble Voting Classifier: Based on the fine-tuned estimators (AdaBoost, random forest, gradient boosting, XGBoost) and the other top-performing estimators (SVC, SGD, logistic regression), an ensemble voting classifier was constructed. This ensemble classifier combined the predictions of multiple models, leveraging their collective knowledge to make a final classification decision.

By following these steps, we conducted a comprehensive analysis and model selection process to generate the most effective machine learning model utilizing the machine-learning algorithms listed above and forming an ensemble learning model for classifying heart disease using the Cleveland Heart Disease dataset. The outcome of the above steps is shared and compared in the Results section and the code is available on GitHub [58].

4. Results

The datasets were analyzed using PyCaret v3.0, AutoGluon v0.7.0, and AutoKeras v1.1.0. Default settings were used for all AutoML tools. Missing values were imputed to the respective attribute's mode, if discrete, and mean, if continuous. Attributes ca, thal, and slope were excluded from the Hungarian data analyses due to missing more than half of each of these attributes. Data were split with 80% for training and 20% for testing, using stratified sampling by sex. Stratified sampling was used due to the difference in representation by sex. This difference was less pronounced in the Cleveland and Hungarian datasets, but it was more significant in the Switzerland and VA datasets. We verified that the representation of heart disease-positive patients was approximately the same for both the training and testing subsets of the Cleveland, Hungarian, and combined datasets: 46%, 36%, and 55%, respectively. We also verified that the data were successfully split using stratified sampling. The testing and training datasets were both approximately 33%, 27%, and 21% female for the Cleveland, Hungarian, and combined datasets, respectively.

As described in the previous Methodology section, we performed traditional steps to develop a well-performing machine learning model using the sklearn libraries on the Cleveland dataset to compare the manually generated models with the models generated by the AutoML tools. The manual steps included cleaning the data, reducing the data based on correlation analysis, exploring the performance of 10 machine learning algorithms, selecting top-performing models and applying hyperparameter fine-tuning, and then ensembling various top-performing models to form a well-performing model. The results of this manual approach are in Table 4.

Table 4. ML model generation using traditional manual steps on the Cleveland dataset.

Machine Learning Algorithm	Accuracy (Correlated)	Accuracy (Unreduced)
Stochastic Gradient Descent (SGD)	0.59	0.58
Logistic Regression	0.59	0.59
Support Vector Machine (SVM) (Linear Kernel)	0.55	0.57
Support Vector Machine (SVC) (RBF Kernel)	0.57	0.56
Decision Tree	0.52	0.49
Random Forest	0.62	0.59
Extra Trees	0.57	0.57
AdaBoost	0.58	0.57
Gradient Boosting	0.60	0.59
XGBoost	0.55	0.56
Ensemble of the following: AdaBoost, Random Forest, Gradient Boosting, XGBoost, SVM-Linear, SGD, Logistic Regression	0.60	0.58

As shown in Table 4, the best-performing models were based on ensemble algorithms such as random forest, gradient boosting, and our custom ensemble model that combined seven models. When the dataset was processed by reduction based on correlated fields, it tended to perform better, as can be noticed by comparing accuracy scores using the correlated and unreduced datasets in Table 4. Results from analyses using the three different AutoML tools on the three different datasets are in Tables 5 and 6. Data in the "correlated" row are for the outcome performed on datasets using only features that correlated with the label of at least 0.2. The "unreduced" data are for the outcome where all features were used. The top three models from the leaderboard are listed for PyCaret and AutoGluon in Tables 5–7. Results from a single analysis for AutoKeras for each dataset are shown. Accuracies for repeat analyses using AutoKeras are shown in Table 8.

PyCaret accuracies were generally in the low eighties with slightly lower F1 scores. AutoGluon accuracies were the highest of all three AutoML tools. Its accuracies for the unreduced dataset were in the mid-to-high eighties and its F1 scores were the same or higher. The correlated dataset results were slightly lower, in the mid-eighties, except for the results achieved by the top model on the leaderboard, which were only around 78%. The accuracy for the unreduced dataset, when analyzed using AutoKeras, was comparable, about 80%, with a slightly higher F1 score. The AutoKeras accuracy for the Cleveland correlated dataset was only 54%. The F1 score was still poor but substantially better at approximately 67%. Other analyses using the same data and input conditions produced much higher accuracies (see Tables 5–7).

Table 5. Cleveland dataset analysis using PyCaret, AutoGluon, and AutoKeras.

	Cleveland		
	Accuracy	F1 Score	Best Model
Unreduced:			
	0.8525	0.8037	1. Linear Discriminant Analysis
PyCaret	0.8215	0.7998	2. Ridge Classifier
	0.8180	0.7939	3. Naïve Bayes
	0.8688	0.8709	1. WeightedEnsemble_L2
AutoGluon	0.8688	0.8709	2. RandomForestGini
	0.8524	0.8524	3. RandomForestEntr
AutoKeras	0.8033	0.8182	N/A
Correlated:			
	0.8137	0.8012	1. Logistic Regression
PyCaret	0.8048	0.7814	2. Linear Discriminant Analysis
	0.8008	0.7775	3. Ridge Classifier
	0.7868	0.7796	1. WeightedEnsemble_L2
AutoGluon	0.8524	0.8474	2. RandomForestGini
	0.8360	0.8333	3. RandomForestEntr
AutoKeras	0.5410	0.6667	N/A

Table 6. Combined dataset analysis using PyCaret, AutoGluon, and AutoKeras.

	Combined		
	Accuracy	F1 Score	Best Model
Unreduced:			
	0.6873	0.6678	1. Logistic Regression
PyCaret	0.6833	0.6839	2. Linear Discriminant Analysis
	0.6832	0.6484	3. Ridge Classifier
	0.8478	0.8691	1. WeightedEnsemble_L2
AutoGluon	0.8478	0.8691	2. RandomForestEntr
	0.8423	0.8651	3. ExtraTreesGini
AutoKeras	0.8152	0.8365	N/A
Correlated:			
	0.7826	0.7311	1. Random Forest Classifier
PyCaret	0.7459	0.7168	2. Ridge Classifier
	0.7432	0.7260	3. Logistic Regression
	0.8423	0.8638	1. WeightedEnsemble_L2
AutoGluon	0.8423	0.8638	2. RandomForestEntr
	0.8369	0.8369	3. RandomForestGini
AutoKeras	0.8315	0.8545	N/A

Table 7. Hungarian dataset analysis using PyCaret, AutoGluon, and AutoKeras.

	Hungarian		
	Accuracy	F1 Score	Best Model
Unreduced:			
	0.6976	0.6465	1. Logistic Regression
PyCaret	0.6806	0.6092	2. Ridge Classifier
	0.6766	0.6334	3. Linear Discriminant Analysis
	0.8475	0.7804	1.WeightedEnsemble_L2
AutoGluon	0.8474	0.7804	2. RandomForestEntr
	0.8305	0.7619	3. ExtraTreesEntr
AutoKeras	0.8305	0.7059	N/A

Table 7. Cont.

	Hungarian		
	Accuracy	F1 Score	Best Model
Correlated:			
	0.8304	0.7516	1. Ridge Classifier
PyCaret	0.8303	0.7506	2. Log. Regression
	0.8263	0.7470	3. Linear Discriminant Analysis
	0.8983	0.8500	1. WeightedEnsemble_L2
AutoGluon	0.8983	0.8500	2. RandomForestEntr
	0.8644	0.8095	3. ExtraTreesGini
AutoKeras	0.8305	0.7059	N/A

Table 8. Run times and accuracies from repeat analyses using AutoKeras.

		Run 1		Run 2		Run 3		Mean σ st. dev.
		Accuracy	Run Time	Accuracy	Run Time	Accuracy	Run Time	
Cleveland	Unreduced	0.8197	40 m 51 s	0.7705	6 m 5 s	0.8033	6 m 35 s	0.7978 σ 0.0251
	Correlated	0.7541	18 m 47 s	0.8197	6 m 29 s	0.7705	11 m 10 s	0.7814 σ 0.0341
Hungarian	Unreduced	0.8644	7 m 36 s	0.7966	10 m 29 s	0.6610	52 m 27 s	0.7740 σ 0.1035
	Correlated	0.8136	5 m 34 s	0.8644	7 m 55 s	0.6610	7 m 23 s	0.7797 σ 0.1059
Combined	Unreduced	0.8478	18 m 24 s	0.8207	15 m 57 s	0.8478	12 m 54 s	0.8388 σ 0.0156
	Correlated	0.7989	35 m 51 s	0.8152	10 m 41 s	0.7880	24 m 02 s	0.8007 σ 0.0137

PyCaret's performance on the unreduced Hungarian dataset was significantly worse than that on the Cleveland dataset, with accuracies in the upper 60% and lower F1 scores. Although PyCaret accuracies for the correlated dataset were back in the eighties, the F1 scores were much lower at only about 75%. Accuracies resulting from AutoGluon were all in the mid-to-upper eighties, but its F1 scores were also lower than was seen when using the Cleveland dataset. AutoKeras results were similar, with 83% accuracies and 71% F1 scores.

When analyzing the combined dataset, PyCaret's results were similar to those it achieved when analyzing the Hungarian dataset and lower than those for the Cleveland. Results were below seventy for the unreduced dataset and in the mid-to-low seventies for the correlated.

AutoGluon performed well, with accuracies around 84% and most F1 scores around 86%. AutoKeras results for these runs were also greater than 80%. The code used to obtain the above results is shared on the GitHub page [58]. The open-source code includes exploratory data analysis; AutoML implementation for AutoGluon, PyCaret, and AutoKeras; as well as the code that performed model generation by following the traditional steps.

5. Discussion

The AutoML tools in question function by autonomously testing various embedded algorithms and subsequently presenting the most effective model. As users, we lacked the facility to specify a particular model for application; instead, the tools independently determined the optimal choice. Our comparative analysis, therefore, did not stem from a selection of models we wished to evaluate side by side. Rather, it arose from assessing the peak-performing model provided by one AutoML tool against the counterpart from another, essentially comparing the pinnacle of what each tool asserted to be its most proficient solution.

Our analysis operated under the assumption that tool developers had carefully chosen the best hyperparameters to enhance their tool's performance. Respecting their expertise, we did not modify these parameters, trusting that the default settings were optimized for peak performance. We analyzed each tool in its default state, mirroring typical user experience without advanced machine learning knowledge. This approach provided valuable insights into the performance of each tool with minimal customization—important for users unfamiliar with algorithm intricacies or specific tuning options. AutoML tools have diverse adjustable settings, complicating any attempt to standardize them with identical algorithms. For example, AutoKeras focuses on neural architecture search (NAS) to find the most effective neural network configuration, but it does not inherently support traditional models like SVM, decision trees, or random forests. This makes a direct comparison using the same algorithms and parameters across different tools both complex and often impractical.

By following examples on the AutoKeras website, building and evaluating a basic model was easy, requiring little to no data preprocessing. However, while model customization and tuning are possible, the website resources could be more in-depth and accessible to an inexperienced user. Performance inconsistency between runs was an issue during the analysis. Repeat analyses took different run times and produced models with different accuracies. Run times and accuracies, including means and standard deviations, obtained from three sets of analyses are shown in Table 8.

The model produced from one of these runs (on the unreduced Cleveland dataset, run 3) is shown in Table 9. The resulting model and number of parameters varied widely for the various runs, sometimes having fewer than 1500 parameters and sometimes more than 50,000. Models always consisted of some dense layers and sometimes also included one or more normalization/batch-normalization layers and/or dropout layers. The number of dense layers varied between models, but ReLU activation functions were always used for the hidden layers. The official website documentation for AutoGluon was fairly easy to follow and contained several tutorials on how to use the tool. However, in-depth explanations of how to use and interpret results were lacking and would require the user to have a prior understanding of machine learning. The user would need to look to other resources for a better understanding of machine learning concepts. AutoGluon also tends to default to the best model when displaying results; however, this can be changed with input options. Models with the best validation scores also did not always provide the best accuracy on the test data; however, with more test data, this may have changed and thus more datasets would be needed for testing. Advanced custom metrics are also possible with AutoGluon, but this requires an in-depth understanding of statistics and machine learning that is likely beyond the basic user. A useful feature with AutoGluon is the leaderboard, which displays models based on validation score by default with no inputs or by accuracy if test data are inputted. An example leaderboard of the AutoGluon tool is presented in Table 10.

Table 9. Example neural network produced by AutoKeras.

Layer (Type)	Output Shape	Param
Input$_1$(InputLayer)	[(None, 13)]	0
MultiCategoryEncoding (MultiCategoryEncoding)	(None, 13)	0
Normalization (Normalization)	(None, 13)	27
Dense (Dense)	0.150825	896
Relu(ReLU)	0.169202	0
Dense$_1$(Dense)	0.223120	16,640
Relu$_1$(ReLU)	0.276816	0
Dense$_2$(Dense)	0.339213	32,896
Relu$_2$(ReLU)	0.414446	0
Dense$_3$(Dense)	0.424510	129
Classificationhead$_1$ (Activation)	0.431894 0.460033	0
Total params:		50,588
Trainable params:		50,561
Non-trainable params:		27

Table 10. Example AutoGluon leaderboard (unreduced combined dataset).

Model	Score_Test	Score_Val	Pred_Time_Tes	Pred_Time_Val	Fit_Time	Pred_Time_Test_Marginal	Pred_Time_Val_Marginal	Fit_Time_Marginal
0	RandomForestEntr	0.847826	0.797297	0.036896	0.024798	0.2945	0.036896	0.024798
1	WeightedEnsemble_L2	0.847826	0.810811	0.123012	0.074949	0.979291	0.001744	0.000401
2	RandomForestGini	0.842391	0.77027	0.037669	0.025544	0.297175	0.037669	0.025544
3	ExtraTreesGini	0.842391	0.783784	0.041508	0.024531	0.28753	0.041508	0.024531
4	ExtraTreesEntr	0.826087	0.77027	0.046702	0.024206	0.282546	0.046702	0.024206
5	XGBoost	0.809783	0.722973	0.005913	0.003386	0.023183	0.005913	0.003386
6	KNeighborsDist	0.690217	0.668919	0.00367	0.001662	0.004442	0.00367	0.001662
7	KNeighborsUnif	0.690217	0.662162	0.014753	0.002047	0.012023	0.014753	0.002047

PyCaret documentation is well labeled and defined, making it quick to understand the capacity of utility that it has available to offer, covering several machine learning techniques (classification, regression, anomalies, clustering, and time series). Opening any one of the tabs for the desired technique immediately gives insight into the higher workings and functions of the chosen function, which makes it appear convoluted, but those familiar with machine learning will be able to understand all that they provide and the freedom of its utility for these AutoML tools. Functionally, when PyCaret runs with the chosen technique, it provides a leaderboard like other AutoML tools, which displays the top-ranked models by various scores (F1, accuracy, etc.) that best apply to the data that it was given. Across the leaderboard, it usefully highlights the best scores in each given category; however, the ranking will sometimes find better scores for different models as opposed to the best model across the leaderboard. Testing the PyCaret AutoML tool with the Heart Disease datasets was proven to have successful results in identifying efficient models that can be utilized, especially after implementing data preprocessing and reducing the dataset to focus on the parameters that matter more. In some circumstances, there have been less promising results, giving lower accuracy, and this could be because of the differing size of the data in some cases, as well as potentially not reducing the datasets to isolate the more correlated features.

The impact of feature selection performed when reducing the datasets based on correlation was not clear. When using AutoGluon, the accuracy, after reducing for correlation, was worse for the Cleveland dataset, better for the Hungarian, and almost the same for the combined. Results for the unreduced and correlated versions were similar for all three datasets when AutoKeras was used. Interestingly, the accuracy obtained by AutoGluon for the "correlated" Cleveland dataset is among the lowest in Table 4. This could be a case of underfitting for this particular dataset and the model combination. Other than this result, AutoGluon produced consistent results and some of the highest accuracies. The best model, based on validation accuracies, for each analysis was WeightedEnsemble-L2.

Unlike PyCaret and AutoGluon, repeat analyses using AutoKeras produced different models and different accuracies. In addition to the disadvantage of inconsistent results, AutoKeras took the longest to run, with some of its shortest run times still longer than those for the other two tools. The datasets used here were small. The time required by AutoKeras could be a prohibitive problem for large datasets.

Traditional manual steps were applied to create ML models utilizing ten machine learning algorithms and an ensemble model that merged seven well-performing models, and the results are presented in Table 4. When these results are compared with the results achieved using the AutoML tools, it can be noticed that the AutoML tools generated ML models that could perform much better than manually created models. The top-performing models created manually performed with around 60% accuracy, while the top-performing AutoML-generated models performed with around 85% accuracy on the same Cleveland dataset.

In addition to comparing results with those of conventional machine learning models that were generated using sklearn libraries, deep learning models could be manually developed using libraries such as Tensorflow, Keras, or PyTorch to compare with them with the AutoKeras AutoML tool's models. This comparison could include a detailed explanation of parameters and FLOPS used during the training. In the literature, researchers have claimed to achieve up to 95% accuracy on heart disease datasets [12–22,59,60]. However, we did not have a chance to repeat the results of these studies since the code and configurations were not shared. To let other researchers compare their results with ours, we open-sourced our code that utilized AutoML tools and applied traditional model generation steps on GitHub [58]. Accuracies and F1 scores are the key metrics in Tables 5–7; however, accuracy alone should not be considered a true metric as it may not provide a complete picture of a model's performance. It does not consider the nuances of different classes, class imbalances, or the cost associated with misclassification. Relying solely on accuracy may lead to misleading conclusions, especially in scenarios where the dataset is imbalanced or the costs of the false positives and false negatives differ significantly.

When utilizing a machine learning tool to aid in medical diagnosis, it is critical that expert knowledge is employed in both judging the soundness of the medical results and the relevance of a wide range of relevant model metrics. While accuracy measured the overall correctness of the predictions, precision focused on the proportion of true positives among all predicted positives, and recall focused on the proportion of true positives among all actual positives. In scenarios where class imbalance exists, optimizing for high accuracy may result in low precision or recall as the model may favor the majority class. Therefore, a trade-off exists between accuracy and precision/recall, and the choice depends on the specific requirements of the application. F1 scores combine precision and recall into a single metric, providing a balance between the two. However, optimizing for F1 score may not be suitable in all scenarios. In some cases, precision or recall may be more important, and a trade-off exists between F1 score and precision/recall. We decided to utilize accuracy and F1 score metrics since many of the comparable studies utilized these metrics. However, sensitivity and specificity are also important metrics generally used in the medical domain. Further studies should consider utilizing sensitivity and specificity as well. In the process of optimizing a model, it is important to consider that as models become more complex and accurate, they often require more computational resources and longer inference times. There is a trade-off between achieving higher accuracy and the computational cost required for inference. There is also the risk of overfitting. Overfitting occurs when a model performs well on the training data but fails to generalize to unseen data, while underfitting occurs when a model is too simple to capture underlying patterns in the data. These represent opposite ends of a trade-off. Increasing model complexity may reduce underfitting but increase the risk of overfitting, while reducing model complexity may reduce overfitting but increase the risk of underfitting.

In addition to model evaluation metrics, essential to account for are the limitations of the data, assumptions made, and constraints applied. We acknowledge and discuss/explain these uncertainties to help readers gain a more nuanced understanding of the limitations and potential sources of error associated with the evaluation metrics. We hope this will promote transparency and help readers interpret the results more accurately. Dataset limitations included size, quality, representativeness, and potential biases. The datasets used in this paper were very small. Although they have been used in numerous other studies, allowing for easier comparison of results, small size means the datasets are not likely to be representative of large populations and may be more susceptible to selection biases. There were also a large number of missing values in all but the Cleveland datasets. A key assumption made during this analysis was that these datasets and tools can be used to effectively predict heart disease. This is a huge assumption, and it should be noted that employing machine learning, particularly black-box tools like AutoML, requires caution and diligence. The data used here included both male and female patients. However, this may have led to the importance of other features being suppressed. Different features may have different levels of importance for male and female patients as well. This is not accounted for in this paper, but female under-representation in medical research is a well-known and persistent problem. Of the 41,622 participants in US government clinical trials analyzed by Mayor et al., only about 27.5% of them were female. [54] Future research should explore how sex impacts feature importance and model performance. Moreover, larger datasets could be used to assess model performances, including accuracies, precision, recall, and inference times.

Some features were excluded from our analyses using the combined dataset due to missing data. The inclusion of these, as well as other previously unused variables, may have had a significant impact on tool performance. The binary classification was used here; however, all three AutoML tools have the ability to perform multilabel classification, and their performances at this task could be compared in the future. Two previous examples we referenced of AutoML tools being used to analyze heart disease data were from 2021 [8,15].

New studies are needed to comprehensively test the performance of these and additional AutoML tools as these tools continue to be developed and improved. Two AutoML tools that were developed specifically for the medical field were found while working on this project [61–63]. AutoPrognosis was first released in 2018 and uses Bayesian optimization to create and optimize pipeline ensembles [60]. An updated version of the tool, AutoPrognosis 2.0, was released in 2022 [63–65]. Pharm-AutoML was developed by Genentech employees Liu, Lu, and Lu in 2020 [65]. If using csv-formatted data, Pharm-AutoML can handle steps from data preprocessing through model selection and evaluation for multiclassification problems [61]. AutoPrognosis 2.0 and Pharm-AutoML are both open-source and have been used to analyze heart disease datasets, though different from the data we used [62–66].

6. Conclusions

This study ventured into the effectiveness of automated machine learning (AutoML) tools for heart disease diagnosis and discovered that AutoGluon consistently outperformed its peers, with accuracy rates ranging from 78% to 86%. PyCaret's performance was found to vary depending on the dataset, with accuracy rates from 65% to 83%, suggesting a nuanced relationship between tool efficacy and dataset characteristics. AutoKeras showed the most variation in results, with accuracies between 54% and 83%, indicating the potential for high performance but also a significant dependency on the dataset used.

Compared to traditional machine learning methods, which yielded accuracy rates of 55% to 60% via standard practices like exploratory data analysis (EDA), data cleaning, feature engineering, and various modeling algorithms from the sklearn library, the advantage of AutoML tools is clear. This discrepancy illustrates the promising potential of AutoML to revolutionize diagnostic accuracy and make sophisticated analyses more accessible to healthcare practitioners.

The insights from this study suggest that AutoML tools, especially AutoGluon, have the capacity to significantly refine and expedite the diagnostic process, with profound implications for the treatment and prevention of heart disease internationally. Nevertheless, this investigation serves as an initial step towards a broader and more detailed exploration of AutoML's capabilities, underscoring the necessity for future research that includes larger and more varied datasets as well as a wider array of AutoML tools, potentially revolutionizing patient care in the process.

Author Contributions: Conceptualization, Methodology, and Writing—Review and Editing: O.T. and T.C.A.; Investigation, Software, Writing Original Draft: L.M.P., A.H. and A.P.; Validation: L.M.P., O.T. and T.C.A.; Supervision: O.T. All authors have read and agreed to the published version of the manuscript.

Funding: This research received no external funding.

Data Availability Statement: Data are contained within the article.

Acknowledgments: The authors would like to thank the creators of the datasets: Andras Janosi, Hungarian Institute of Cardiology, Budapest; William Steinbrunn, University Hospital, Zurich, Switzerland; Matthias Pfisterer, University Hospital, Basel, Switzerland; and Robert Detrano, V.A. Medical Center, Long Beach and Cleveland Clinic Foundation. We would like to express our sincere gratitude to all who provided insights and constructive feedback, which contributed to the improvement of this article.

Conflicts of Interest: The authors declare no conflict of interest.

References

1. Gaidai, O.; Cao, Y.; Loginov, S. Global Cardiovascular Diseases Death Rate Prediction. *Curr. Probl. Cardiol.* **2023**, *48*, 101622. [CrossRef]
2. Laslett, L.J.; Alagona, P.; Clark, B.A.; Drozda, J.P.; Saldivar, F.; Wilson, S.R.; Poe, C.; Hart, M. The Worldwide Environment of Cardiovascular Disease: Prevalence, Diagnosis, Therapy, and Policy Issues. *J. Am. Coll. Cardiol.* **2012**, *60*, S1–S49. [CrossRef]
3. Luo, C.; Tong, Y. Comprehensive study and review of coronary artery disease. In Proceedings of the Second International Conference on Biological Engineering and Medical Science (ICBioMed 2022), Oxford, UK, 7–13 November 2022. [CrossRef]

4. Absar, N.; Das, E.K.; Shoma, S.N.; Khandaker, M.U.; Miraz, M.H.; Faruque, M.R.I.; Tamam, N.; Sulieman, A.; Pathan, R.K. The Efficacy of Machine-Learning-Supported Smart System for Heart Disease Prediction. *Healthcare* **2022**, *10*, 1137. [CrossRef]
5. Rani, U. Analysis of Heart Diseases Dataset Using Neural Network Approach. *Int. J. Data Min. Knowl. Manag. Process* **2011**, *1*, 1–8. [CrossRef]
6. Singh, P.; Singh, S.; Pandi-Jain, G.S. Effective heart disease prediction system using data mining techniques. *Int. J. Nanomed.* **2018**, *13*, 121–124. [CrossRef]
7. Ismail, A.; Ravipati, S.; Gonzalez-Hernandez, D.; Mahmood, H.; Imran, A.; Munoz, E.J.; Naeem, S.; Abdin, Z.U.; Siddiqui, H.F. Carotid Artery Stenosis: A Look into the Diagnostic and Management Strategies, and Related Complications. *Cureus* **2023**, *15*, e38794. [CrossRef]
8. Pol, U.R.; Sawant, T.U. Automl: Building a classification model with PyCaret. *YMER* **2021**, *20*, 547–552. [CrossRef]
9. Ferreira, L.; Pilastri, A.; Martins, C.M.; Pires, P.M.; Cortez, P. A Comparison of AutoML Tools for Machine Learning, Deep Learning and XGBoost. In Proceedings of the 2021 International Joint Conference on Neural Networks (IJCNN), Shenzhen, China, 18–22 July 2021; pp. 1–8. [CrossRef]
10. Lenkala, S.; Marry, R.; Gopovaram, S.R.; Akinci, T.C.; Topsakal, O. Comparison of Automated Machine Learning (AutoML) Tools for Epileptic Seizure Detection Using Electroencephalograms (EEG). *Computers* **2023**, *12*, 197. [CrossRef]
11. Topsakal, O.; Akinci, T.C. Classification and Regression Using Automatic Machine Learning (AutoML)–Open Source Code for Quick Adaptation and Comparison. *Balk. J. Electr. Comput. Eng.* **2023**, *11*, 257–261. [CrossRef]
12. Hazra, A.; Mandal, S.K.; Gupta, A.; Mukherjee, A.; Mukherjee, A. Heart disease diagnosis and prediction using machine learning and data mining techniques: A review. *Adv. Comput. Sci. Technol.* **2017**, *10*, 2137–2159.
13. Khan, Y.; Qamar, U.; Yousaf, N.; Khan, A. Machine learning techniques for heart disease datasets: A survey. In Proceedings of the 2019 11th International Conference on Machine Learning and Computing (ICMLC '19), Zhuhai, China, 22–24 February 2019; ACM: New York, NY, USA, 2019; pp. 27–35. [CrossRef]
14. Marimuthi, M.; Abinaya, M.; Hariesh, K.S.; Madhankumar, K.; Pavithra, V. A review on heart disease prediction using machine learning and data analytics approach. *Int. J. Comput. Appl.* **2018**, *181*, 20–25. [CrossRef]
15. Nagavelli, U.; Samanta, D.; Chakraborty, P. Machine Learning Technology-Based Heart Disease Detection Models. *J. Healthc. Eng.* **2022**, *2022*, 7351061. [CrossRef] [PubMed]
16. Li, Y.; Shen, F.; Hu, L.; Lang, Z.; Liu, L.D.; Cai, F.; Fu, L. A Stare-Down Video-Rate High-Throughput Hyperspectral Imaging System and Its Applications in Biological Sample Sensing. *IEEE Sens. J.* **2023**, *23*, 23629–23637. [CrossRef]
17. Shen, F.; Deng, H.; Yu, L.; Cai, F. Open-source mobile multispectral imaging system and its applications in biological sample sensing. *Spectrochim. Acta Part A Mol. Biomol. Spectrosc.* **2022**, *280*, 121504. [CrossRef] [PubMed]
18. Squiers, J.J.; Thatcher, J.E.; Bastawros, D.S.; Applewhite, A.J.; Baxter, R.D.; Yi, F.; Quan, P.; Yu, S.; DiMaio, J.M.; Gable, D.R. Machine learning analysis of multispectral imaging and clinical risk factors to predict amputation wound healing. *J. Vasc. Surg.* **2022**, *75*, 279–285. [CrossRef]
19. Staszak, K.; Tylkowski, B.; Staszak, M. From Data to Diagnosis: How Machine Learning Is Changing Heart Health Monitoring. *Int. J. Environ. Res. Public Health* **2023**, *20*, 4605. [CrossRef]
20. Padmanabhan, M.; Yuan, P.; Chada, G.; Nguyen, H.V. Physician-friendly machine learning: A case study with cardiovascular disease risk prediction. *J. Clin. Med.* **2019**, *8*, 1050. [CrossRef]
21. Valarmathi, R.; Sheela, T. Heart disease prediction using hyperparameter optimization (HPO) tuning. *Biomed. Signal Process. Control* 2021. [CrossRef]
22. Romero, R.A.A.; Deypalan, M.N.Y.; Mehrotra, S.; Jungao, J.T.; Sheils, N.E.; Manduchi, E. Benchmarking AutoML frameworks for disease prediction using medical claims. *BioData Min.* **2022**, *15*, 15. [CrossRef]
23. Wang, X.; Zhang, Z.; Zhu, W. Automated graph machine learning: Approaches, libraries, and directions. *arXiv* **2022**, arXiv:2201.01288. [CrossRef]
24. Bu, C.; Lu, Y.; Liu, F. Automatic Graph Learning with Evolutionary Algorithms: An Experimental Study. In *PRICAI 2021: Trends in Artificial Intelligence. PRICAI 2021, Hanoi, Vietnam, 8–12 November 2021*; Pham, D.N., Theeramunkong, T., Governatori, G., Liu, F., Eds.; Lecture Notes in Computer Science; Springer: Cham, Switzerland, 2021; Volume 13031. [CrossRef]
25. Alamin, M.A. Democratizing Software Development and Machine Learning Using Low Code Applications. Master's Thesis, University of Calgary, Calgary, AB, Canada, 2022.
26. Topsakal, O.; Dobratz, E.J.; Akbas, M.I.; Dougherty, W.M.; Akinci, T.C.; Celikoyar, M.M. Utilization of Machine Learning for the Objective Assessment of Rhinoplasty Outcomes. *IEEE Access* **2023**, *11*, 42135–42145. [CrossRef]
27. Madhugiri, D. Beginner's Guide to AutoML with an Easy AutoGluon Example. Analytics Vidhya, 18 September 2022. Available online: https://www.analyticsvidhya.com/blog/2021/10/beginners-guide-to-automl-with-an-easy-autogluon-example/ (accessed on 9 September 2023).
28. Jin, H.; Chollet, F.; Song, Q.; Hu, X. AutoKeras: An AutoML Library for Deep Learning. *J. Mach. Learn. Res.* **2023**, *24*, 1–6.
29. Budjac, R.; Nikmon, M.; Schreiber, P.; Zahradnikova, B.; Janacova, D. Automated machine learning overview. *Sciendo* **2019**, *27*, 107–112. [CrossRef]
30. Koh, J.C.O.; Spangenberg, G.; Kant, S. Automated Machine Learning for High-Throughput Image-Based Plant Phenotyping. *Remote Sens.* **2021**, *13*, 858. [CrossRef]

31. Singh, V.K.; Josh, K. Automated Machine Learning (AutoML): An overview of opportunities for application and research. *J. Inf. Technol. Case Appl. Res.* **2022**, *24*, 75–85. [CrossRef]
32. Lee, S.; Kim, J.; Bae, J.H.; Lee, G.; Yang, D.; Hong, J.; Lim, K.J. Development of Multi-Inflow Prediction Ensemble Model Based on Auto-Sklearn Using Combined Approach: Case Study of Soyang River Dam. *Hydrology* **2023**, *10*, 90. [CrossRef]
33. Pushparaj, S.N.; Sivasankaran, S.M.; Thamizh Chem-mal, S. Prediction of Heart Disease Using a Hybrid of CNN-LSTM Algorithm. *J. Surv. Fish. Sci.* **2023**, *10*, 5700–5710.
34. Ferreira, L.; Pilastri, A.L.; Henrique, C.; Santos, P.A.; Cortez, P. A Scalable and Automated Machine Learning Framework to Support Risk Management. *Lect. Notes Comput. Sci.* **2020**, *12613*, 291–307. [CrossRef]
35. Egger, R. Machine Learning in Tourism: A Brief Overview. In *Applied Data Science in Tourism*; Spring: Berlin/Heidelberg, Germany, 2022. [CrossRef]
36. Yang, S.; Bhattacharjee, D.; Kumar, V.B.Y.; Chatterjee, S.; De, S.; Debacker, P.; Verkest, D.; Mallik, A.; Catthoor, F. AERO: Design Space Exploration Framework for Resource-Constrained CNN Mapping on Tile-Based Accelerators. *IEEE J. Emerg. Sel. Top. Circuits Syst.* **2022**, *12*, 508–521. [CrossRef]
37. Sarangpure, N.; Dhamde, V.; Roge, A.; Doye, J.; Patle, S.; Tamboli, S. Automating the Machine Learning Process using PyCaret and Streamlit. In Proceedings of the 2023 2nd International Conference for Innovation in Technology (INOCON), Bangalore, India, 3–5 March 2023; pp. 1–5. [CrossRef]
38. Vinicius, M.; Paulo, N.; Cecilia, M. Auto machine learning to predict pregnancy after fresh embryo transfer following in vitro fertilization. *World J. Adv. Res. Rev.* **2022**, *16*, 621–626. [CrossRef]
39. Olson, R.S. TPOT. Available online: http://epistasislab.github.io/tpot/ (accessed on 3 March 2023).
40. Gurdo, N.; Volke, D.C.; McCloskey, D.; Nikel, P.I. Automating the design-build-test-learn cycle towards next-generation bacterial cell factories. *New Biotechnol.* **2023**, *74*, 1–15. [CrossRef] [PubMed]
41. Erickson, N.; Mueller, J.; Shirkov, A.; Zhang, H.; Larroy, P.; Li, M.; Smola, A. AutoGluon-Tabular: Robust and Accurate AutoML for Structured Data. *arXiv* **2020**, arXiv:2003.06505.
42. Ali, A.A.; Khedr, A.M.; El-Bannany, M.; Kanakkayil, S. A Powerful Predicting Model for Financial Statement Fraud Based on Optimized XGBoost Ensemble Learning Technique. *Appl. Sci.* **2023**, *13*, 2272. [CrossRef]
43. Gaur, S.; Kalani, P.; Mohan, M. Harmonic-to-noise ratio as a speech biomarker for fatigue: K-nearest neighbour machine learning algorithm. *Med. J. Armed Forces India* **2023**. [CrossRef]
44. Jawad, B.J.; Shaker, S.M.; Altintas, I.; Eugen-Olse, J.; Nehlin, J.; Andersen, O.; Kallemose, T. Development and validation of prognostic machine learning models for short- and long-term mortality among acutely hospitalized patients. *Eur. PMC* **2023**. [CrossRef]
45. Suresh, K.; Elkahwagi, M.A.; Garcia, A.; Naples, J.G.; Corrales, C.E.; Crowson, M.G. Development of a Predictive Model for Persistent Dizziness Following Vestibular Schwannoma Surgery. *Laryngoscope* **2023**, *133*, 3534–3539. [CrossRef] [PubMed]
46. Ortiz-Perez, A.; Izquierdo Lozano, C.; Meijers, R.; Grisoni, F.; Albertazzi, L. Identification of fluorescently-barcoded nanoparticles using machine learning. *Nanoscale Adv.* **2023**, *5*, 2307–2317. [CrossRef]
47. Ehlers, M.R.; Lonsdorf, T.B. Data sharing in experimental fear and anxiety research: From challenges to a dynamically growing database in 10 simple steps. *Neurosci. Biobehav. Rev.* **2022**, *143*, 104958. [CrossRef]
48. Lu, P.J.; Chuang, J.-H. Fusion of Multi-Intensity Image for Deep Learning-Based Human and Face Detection. *IEEE Access* **2022**, *10*, 8816–8823. [CrossRef]
49. Maghfour, J.; Ceresnie, M.; Olson, J.; Lim, H.W. The association between frontal fibrosing alopecia, sunscreen, and moisturizers: A systematic review and meta-analysis. *J. Am. Acad. Dermatol.* **2022**, *87*, 395–396. [CrossRef]
50. Datasets | Kaggle. Kaggle.com. 2019. Available online: https://www.kaggle.com/datasets (accessed on 25 April 2023).
51. UCI Machine Learning Repository: Data Sets. Uci.edu. 2009. Available online: https://archive.ics.uci.edu/dataset/45/heart+disease (accessed on 18 April 2023).
52. Price, W.N., II; Cohen, I.G. Privacy in the age of medical big data. *Nat. Med.* **2019**, *25*, 37–43. [CrossRef] [PubMed]
53. Cleveland, Hungarian, Switzerland, and VA Datasets. Available online: https://archive.ics.uci.edu/ml/datasets/heart+disease (accessed on 9 September 2023).
54. Pathare, A.; Mangrulkar, R.; Suvarna, K.; Parekh, A.; Thakur, G.; Gawade, A. Comparison of tabular synthetic data generation techniques using propensity and cluster log metric. *Int. J. Inf. Manag. Data Insights* **2023**, *3*, 100177. [CrossRef]
55. El-Bialy, R.; Salamay, M.A.; Karam, O.H.; Khalifa, M.E. Feature analysis of coronary artery heart disease data sets. *Procedia Comput. Sci.* **2015**, *65*, 459–468. [CrossRef]
56. Sarra, R.R.; Dinar, A.M.; Mohammed, M.A.; Abdulkareem, K.H. Enhanced heart diseaseprediction based on machine learning and X2 statistical optimal feature selection model. *Designs* **2022**, *6*, 87. [CrossRef]
57. Ahmed, I. A Study of Heart Disease Diagnosis Using Machine Learning and Data Mining. Master's Thesis, California State University, San Bernardino, CA, USA, 2022. Volume 1591. Available online: https://scholarworks.lib.csusb.edu/etd/1591 (accessed on 9 September 2023).
58. AutoML Comparison for Heart Disease Diagnosis GitHub Page. Available online: https://github.com/researchoutcome/automl-comparison-heart/ (accessed on 4 July 2023).
59. Chandrasekhar, N.; Peddakrishna, S. Enhancing Heart Disease Prediction Accuracy through Machine Learning Techniques and Optimization. *Processes* **2023**, *11*, 1210. [CrossRef]

60. Mayor, J.M.; Preventza, O.; McGinigle, K.; Mills, J.L.; Montero-Baker, M.; Gilani, R.; Pallister, Z.; Chung, J. Persistent under-representation of female patients in United States trials of common vascular diseases from 2008 to 2020. *J. Vasc. Surg.* **2022**, *75*, 30–36. [CrossRef] [PubMed]
61. Finkelhor, R.S.; Newhouse, K.E.; Vrobel, T.R.; Miron, S.D.; Bahler, R.C. The ST segment/heartrate slope as a predictor of coronary artery disease: Comparison with quantitative thallium imaging and conventional ST segment criteria. *Am. Heart J.* **1986**, *112*, 296–304. [CrossRef]
62. Islam, M.M.; Haque, M.R.; Iqbal, H.; Hasan, H.M.M.; Hasan, M.; Kabir, M.N. Breast cancer prediction: A comparative study using machine learning techniques. *SN Comput. Sci.* **2020**, *1*, 290. [CrossRef]
63. Alaa, A.M.; van der Schaar, M. AutoPrognosis: Automated clinical prognostic modeling via Bayesian optimization with structured kernel learning. *arXiv* **2018**, arXiv:1802.07207. [CrossRef]
64. Imrie, F.; Cebere, B.; McKinney, E.F.; van der Schaar, M. AutoPrognosis 2.0: Democratizing diagnostic and prognostic modeling in healthcare with automated machine learning. *arXiv* **2022**, arXiv:2210.12090. [CrossRef]
65. Liu, G.; Lu, D.; Lu, J. Pharm-AutoML: An open-source, end-to-end automated machine learning package for clinical outcome prediction. *CPT Pharmacomet. Syst. Pharmacol.* **2021**, *10*, 478–488. [CrossRef] [PubMed]
66. Alaa, A.M.; van der Schaar, M. Cardiovascular disease risk prediction using automated machine learning: A prospective study of 423,604 UK Biobank participants. *PLoS ONE* **2019**, *14*, e0213653. [CrossRef] [PubMed]

Disclaimer/Publisher's Note: The statements, opinions and data contained in all publications are solely those of the individual author(s) and contributor(s) and not of MDPI and/or the editor(s). MDPI and/or the editor(s) disclaim responsibility for any injury to people or property resulting from any ideas, methods, instructions or products referred to in the content.

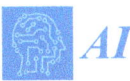

Article

Convolutional Neural Networks in the Diagnosis of Colon Adenocarcinoma

Marco Leo [1], Pierluigi Carcagnì [1], Luca Signore [2], Francesco Corcione [3], Giulio Benincasa [4], Mikko O. Laukkanen [5,*] and Cosimo Distante [1,2]

1. Institute of Applied Sciences and Intelligent Systems (ISASI), National Research Council (CNR) of Italy, 73100 Lecce, Italy; marco.leo@cnr.it (M.L.); pierluigi.carcagni@cnr.it (P.C.); cosimo.distante@cnr.it (C.D.)
2. Dipartimento di Ingegneria per L'Innovazione, Università del Salento, 73100 Lecce, Italy; luca.signore@unisalento.it
3. Clinica Mediterranea, 80122 Naples, Italy; francesco.corcione@unina.it
4. Italo Foundation, 20146 Milano, Italy; giulio.benincasa@pinetagrande.it
5. Department of Translational Medical Sciences, University of Naples Federico II, 80131 Naples, Italy
* Correspondence: mikko.laukkanen@utu.fi

Abstract: Colorectal cancer is one of the most lethal cancers because of late diagnosis and challenges in the selection of therapy options. The histopathological diagnosis of colon adenocarcinoma is hindered by poor reproducibility and a lack of standard examination protocols required for appropriate treatment decisions. In the current study, using state-of-the-art approaches on benchmark datasets, we analyzed different architectures and ensembling strategies to develop the most efficient network combinations to improve binary and ternary classification. We propose an innovative two-stage pipeline approach to diagnose colon adenocarcinoma grading from histological images in a similar manner to a pathologist. The glandular regions were first segmented by a transformer architecture with subsequent classification using a convolutional neural network (CNN) ensemble, which markedly improved the learning efficiency and shortened the learning time. Moreover, we prepared and published a dataset for clinical validation of the developed artificial neural network, which suggested the discovery of novel histological phenotypic alterations in adenocarcinoma sections that could have prognostic value. Therefore, AI could markedly improve the reproducibility, efficiency, and accuracy of colon cancer diagnosis, which are required for precision medicine to personalize the treatment of cancer patients.

Keywords: colon cancer; histological diagnosis; artificial intelligence; deep learning; transformer networks; dataset

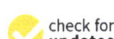

Citation: Leo, M.; Carcagnì, P.; Signore, L.; Corcione, F.; Benincasa, G.; Laukkanen, M.O.; Distante, C. Convolutional Neural Networks in the Diagnosis of Colon Adenocarcinoma. *AI* **2024**, *5*, 324–341. https://doi.org/10.3390/ai5010016

Academic Editors: Tim Hulsen and Hiroyuki Yoshida

Received: 9 November 2023
Revised: 5 January 2024
Accepted: 24 January 2024
Published: 29 January 2024

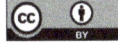

Copyright: © 2024 by the authors. Licensee MDPI, Basel, Switzerland. This article is an open access article distributed under the terms and conditions of the Creative Commons Attribution (CC BY) license (https://creativecommons.org/licenses/by/4.0/).

1. Introduction

Colorectal carcinoma (CRC) is a well-characterized heterogeneous disease induced by different tumorigenic modifications in colon cells [1]. CRC contains several stromal and epithelial tissue types representing different differentiation stages, including benign residual adenoma, that collectively support carcinogenesis and serve as diagnostic components. Malignant transformation modifies the morphology of the intestinal crypt structure in the mucosa, replacing it with irregular tissue composed of cells with an increased nucleus/cytoplasm ratio, thereby disrupting the normal glandular structure of colon tissue [2].

Malignant transformation of immortalized cells in high-grade adenomas is the earliest form of clinically relevant colorectal cancer, pT1, in which cancer cells have invaded the submucosa but not the muscular layer. At stage pT2, the tumor has invaded through muscularis propria, the muscle layer, but it has not migrated to nearby lymph nodes or distant organs. Stage pT3 cancer has grown through the muscularis propria into the subserosa, a thin layer of connective tissue covering the muscle layer, and often invades into tissues surrounding the colon. At stage pT4, the tumor has grown through all layers of the colon, invaded the visceral peritoneum, and commonly metastasized to distant organs. Metastatic colon cancer typically invades through the muscularis mucosa into the submucosa and occasionally into the proximity of blood vessels. A second distinctive histological feature indicating metastasis is a desmoplastic reaction in the tumor stroma, and the third nominator of possible metastasis is the presence of necrotic debris in the glandular lumina [3–5].

In addition to staging, colon cancer is classified based on grading, which is determined by the stage of undifferentiation of the cells, i.e., the number of abnormalities in the cellular phenotype. Colon cancer is usually divided into three grades: well-differentiated (low grade, G1), moderately differentiated (intermediate grade, G2), and poorly differentiated (high grade, G3) [6]. A well-differentiated (G1) adenocarcinoma has conserved more than 95% of the normal glandular formation, whereas in moderately differentiated colon cancer (G2), the colon has 50–95% glandular formation, and poorly differentiated (G3) has less than 50% glandular formation [6].

The current histologic diagnosis has several deficiencies, which may affect the therapy decisions, consequent recovery, and survival of patients. Artificial intelligence (AI), especially recently developed computer vision methodologies based on deep learning and digital pathology, can recognize and mark pixels in the image, distinguish the pixels based on their characteristics, and detect the differences and grade cancers [7]. The computer-based analysis of colon digital histologic images involves different tasks [7,8], such as the normalization of histologic staining, to match the staining colors with a given template to eliminate the variability of histological sample staining [9]. Other tasks include the segmentation of cells to identify cellular structures and organelles [10]; the division of tissues into the tumor, stroma, and adipose tissue [11]; the detection of the parameters indicating cancer progression, e.g., lymphocyte migration and cellular proliferation [12]; and the prediction of consequent survival by combining the information of patient's age, gender, medical status, and physical condition [13].

In the current work, we used subclasses of artificial neural networks that learn directly from data: ResidualNet, DenseNet, EfficientNet, and Squeeze-and-ExcitationNet. Neural networks are simplified artificial models of human brain physiology that can be used for the analysis of histologic sections in the diagnosis of cancer. The CNNs used in this work were combined as ensembles to improve the stability and predictivity of the final output [14]. To further improve machine learning, we introduced transformer models to adopt the mechanism of cognitive attention and classify the observed and unobserved data by predicting the latter [15]. Lastly, we introduced an optimal network model to improve network performance [16].

To train the algorithm, we used the CRC-Dataset [17], extended CRC dataset [1], and GLA dataset [18] that contain 484 visual fields, which were then further divided into subfigures. The trained algorithm was used to diagnose patients with low-grade (G1), intermediate-grade (G2), and high-grade (G3) colon adenocarcinomas. The algorithm demonstrated high accuracy in the diagnosis of colon cancer.

The innovation of this study is to propose a two-stage CNN model for glandular region classification that mimics the work of a pathologist. In this new data flow, we characterized which CNN model is most suited to extract information from glandular regions and how different models could be combined to further improve cancer staging capabilities.

The main contributions of this study are as follows:

- This is an innovative two-stage pipeline approach, as opposed to previous approaches that grade carcinoma initiating from patches containing glandular regions and other indiscriminative areas (e.g., epithelium).
- This is among the first clinical approaches of this type of pipeline. This study provides early evidence of its suitability for clinical practice and a systematic report of the capabilities of the proposed model.
- In this new data flow, we attempted to understand which CNN model is most suited to extract information from glandular regions and how different models could be

combined to further improve cancer staging capabilities. The current work represents a few attempts at applying machine learning strategies in actual clinical practice for colon cancer grading.
- This is among the first attempts to concentrate classification only on glandular regions, which shows a focus of attention similar to the diagnosis of a pathologist. This is one of the most important contributions of the self-attention mechanism learning approach.

2. Related Work

Extracting information from small datasets of biased and tagged data is challenging because of variation and similarities between or within classes that result from the continuum created by the various grade levels. Shallow classifiers and manually created features were the mainstays of early attempts to use AI in colon cancer grading [19]. Recently, deep learning-based methods have proven to be superior in the grading of colon cancer because of computational and memory constraints; CNNs are typically used for representation learning from small image patches (e.g., 224×224) recovered from digital histological images [20].

To aggregate predictions and model the reality that not all patches will be discriminative, patch-level classification results must be aggregated [21]. Based on images of tumor samples, the authors of [20] trained a deep network to forecast colorectal cancer outcomes by combining convolutional and recurrent architectures. In a novel cell graph convolutional neural network (CGC-Net), the increased accuracy of computational models was achieved by integrating contextual information with feature sharing and learning dependencies across and between scales using a long short-term memory (LSTM) unit [22].

In this model, large images are presented as a graph, where each node is represented by a nucleus within the original image, and cellular interactions are indicated as edges between these nodes based on node similarity. More recently, a proposed method for learning histological images uses a local-aware region CNN (LR-CNN) to first train the local representation and then a representation aggregation CNN (RA-CNN) to aggregate contextual data [23].

However, because there is often an insufficient amount of data available for robust knowledge generalization, a recent study [24] examined multiple CNN architectures and demonstrated that classical network models created for image classification have higher performance than those incorporating domain-specific solutions. Furthermore, it was shown that the EfficientNet-B1 and EfficientNet-B2 architectures [25] perform better than all previous state-of-the-art methods for CRC grading. Lastly, CNN has recently been suggested to effectively assist in completing knowledge extraction tasks from large histological images when an attention mechanism is applied in parallel to capture key features that aid network categorization [26].

Most of the existing approaches have been tested on benchmark datasets [27,28], but it is unclear whether there are enough data to support their implementation in current evidence-based clinical practice [29]. Advanced studies reporting clinical trials have been conducted only for colon tissue or nucleus segmentation [30].

3. Methods

The main aim of this paper was to introduce a two-stage colon adenocarcinoma grading pipeline. The first stage aimed at segmenting glandular regions, whereas the second step was devoted to grading regions retained after segmentation. The second contribution was to merge the advantages of CNN and transformer architectures. Transformers were exploited for the segmentation step to precisely determine glandular boundaries to be supplied to the following multiclass grading problem, relying on the CNN to extract local patterns of cells' configurations.

3.1. Patients

Human adenocarcinoma sections were stained with hematoxylin–eosin (Sigma-Aldrich, St. Louis, MO, USA) and prepared for microscopy and imaging (Leica DMI3000B microscope and Leica Application Suite X 1.1.0.12420 camera software, Leica, Wetzlar, Germany). The ethical permissions for the study were approved by the Monaldi Hospital ethical committee, the University of Naples Federico II ethical committee, and the Clinica Mediterranea ethical committee. Inform consent was asked from all patients.

3.2. Development of the Algorithm

In this study, a transformer-based model with an additional control mechanism in the self-attention module was preliminarily exploited to understand discriminative regions in large histological images.

The development of the deep learning diagnosis tool was performed a workstation equipped with an Intel(R) Xeon(R) E5-1650 @ 3.20 GHz CPU, one GeForce GTX 1080 Ti with 11 GB of RAM GPU, and the Ubuntu 16.04 Linux operating system. In this study, we used the most advanced architectures that have demonstrated significant performance in the ImageNet Large Scale Visual Recognition Challenge (ILSVRC) [19] and in solving vanishing gradient architectures caused by the analysis of several layers. In the selection process, we used a generalization combined with a low memory footprint during the interference in the related problems [31]: ResidualNet [32], DenseNet [33], Squeeze-and-ExcitationNet [34], and EfficientNet [35]. All networks were modified to adapt to a 3-class inference problem.

Data augmentation was applied to the original data in terms of operations of horizontal and vertical image flipping, rotation with a value of $\pm 45°$ and $\pm 90°$, and shearing between $-20°$ and $20°$. For the validation set, we used a stochastic gradient descent optimizer with a learning rate of 0.001, momentum of 0.9, and weight decay of 0.001. For the training process, we used an early stopping strategy of 22 epochs (the number of times a dataset passes through an algorithm), with a maximum of 100 training epochs.

In this work, we used a RegNet architecture, a network design space needed for architectures to function, integrating the Squeeze-and-ExcitationNet across a wide range of floating point operations (FLOPs) per second regimes, i.e., the number of multiply–add operations per processed image. For the identification of the generated models, the corresponding FLOP regime was marked on the basis of its construction; e.g., RegNetY-400MF means that the RegNet architecture built a 400 mega-FLOP model.

To extract information from both the entire image and local patches, where finer details can be found, visual fields were fed as inputs to a transformer network that combines local and global training [12]. They employ a deep local branch and a shallow global branch to gather data for their local–global training strategy. The feature maps, which were extracted from the first convolution block with three convolution layers each followed by batch normalization and ReLU activation, were fed into both branches. The encoder bottleneck was composed of two layers of multi-head attention layers, one operating along the width axis and the other along the height axis, after normalization and a 1×1 convolution layer.

Each multi-head attention block consisted of an axial attention layer. To create the output attention maps, the output from the multi-head attention blocks was concatenated, run through an additional 1×1 convolution, and then added to the residual input maps. The convolution layer, upsampling layer, and ReLU comprised the decoder block, consisting of two encoding blocks and two decoding blocks in the global branch. In the local branch, there were five encoding blocks and five decoding blocks.

In the grading of colon carcinomas, the transformer architecture aids in determining which regions of the large-scale histology images can aid in the discrimination of different grades of carcinomas by the subsequent CNN architectures, which enables higher performance using less data. The transformer was trained to extract glandular structures from the rest of the visual field content. These structures are currently considered to be one of the key biomarkers for determining tumor grade [17].

In subsequent training, the structures can produce matching binary masks that identify glandular regions on unseen visual fields. These masks can then be used to retain only the relevant portion for further processing by CNN models. EfficientNet architectures [10], which uniformly scale the width, depth, and resolution of the network using a compound coefficient, are most commonly used for CRC grading tasks.

3.3. Training of the Algorithm

For machine learning, we used three open-source datasets. Firstly, we used the CRC-Dataset [17], which comprises 139 visual fields extracted from 38 hematoxylin–eosin-stained whole-slide images with an average size of 4548 × 7520 pixels obtained at 20× magnification. These visual fields were classified into three different classes; normal tissue, low-grade cancer, and high-grade cancer, based on the histological structure of the glands. Second, the extended CRC dataset, which has been extracted from 68 hematoxylin-eosin-stained whole-slide images, consists of 300 visual fields with an average size of 5000 × 7300 pixels [1]. Third, the GLAs dataset [36] consists of 165 images derived from 16 hematoxylin–eosin-stained sections representing stage T3 or T4 colorectal adenocarcinoma. Because the histological images originate from different sources, the datasets exhibit high inter-subject variability in both stain distribution and tissue architecture. The digitization of these histological sections to whole-slide images was performed using a Zeiss MIRAX MIDI Slide Scanner with a pixel resolution of 0.465 µm. The whole-slide images were subsequently rescaled to a pixel resolution equivalent to 20× magnification. A total of 52 visual fields from both malignant and benign areas across the entire set of whole-slide images were selected to cover the tissue architectures. Manual annotation of glandular regions as normal, low grade, and high grade was used as a "ground truth" for training the transformer network (Table 1). Because of interobserver variation, G1 and G2 were combined to a low grade, and G3 was considered a high grade.

Table 1. The number of images in CRC and in extended CRC datasets used in the design of the "ground truth".

Dataset	Normal	Low Grade	High Grade	Total
CRC	71	33	35	139
Extended CRC	120	120	60	300

3.4. Diagnosis of Patients

The developed algorithm was used to diagnose images covering the whole tissue section (1824 × 1368 pixels, 20× magnification) of 11 patients with different stages of colon adenocarcinoma. From the images, we prepared a dataset consisting of 11,089 hematoxylin–eosin-stained images that were divided into 11 directories, each representing one patient (Table 2).

Table 2. Classification and the number of the images used in the testing of the algorithm.

Directory ID	Clinical Diagnosis	Number of Images
Patient 1	Intermediate	202
Patient 2	High	192
Patient 3	Low	146
Patient 4	Low	240
Patient 5	Intermediate	242
Patient 6	Intermediate	156
Patient 7	High	270
Patient 8	High	180
Patient 9	High	189
Patient 10	Intermediate	328
Patient 11	High	110

Correspondingly to datasets used for machine learning, the diagnosis aimed to classify the adenocarcinomas as well-differentiated (low grade), moderately differentiated (intermediate grade), and poorly differentiated (high grade). The selected patients represented advanced pT3 and pT4 stages of adenocarcinoma with neoplastic infiltration into neighboring tissues, excluding samples from patients 1 and 3. The sample from patient 1 was isolated from a liver metastasis, whereas patient 3 had a pathological stage pT1 adenocarcinoma with no metastasis. The dataset of image directories is available at https://dataset.isasi.cnr.it/2021/10/18/cnr-crc/ (accessed on 24 January 2024).

The main limitations of this study are as follows: (1) the number samples used for real clinical experimentation and (2) the necessity to start large training sessions when additional examples from different patients become available.

4. Results

4.1. Development of the Algorithm

Deep learning-based colon carcinoma grading is an emerging diagnostic method that can improve the overall grading accuracy in tumors with several grading levels and reduce person-related alterations in the diagnosis. To use artificial intelligence in patch-based approaches of histological diagnosis, tissue sections are generally divided into single patches, e.g., size 224 × 224 pixels, for the primary analysis, which are then combined to cover the whole section for classification of the informative content of each patch and for predictions to label the whole image. Deep CNNs have inherent inductive biases without the ability to calculate long-range dependencies, whereas transformer-based network architectures [37] developed for language tasks can be used for image segmentation analysis [38].

In this paper, a transformer-based model equipped with an additional control mechanism in the self-attention module was used to analyze discriminative regions in histological images. During the training process, the transformer gained binary masks, which marked the glandular regions used in the CNN model (Figure 1).

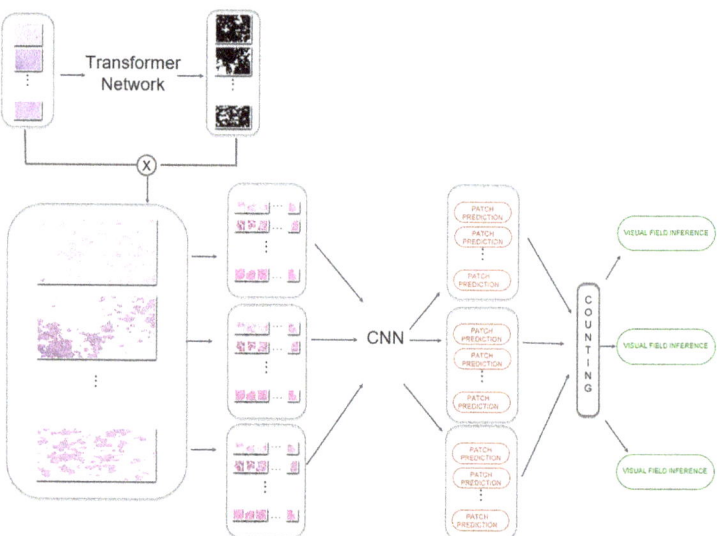

Figure 1. A schematic representation of the proposed pipeline exploiting a transformer architecture to initially segment glandular regions, which are then processed to determine the disease grade.

The algorithm comprised ResidualNet, DenseNet, Squeeze-and-ExcitationNet, and EfficientNet [32–35] architectures that minimize the vanishing problem and have high generalization capacity and a low memory footprint. ResidualNet addresses the vanishing gradient and training degradation problems by introducing a deep residual learning approach, in which each of the stacked layers of the entire network was analyzed using skip connections. Once ResidualNet had created the infrastructure, the DenseNet architecture was used to connect each layer in a feed-forward fashion, collecting information from all previous layers as input to all subsequent layers. Squeeze-and-ExcitationNet was used to improve the interdependences of the convolutional channels to emphasize the informative features and suppress irrelevant noise. EfficientNet was used to optimize and uniformly scale the network width, depth, and resolution.

Next, to reduce the inaccuracy and bias created by single neural networks, we assembled them as a Max-Voting ensemble and Argmax ensemble, which combine neural networks that have been trained with different parameters [20]. The Max-Voting ensemble combines the network predictions from each patch and assigns the most voted label to the final result. The Argmax ensemble computes the total number of patches produced by the combined networks and assigns to each patch a vector of labels equal to the number of networks involved in the ensemble.

4.2. Training of the Algorithm

The training addressed two classifications: first, the binary problem to distinguish normal tissue from tumor tissue in which intermediate and high grades have been put together and considered as a unique class against the class including only examples of lower-grade cancer, and second, the ternary three-class problem of grading tissues to normal tissue, low-grade cancer, and high-grade cancer. Because all the previous approaches have used cross-validation of the same split to avoid data leakage (i.e., the patches of each subject were in the same fold without using the subject for training or testing), we used three-fold cross-validation for a fair comparison of existing approaches.

To avoid overfitting, we split 92 visual fields for fold 1, 92 visual fields for fold 2, and 89 visual fields for fold 3. From each visual field, we extracted 224 × 224-pixel non-overlapping size-16 patches, which were labeled according to the label of the corresponding visual field or the background. These were then used as inputs to the subsequent machine-learning strategies with a batch size of 16. The patch distribution per fold and class extracted from the extended CRC dataset are shown in Table 3. We excluded approximately 11% of patches representing the crypts or lamina propria from further analysis because of their irrelevant informative content. These background batches had an average radiometric value higher than 235 in the three-color channels and appeared white in the images.

Table 3. Patch distribution per fold and class: no tumor, low grade, and high grade. Background represents the excluded patches.

	No Tumor	Low Grade	High Grade	Background
Fold 1	20911	28298	13084	8799
Fold 2	22430	29042	12412	8768
Fold 3	22879	28388	13495	6302

The metrics used for the evaluation were average accuracy, which refers to the correct classification percentage of the visual fields, and weighted accuracy, which is the sum of the accuracies in each class weighted by the number of samples in that class. For each fold j in the range $[1, k]$ ($k = 3$ in the following experiments), the average accuracy was computed as follows:

$$acc_j = \frac{\sum_{i=1}^{c} TP_i}{\sum_{i=1}^{c} N_i} \qquad (1)$$

Similarly, the weighted accuracy was computed as the average of

$$acc_{c_j} = \frac{\sum_{i=1}^{C} \frac{TP_i}{N_i}}{C} \qquad (2)$$

where C indicates the number of classes (2 or 3), N_i is the number of elements in class i, and TP_i is the number of true positives for class i. Once the patches were analyzed with

ResidualNet, DenseNet, Squeeze-and-ExcitationNet, and EfficientNet architectures, we combined them with the Max-Voting ensemble to improve the prediction result.

In the training process, we first analyzed the average and weighted classification of the binary and ternary three-class problems, and then the variance of the folding scores on the extended CRC dataset (Table 4).

Table 4. Average and weighted classification results on the extended CRC dataset using advanced deep learning architectures. D121 = DenseNet121; EffB* = EfficientNet-B*; SER50 = Squeeze-and-ExitationNet-ResidualNet50.

Model	Average (%) (Binary)	Weighted (%) (Binary)	Average (%) (3-Classes)	Weghted (%) (3-Classes)
D121	94.98 ± 2.14	95.69 ± 1.99	87.24 ± 2.94	83.33 ± 2.04
EffB0	93.63 ± 0.94	93.80 ± 1.10	85.89 ± 3.64	83.55 ± 3.54
EffB1	95.64 ± 1.23	94.79 ± 1.15	85.89 ± 3.64	83.56 ± 3.39
EffB2	96.99 ± 2.94	96.65 ± 3.11	87.58 ± 3.36	85.54 ± 2.21
EffB3	96.65 ± 2.05	96.22 ± 2.22	86.57 ± 2.68	83.31 ± 1.82
EffB4	95.31 ± 1.24	94.36 ± 1.27	84.89 ± 2.91	82.44 ± 1.84
EffB5	95.98 ± 1.62	95.66 ± 1.72	87.57 ± 3.37	84.98 ± 3.80
EffB7	95.98 ± 1.62	95.36 ± 1.68	86.90 ± 3.01	84.41 ± 2.78
ResNet-50	94.96 ± 0.79	95.45 ± 1.20	86.57 ± 2.43	80.60 ± 1.73
Res152	95.64 ± 0.94	95.82 ± 1.01	84.22 ± 4.58	79.99 ± 4.13
SER50	93.30 ± 2.47	93.14 ± 2.54	84.89 ± 3.02	81.63 ± 2.08

ResNet50 was used as a PIVOT tool to verify the implementation of the data handling process. EfficientNet-B2 and DenseNet121 models demonstrated the highest accuracy scores for both the binary and ternary three-class problems. The training time for EfficientNet-B2 was 477 min, for DenseNet121 746 min, for EfficientNet-B0 224 min, for EfficientNet-B1 452 min, for EfficientNet-B3 481 min, EfficientNet-B4 518 min, for EfficientNet-B5 677 min, for EfficientNet-B7 1188 min, for ResidualNet50 276 min, for ResidualNet152 493 min, and for Squeese-and-ExitationNet-ResidualNet50 4496 min.

Next, we trained the classification and grading on the extended CRC dataset (Table 5). When optimally designed network models, RegNetY-4.0GF and RegNetY-6.4GF, were used, the training time demonstrated improved performance of 273 min and 337 min, respectively.

Table 5. Classification and grading of the extended CRC dataset using optimally designed network models. The model refers to floating point operations per second (FLOPS).

Model	Average (%) (Binary)	Weighted (%) (Binary)	Average (%) (3-Classes)	Weighted (%) (3-Classes)
200MF	92.97 ± 3.73	93.87 ± 2.92	83.90 ± 0.76	80.54 ± 1.03
400MF	93.97 ± 2.94	93.99 ± 3.11	84.23 ± 2.62	81.92 ± 1.74
800MF	93.65 ± 4.77	94.15 ± 4.17	84.24 ± 1.63	81.10 ± 1.41
4.0GF	95.64 ± 0.94	95.37 ± 1.52	84.55 ± 2.57	81.36 ± 1.43
6.4GF	94.31 ± 2.48	94.26 ± 2.15	86.57 ± 2.12	83.58 ± 2.21
8.0GF	91.95 ± 2.15	92.19 ± 2.40	82.55 ± 1.70	80.81 ± 2.06
12GF	93.97 ± 2.93	94.28 ± 2.93	84.22 ± 2.41	82.21 ± 3.09
16GF	94.97 ± 1.62	94.24 ± 2.08	85.22 ± 3.93	83.29 ± 3.45
32GF	94.64 ± 2.49	94.55 ± 2.79	84.56 ± 2.68	81.65 ± 2.39

To train the images and binary mask of the transformer network, we used GLA dataset histological images. Subsequently, the learned configuration was used to extract a binary mask for the extended CRC dataset. The patches corresponding to the predicted glandular regions were then used as inputs to the subsequent CNN-based colon carcinoma grading (Figure 2).

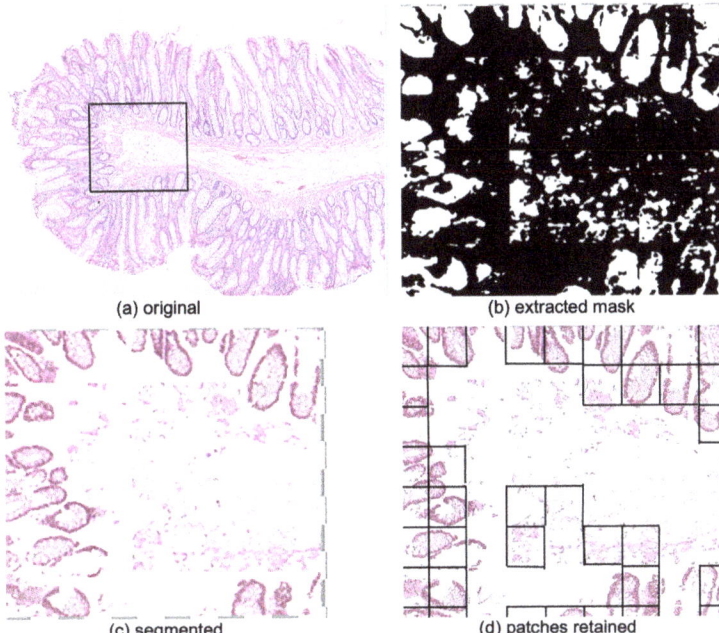

Figure 2. An example of how transformer networks accept only patches related to glandular regions for subsequent classifiers used for colon carcinoma. The transformer network focuses on the regions relevant for grading, discarding the patches that introduce noise in the learning process. (**a**) Original visual field with superimposed ROI. (**b**–**d**) ROI in a histological image of intermediate-grade (grade 1) colon carcinoma. (**b**) The extracted mask depicts the corresponding binary mask extracted by the transformer network. The glandular regions are shown in white. (**c**) The segmented image was obtained using the average and logical mask values. (**d**) Retained patches (squares) for subsequent steps and discarded areas (no squares) in the CNN analysis of carcinoma grading.

The workstation used for the experiments had an Intel(R) Xeon(R) CPU E5-1650 @ 3.20 GHz, a GeForce GTX 1080 Ti GPU, 11 GB of RAM-GPU, and SO Ubuntu 16.04 Linux. All the examined CNNs were optimized by initiating from the pre-trained ImageNet models that come with the reference implementations. Next, we employed data augmentation techniques to restrict the number of visual fields. More specifically, horizontal and vertical flipping, as well as rotation using a random value, was selected from the list (−90, −45, 45, 90), whereas random x-axis shearing ranged from −20 to 20 degrees.

Lastly, we used learning rate = 0.001, momentum = 0.9, weight decay = 0.001, batch = 16 parameters, an early stopping strategy of 10 epochs on the validation set with a maximum number of 100 training epochs, and the stochastic gradient descent (SGD) optimizer, followed by the training configuration for the transformer architecture, which included an Adam optimizer, a batch size of 4, and a learning rate of 0.001. The network was trained for 400 epochs.

To analyze and mark the background from the experimental batches, we analyzed the per fold and class of the patch distribution, which were extracted from the visual fields of the extended CRC database (Table 6). The analysis reduced approximately 46% of (1) sporadic noise regions and (2) regions delineating the border of the experimental batches in the initial study area. As a result, the workload of the CNN models was reduced from 89% to 40%. Importantly, the reduction affected only the number of patches contributing to the final labeling, whereas the number (300) of visual fields classified in the extended CRC dataset remained the same (Supplemental Table S1).

Table 6. The ensembles strategies and network architectures. (a) Label refers to the labeling of the network combinations, models refer to network models, and strategy refers to the type of ensemble used. (b) Results of detection and grading using ensembles of deep learning architectures.

(a)

Label	Models	Strategy
E1	DenseNet121 EfficientNet-B7 RegNetY16GF	Max-Voting
E2	DenseNet121 EfficientNet-B7 RegNetY16GF SE-ResNet50	Max-Voting
E3	DenseNet121 EfficientNet-B7 RegNetY16GF RegNetY6.4GF	Max-Voting
E4	DenseNet121 EfficientNet-B7 RegNetY6.4GF	Max-Voting
E5	DenseNet121 EfficientNet-B2 RegNetY16GF	Max-Voting
E6	DenseNet121 EfficientNet-B2 RegNetY16GF	Max-Voting
E7	DenseNet121 EfficientNet-B2	Argmax
E8	DenseNet121 EfficientNet-B7 RegNetY16GF SE-ResNet50	Argmax
E9	EfficientNet-B7 RegNetY16GF SE-ResNet50	Argmax
E10	DenseNet121 EfficientNet-B2 RegNetY16GF	Argmax
E11	DenseNet121 EfficientNet-B2 RegNetY16GF	Argmax
E12	EfficientNet-B1 EfficientNet-B2	Argmax

(b)

Model	Average (%) (Binary)	Weighted (%) (Binary)	Average (%) (3-classes)	Weighted (%) (3-classes)
E1	95.65 ± 1.87	95.52 ± 1.85	86.90 ± 4.16	84.15 ± 3.81
E2	95.31 ± 2.48	95.68 ± 2.41	87.24 ± 3.37	83.88 ± 3.08
E3	95.31 ± 1.68	95.40 ± 1.89	87.23 ± 4.18	84.15 ± 4.10
E4	94.98 ± 1.62	95.12 ± 1.88	87.23 ± 1.18	84.15 ± 4.10
E5	95.98 ± 2.45	95.81 ± 2.72	86.90 ± 4.39	84.15 ± 3.81
E6	95.31 ± 2.34	95.40 ± 2.37	86.23 ± 3.37	83.32 ± 2.74
E7	95.65 ± 2.05	95.82 ± 2.23	87.91 ± 3.33	84.72 ± 3.43
E8	95.98 ± 2.15	95.95 ± 2.26	87.57 ± 3.75	84.71 ± 3.44
E9	97.32 ± 1.26	97.33 ± 1.57	88.24 ± 4.26	85.53 ± 3.76
T + E5	99.00 ± 0.82	99.02 ± 0.71	89.24 ± 4.09	87.49 ± 3.61
T + E7	99.33 ± 0.94	99.44 ± 0.79	89.58 ± 3.83	87.22 ± 3.87
T + E10	98.33 ± 1.25	98.46 ± 1.10	88.24 ± 4.10	85.52 ± 3.88
T + E11	99.33 ± 0.94	99.44 ± 0.79	90.25 ± 3.74	88.06 ± 3.14
T + E12	99.00 ± 0.82	99.02 ± 0.71	89.92 ± 3.00	87.49 ± 2.36

The results obtained from patch distribution were confirmed by quantitative results (Supplemental Table S2) that showed grading data using transformer networks to discard discriminative regions.

The use of the transformer network corroborated the CNN classification for all models, most prominently for EfficientNet, and improved the performance. The EfficientNet-B1 model demonstrated the highest performance in binary classification, whereas the EfficientNet-B2 model was the most efficient in solving the ternary three-class problem. Furthermore, the use of the transformer network reduced the number of patches included in the analysis, consequently shortening the training time. The training times of T + EfficientNet-B1 and T + EfficientNet-B2 were 121 and 133 min, respectively, demonstrating a marked 70% reduction compared with to training without the transformer network. The ensembles built for testing the extended CRC dataset demonstrated robust performance in analyzing the average and weighted accuracy of the ternary three-class problem (Table 6a).

The preliminary application of the transformer network allowed the analysis chain (Figure 1) to utilize the ensemble of networks to gain increased accuracy in colon carcinoma grading in the extended CRC dataset. The ensembling markedly increased the scores compared with the performance of single network architectures (Table 6b), most prominently ensembling EfficientNet-B1, EfficientNet-B2, and RegNetY16GF E11 (Table 6a), which resulted in the highest performance in both binary and ternary classification problems.

Finally, we performed an ablation study to assess the contribution of transformer architecture. In the same pipeline, a CNN-based segmentation model was used instead of a transformer in the first stage of the pipeline. For this purpose, we used a faster region-based convolutional neural network (fRCNN) architecture for segmentation with a ResNet-101 feature extraction backbone, as previously reported in [39]. The network was trained on the GLAs dataset and validated on the extended CRC. The extracted patches were then split in folds and given as inputs to the E11 ensemble (Table 6). The binary (average and weighted) and ternary (average and weighted) classification outcomes were 97.21 ± 0.35, 96.32 ± 3.41, 88.95 ± 3.45, and 87.88 ± 2.45, respectively. The data suggested that by exploiting CNN-based segmentation, the classification accuracy decreased in cases in which the proposed transform was used for the segmentation of glandular regions.

4.3. Diagnosis of Patients

The neural networks graded cancer using images (20× magnification) divided into patches. For each visual field, the proposed pipeline created a map in which colon grading in each selected patch was highlighted by the transformer (green, blue, and red for grades 0, 1, and 2, respectively) (Figure 3).

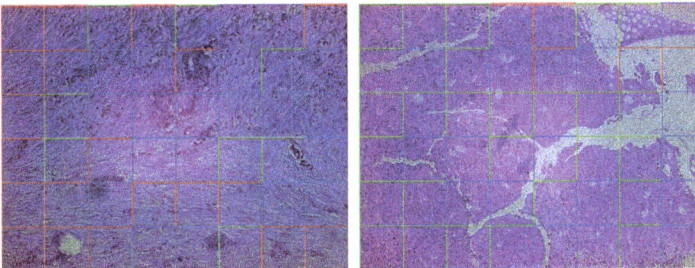

Figure 3. Visual representation of the path-based classification provided by the proposed model. These intermediate outcomes clarify how the system functions and which portions of the visual field are used for the final decision.

To quantitatively validate the deep learning procedure, the developed network was tested using our colon adenocarcinoma patient dataset. A pathologist diagnosed the patients based on their personal data (gender, age, medical history), surgical information, microsatellite analysis, oncogene (*EGFR, NRAS, KRAS, BRAS*) mutation analysis, and histological information, such as glandular structure, tumor budding, inflammatory cell staining, local invasion and infiltration, lymph node/liver metastasis, mismatch protein staining, and differentiation marker staining (Table 7).

Table 7. The histopathological diagnosis of patients.

Patient 1	Hepatic metastasis from moderately differentiated adenocarcinoma. Pathological stage: pTx, pNx, pM1a. Observations: Residues of mild hepatic steatosis, surgical margins free of neoplasia, KRas mutation at exon 2.
Patient 2	Poorly differentiated adenocarcinoma. Pathological stage: pT4a, pNx. Observations: Diffuse infiltration to omental tissue, positive immunohistochemical staining for cytokeratin 20 and CDX2 but negative for cytokeratin 7, suggesting large intestine origin for the pathology.
Patient 3	Well-differentiated adenocarcinoma. Pathological stage: pT1, pNx. Observations: No metastasis, KRas mutation at exon 2.

Table 7. Cont.

Patient 4	Poorly differentiated adenocarcinoma. Pathological stage: pT3, pN0. Observations: Neoplastic infiltration to the muscular layer and to perivisceral fat, no lymphovascular infiltration, nine tumor buds observed suggesting an intermediate risk of vascular metastasis, lymph nodes free of neoplasia, omemtum free of neoplasia, surgical margins free of neoplasia. KRas mutation at exon 2.
Patient 5	Moderately differentiated colloid adenocarcinoma and tubulovillous adenoma with low-grade epithelial dysplasia. Pathological stage: pT3 pN0. Observations: Neoplastic infiltration to the perivisceral fat, 19 lymph nodes have metastasis, no lymphovascular infiltration, appendix free of neoplasia, surgical margins free of neoplasia. KRas mutation at exon 2.
Patient 6	Moderately differentiated adenocarcinoma. Pathological stage: pT3 pN1a. Observations: Neoplastic invasion to muscle layer and to visceral fat, one lymph node has metastasis suggesting low risk of vascular metastasis.
Patient 7	Poorly differentiated adenocarcinoma. Pathological stage: pT3, pN0. Observations: Neoplastic infiltration to muscle layer and to visceral fat, one tumor bud observed suggesting low risk of vascular metastasis, lymph nodes free of metastasis, surgical margins free of neoplasia.
Patient 8	Poorly differentiated adenocarcinoma. Pathological stage: pT4b pNx. Observations: Neoplastic infiltration to ovary capsule and extrinsically to colon wall, fallopian tubes free of infiltration, atrophic endometrium, chronic cervicitis. Positive immunohistochemical staining for CDX2 and cytokeratin 20 but negative for PAX8, cytokeratin 7, WT1, and p53, suggesting large intestine origin for the pathology.
Patient 9	Poorly differentiated adenocarcinoma. Pathological stage: pT4b, pN1b. Observations: The neoplasm infiltrates the muscular layer up to the perivisceral fat. Over ten tumor buds observed suggesting a high risk of vascular metastasis, neoplastic infiltration at omentum, extrinsic neoplastic infiltration on the serosa of the bowel, no lymphovascular infiltration, three lymph nodes have metastasis, mucosa of the small intestine free of neoplasia, surgical margins free of neoplasia. KRas mutation at exon 2.
Patient 10	Moderately differentiated adenocarcinoma. Pathological stage: pT3, pN0. Observations: The neoplasm infiltrates the muscular layer up to the perivisceral fat. Over ten tumor buds observed suggesting a high risk of vascular metastasis, a moderate peritumoral infiltration, no lymphovascular infiltration, lymph nodes free of neoplasia, surgical margins free of neoplasia.
Patient 11	Poorly differentiated adenocarcinoma with hepatic metastasis. Pathological stage: pT3 pN2p pM1a Observations: Neoplastic infiltration to muscle layer and to visceral fat, chronic lithiasic cholecystitis, surgical margins free of neoplasia. KRas mutation at exon 2. Observations: Neoplastic infiltration to muscle layer and to visceral fat, chronic lithiasic cholecystitis, surgical margins free of neoplasia. KRas mutation at exon 2.

TNM staging system: T = size of the tumor (0–4), N = metastasis to lymph nodes, number of lymph nodes metastasized, M = metastasis to other organs.

Table 8 shows a comparison of the grading performed by the pathologist and the algorithm.

Patient 1's sample was isolated from a hepatic metastasis derived from colon adenocarcinoma. Histopathological grading suggested a moderately differentiated tumor, whereas AI predicted poorly differentiated grading. The discrepancy between the histopathological diagnosis and algorithm-predicted grading of the patient 1 tumor may suggest that the aggressive metastasized cancer had been able to maintain the moderately differentiated glandular status even at a distant organ but had gained other phenotypic characteristics of aggressive cancer. Patient 2 had pT4 stage adenocarcinoma that had infiltrated the omental tissue. The pathological stage and histological grading, which were poorly differentiated, supported the grading calculated by the ensemble transformer networks. Patient

3, diagnosed with pT1 stage cancer without metastasis, demonstrated well-differentiated adenocarcinoma by both the pathologist and the network. The data from patient 3 demonstrated that the algorithm created in the current study can separate well-differentiated cancers from advanced-stage tumors.

Table 8. Diagnosis of clinical grading and grading performed by the ensemble transformer network. G1 (well differentiated) corresponds to low grade; G2 (moderately differentiated) corresponds to intermediate grade; and G3 (poorly differentiated) corresponds to high grade.

Patient	Clinical Diagnosis	Algorithm Well-Differentiated	Algorithm Moderately Differentiated	Algorithm Poorly Differentiated
Patient 1	Moderately differentiated	2% (4)	19% (38)	79% (160)
Patient 2	Poorly differentiated	4% (8)	14% (27)	82% (157)
Patient 3	Well differentiated	61% (89)	21% (30)	18% (27)
Patient 4	Poorly differentiated	5% (12)	22% (53)	73% (175)
Patient 5	Moderately differentiated	0% (0)	48% (115)	52% (126)
Patient 6	Moderately differentiated	0% (0)	52% (81)	48% (75)
Patient 7	Poorly differentiated	0% (0)	21% (57)	79% (213)
Patient 8	Poorly differentiated	0% (0)	3% (5)	97% (178)
Patient 9	Poorly differentiated	0% (0)	6% (11)	94% (178)
Patient 10	Moderately differentiated	0% (0)	38% (124)	62% (204)
Patient 11	Poorly differentiated	3% (3)	74% (81)	13% (26)

The grading diagnosis of patient 4, suggesting poorly differentiated stage pT3 adenocarcinoma, was the same as that by the pathologist and algorithm. The patient had intratumoral cancer cell migration that reached the muscular layer and perivisceral fat. The histopathological diagnosis of patient 5 suggested moderately differentiated colon adenocarcinoma, whereas the transformer network-predicted analysis suggested poorly differentiated cancer. Interestingly, the predicted diagnosis was a borderline case in which 48% of the analyzed high-power fields suggested moderately differentiated and 52% suggested poorly differentiated grading. The patient had 19 metastatic lymph nodes and intratumoral infiltration of neoplastic cells into the perivisceral fat, indicating the progression of tumorigenesis toward a more aggressive phase. In addition, the diagnosis suggested a rare colloid adenocarcinoma, which results in a lower 5-year survival (71%) rate than the survival rate of a common form of adenocarcinoma (81%). Therefore, the algorithm predicted differentiation grading, which may have identified morphological features characteristic of high-risk cancer and decreased survival.

Similarly, for patient 5, the algorithm-predicted differentiation of patient 6 was divided between moderately differentiated (52%) and poorly differentiated grades (48%). The histopathological diagnosis of moderately differentiated adenocarcinoma was based on the invasion of neoplastic cells into the muscle layer and visceral fat and metastasis in one lymph node. Therefore, the algorithm-predicted diagnosis may suggest that the tumor is transitioning from a moderately to poorly differentiated grade. Patients 7, 8, and 9 were all diagnosed with poorly differentiated adenocarcinoma by both the histological analysis and transformer network calculation.

The grading of adenocarcinoma in patient 10 was diagnosed as moderately differentiated by histopathological analysis. However, the neoplastic region had more than ten tumor buds, and the transformed cells had filtrated to the muscular layer and visceral fat, thereby suggesting a high risk of vascular metastasis, although no lymphovascular infiltration was observed. The algorithm predicted grading and a poor differentiation level, thus challenging the histological diagnosis, which may suggest the presence of morphological characteristics other than changes in gland formation. According to histological grading analysis, patient 11 had a poorly differentiated adenocarcinoma that had metastasized to two nearby lymph nodes and the liver, demonstrating a highly aggressive advanced disease stage. Histological analysis detected neoplastic infiltration into the muscle layer and visceral fat. However, nearly all images, 74%, diagnosed by AI suggested a moderately differentiated grading for the tumor (Table 8).

5. Discussion

Most colon adenocarcinomas have residual adenoma regions, illustrating a high degree of intratumoral heterogeneity of CRCs that complicates histological diagnosis. The conventional diagnosis of colon cancer is based on endoscopic, radiological, and histopathological images [40]. Histological sample isolation by endoscopic biopsy or polypectomy for the initial diagnosis of colon adenocarcinoma may result in compromises caused by superficial or poorly oriented tissue collection. In addition, grading based on glandular differentiation is sensitive to artifacts caused by the subjective definition of poorly differentiated CRC, the inability to apply grading of CRC histotypes other than adenocarcinoma not otherwise specified (adenocarcinoma NOS), the dependence of grading analysis on microsatellite instability, and inter- and intra-observer variability, especially between G1 and G2 grading [41,42].

While colon cancer grading refers to the aggressiveness of the cancer, tumor staging indicates the size and spread of the tumor. Although tumor staging has its weaknesses, particularly in pT3 and pT4 cancers, it remains the most significant prognostic method in deciding the clinical treatment of a patient [6,43]. However, this is hampered by peritoneal involvement, which causes marked diagnostic variation even within the same tumor stage [44]. Based on peritoneal penetration, stage pT4 colon adenocarcinoma is divided into pT4a, penetration to the visceral peritoneum, and pT4b, penetration to adjacent organs, both of which have a high probability of developing into peritoneal metastasis. The probability of pT4 stage cancer developing peritoneal metastasis has significant variability, from 8% to 50%, because of the heterogeneity of pT4 adenocarcinomas [45]. Therefore, tumor staging is fortified by lymph node metastasis staging to support the prognostic value of the diagnosis, which is commonly subjective, poorly reducible, and often affected by cancer cell clusters in the pericolic fat disconnected from the primary tumor (tumor deposits), which can be satellite tumor nodules or lymph node metastases [45].

Tumor budding (cancer cell aggregates in the invasive part of tumor stroma) has significant prognostic value in predicting lymph node metastasis, local recurrence, and vascular invasion [45]. The cells in the aggregates have been demonstrated to have reduced epithelial marker cytokeratin staining and increased mesenchymal vimentin positivity, suggesting epithelial–mesenchymal transition with subsequently acquired increased invasive potential, cancer stem cell characteristics, and resistance to cancer drugs [46]. Vascular invasion observed at tumor buds identifies an increased risk of poor survival but has high interobserver variability, especially when the diagnosis relies only on hematoxylin–eosin staining of the histological sections without using CD31 or CD34 endothelial cell antibodies [18]. Another important prognostic marker suggesting aggressive features and poor prognosis is the perineural invasion of cancer cells around nerve fibers and nerve sheaths. It does not correlate with the pT staging classification, although it can correlate with vascular invasion and lymph node metastasis [47].

Histological diagnosis can be strengthened with molecular pathology to identify microsatellite instability, chromosomal instability, CpG island methylation phenotype, and mutations in *EGFR*, *KRAS*, *NRAS*, and *BRAF* oncogenes. Molecular pathology is important in the support of histological diagnosis, the identification of hereditary forms of colon tumorigenesis, and treatment decisions [48].

Although the current diagnosis of colon cancer relies on several different techniques, there is a need for further development of an examination methodology to create more reliable prognostic and predictive diagnoses to support the therapy options. In our study, the diagnosis of histological patient samples (Table 7) using the developed network architectures corroborates previous observations that the current grading of colon adenocarcinoma based on glandular differentiation is not adequately accurate [49]. The discrepancy between the histopathological diagnosis and algorithm-predicted grading of the tumors of patients

1, 5, 10, and 11 suggests that during the deep learning process, the network architectures omitted additional criteria from the morphology of hematoxylin–eosin-stained tissue sections that characterize aggressive cancer type. The data demonstrate that CNNs equipped with transformers can perform the diagnosis with similar accuracy to a pathologist using only images of hematoxylin–eosin-stained tissue sections. Therefore, histopathological digital image patch processing by computer vision deep learning could provide healthcare professionals with a reproducible and reliable automatic diagnosis of colon carcinoma.

Although CNNs have been used for image segmentation, they originally learned only short-range spatial dependencies [50]. The segmentation approach based on transformers, which relies on self-attention mechanisms and pre-training between neighboring image patches without any convolution operations, has been demonstrated to be more efficient than CNNs [51]. Other advantages include the ability of transformers to introduce a loss of feature resolution that is absent in CNN-based analysis and an additional control mechanism in the self-attention module that improves the image segmentation in medical applications [52]. However, transformer-based models function adequately only when they are trained on large-scale datasets or when a set of pre-learned weights is available.

The solution proposed demonstrated a higher potential for two- and three-class classification tasks than previously published solutions. The data demonstrated higher performance in achieving classification scores for the transformer networks EfficientNet-B1, EfficientNet-B2, and RegNetY16GF. The accuracy scores showed a significant increase of 2% for the average two classes, 2.08% for the weighted two classes, 3.58% for the average three classes, and 3.89% for the weighted three classes (Table 9).

Table 9. Comparisons of current ensemble CNN to previous literature.

Model	Average (%) (Binary)	Weight (%) (Binary)	Average (%) (3-Classes)	Weight (%) (3-Classes)
Proposed Solutions				
EffB2	96.99 ± 2.94	96.65 ± 3.11	87.58 ± 3.36	85.54 ± 2.21
4.0GF	95.64 ± 0.94	95.37 ± 1.52	84.55 ± 2.57	81.36 ± 1.43
6.4GF	94.31 ± 2.48	94.26 ± 2.15	86.57 ± 2.12	83.58 ± 2.21
T + EffB1	99.67 ± 0.47	99.72 ± 0.39	89.58 ± 4.17	87.50 ± 3.54
T + EffB2	98.66 ± 0.95	98.74 ± 0.91	89.92 ± 2.50	87.22 ± 2.08
T + E11	99.33 ± 0.94	99.44 ± 0.79	90.25 ± 3.74	88.06 ± 3.14
Previous Work				
ResNet50 [24]	95.67 ± 2.05	95.69 ± 1.53	86.33 ± 0.94	80.56 ± 1.04
LR+LA-CNN [24]	97.67 ± 0.94	97.64 ± 0.79	86.67 ± 1.70	84.17 ± 2.36
CNN-LSTM [26]	95.33 ± 2.87	94.17 ± 3.58	82.33 ± 2.62	83.89 ± 2.08
CNN-SVM [20]	96.00 ± 0.82	96.39 ± 1.37	82.00 ± 1.63	76.67 ± 2.97
CNN-LR [20]	96.33 ± 1.70	96.39 ± 1.37	86.67 ± 1.25	82.50 ± 0.68

In conclusion, in this study, we developed a novel AI-based colon cancer diagnostic method. For this purpose, we used manually and automatically designed convolutional architectures in classification tasks in the deep learning of colon adenocarcinoma grading from histological images. Transformer architectures further introduced an attention mechanism to highlight the most discriminative areas. Finally, we tested the developed ensembling of networks using patient material. The data demonstrated a substantial improvement in the learning time and quality of the final diagnosis. The introduced machine learning strategies could provide healthcare professionals with a computational tool to objectively evaluate carcinoma, thereby avoiding a bias introduced by different circumstances.

The current data create a foundation for improved cancer diagnosis. Future research directions will address a larger recruitment of patients to allow for a better assessment of the proposed methodology. New end-to-end strategies will be studied, including few-shot and incremental learning strategies, to increase the amount of extracted knowledge in the process to avoid the need to restart training. Furthermore, knowledge and model distillation processes will be used to improve the transfer of knowledge from a large model to a smaller one, which could also be implemented in mobile and low-power devices, thereby enabling remote diagnoses for medical professionals. For the future improvement of visual convolutional networks, we will evaluate the proposed model in the diagnosis and prognosis of other pathologies, such as neuronal degeneration.

Supplementary Materials: The following supporting information can be downloaded at: https://www.mdpi.com/article/10.3390/ai5010016/s1, Supplemental Table S1. Patch distribution per fold and class in the transformer network. Supplemental Table S2. Results for the extended CRC dataset while integrating the transformer networks.

Author Contributions: Methodology, M.L., P.C., L.S., G.B., M.O.L. and C.D.; Software, M.L., P.C., L.S. and C.D.; Validation, M.L., P.C., L.S., F.C., G.B., M.O.L. and C.D.; Formal analysis, P.C., L.S., F.C., G.B. and C.D.; Investigation, M.L., G.B. and M.O.L.; Resources, F.C. and G.B.; Writing—original draft, M.L., P.C., M.O.L. and C.D.; Writing—review and editing, M.O.L.; Supervision, L.S. and C.D.; Project administration, F.C. and C.D.; Funding acquisition, M.O.L. All authors have read and agreed to the published version of the manuscript.

Funding: This research and APC was funded by Campania Region POR CUP B63D18000210007 and Future Artificial Intelligence Research—FAIR CUP B53C220036 30006 grant number PE0000013.

Institutional Review Board Statement: The study with patient samples was conducted in accordance with the Declaration of Helsinki and approved by the Institutional Review Board of the Clinica Mediterranea ethical committee, Naples, Italy, Monaldi Hospital ethical committee (Deliberazione del Direttore Generale n:o 1239), Naples, Italy, and by the University of Naples Federico II ethical committee (protocol number 394/19), Naples, Italy.

Informed Consent Statement: Informed consent was obtained from all subjects involved in the study.

Data Availability Statement: Data is contained within the article and Supplementary Material.

Conflicts of Interest: The authors declare no conflict of interest.

References

1. Testa, U.; Pelosi, E.; Castelli, G. Colorectal cancer: Genetic abnormalities, tumor progression, tumor heterogeneity, clonal evolution and tumor-initiating cells. *Med. Sci.* **2018**, *6*, 31. [CrossRef]
2. Hermanek, P. Colorectal carcinoma: Histopathological diagnosis and staging. *Bailliere's Clin. Gastroenterol.* **1989**, *3*, 511–529. [CrossRef]
3. Lanza, G.; Messerini, L.; Gafa, R.; Risio, M.; Gruppo Italiano Patologi Apparato Digerente (GIPAD); Societa Italiana di Anatomia Patologica e Citopatologia Diagnostica/International Academy of Pathology, Italian Division. Colorectal tumors: The histology report. *Dig. Liver Dis.* **2011**, *43* (Suppl. S4), S344–S355. [CrossRef]
4. Tong, Y.; Liu, D.; Zhang, J. Connection and distinction of tumor regression grading systems of gastrointestinal cancer. *Pathol. Res. Pract.* **2020**, *216*, 153073. [CrossRef]
5. Cammarota, F.; Laukkanen, M.O. Mesenchymal Stem/Stromal Cells in Stromal Evolution and Cancer Progression. *Stem Cells Int.* **2016**, *2016*, 4824573. [CrossRef]
6. Fleming, M.; Ravula, S.; Tatishchev, S.F.; Wang, H.L. Colorectal carcinoma: Pathologic aspects. *J. Gastrointest. Oncol.* **2012**, *3*, 153–173. [CrossRef] [PubMed]
7. Deng, S.; Zhang, X.; Yan, W.; Chang, E.I.; Fan, Y.; Lai, M.; Xu, Y. Deep learning in digital pathology image analysis: A survey. *Front. Med.* **2020**, *14*, 470–487. [CrossRef] [PubMed]
8. Salvi, M.; Acharya, U.R.; Molinari, F.; Meiburger, K.M. The impact of pre- and post-image processing techniques on deep learning frameworks: A comprehensive review for digital pathology image analysis. *Comput. Biol. Med.* **2021**, *128*, 104129. [CrossRef] [PubMed]
9. Ciompi, F.; Geessink, O.; Bejnordi, B.E.; de Souza, G.S.; Baidoshvili, A.; Litjens, G.; van Ginneken, B.; Nagtegaal, I.; van der Laak, J. The Importance of Stain Normalization in Colorectal Tissue Classification with Convolutional Networks. In Proceedings of the 2017 IEEE 14th International Symposium on Biomedical Imaging (ISBI 2017), Melbourne, Australia, 18–21 April 2017; pp. 160–163. [CrossRef]
10. Wang, E.K.; Zhang, X.; Pan, L.; Cheng, C.; Dimitrakopoulou-Strauss, A.; Li, Y.; Zhe, N. Multi-Path Dilated Residual Network for Nuclei Segmentation and Detection. *Cells* **2019**, *8*, 499. [CrossRef] [PubMed]
11. Tsai, M.J.; Tao, Y.H. Deep Learning Techniques for the Classification of Colorectal Cancer Tissue. *Electronics* **2021**, *10*, 662. [CrossRef]
12. Swiderska-Chadaj, Z.; Pinckaers, H.; van Rijthoven, M.; Balkenhol, M.; Melnikova, M.; Geessink, O.; Manson, Q.; Sherman, M.; Polonia, A.; Parry, J.; et al. Learning to detect lymphocytes in immunohistochemistry with deep learning. *Med. Image Anal.* **2019**, *58*, 101547. [CrossRef] [PubMed]

13. Gupta, P.; Chiang, S.F.; Sahoo, P.K.; Mohapatra, S.K.; You, J.F.; Onthoni, D.D.; Hung, H.Y.; Chiang, J.M.; Huang, Y.; Tsai, W.S. Prediction of Colon Cancer Stages and Survival Period with Machine Learning Approach. *Cancers* **2019**, *11*, 2007. [CrossRef] [PubMed]
14. Zhang, L.; Suganthan, P.N. Visual Tracking With Convolutional Random Vector Functional Link Network. *IEEE Trans. Cybern.* **2017**, *47*, 3243–3253. [CrossRef] [PubMed]
15. Khan, S.; Naseer, M.; Hayat, M.; Zamir, S.W.; Khan, F.S.; Shah, M. Transformers in Vision: A Survey. *ACM Comput. Surv.* **2022**, *54*, 1–41. [CrossRef]
16. Radosavovic, I.; Johnson, J.; Xie, S.N.; Lo, W.Y.; Dollár, P. On Network Design Spaces for Visual Recognition. In Proceedings of the 2019 IEEE/CVF International Conference on Computer Vision (ICCV), Seoul, Republic of Korea, 27 October 27–2 November 2019; pp. 1882–1890. [CrossRef]
17. Awan, R.; Sirinukunwattana, K.; Epstein, D.; Jefferyes, S.; Qidwai, U.; Aftab, Z.; Mujeeb, I.; Snead, D.; Rajpoot, N. Glandular Morphometrics for Objective Grading of Colorectal Adenocarcinoma Histology Images. *Sci. Rep.* **2017**, *7*, 16852. [CrossRef] [PubMed]
18. Liang, P.; Nakada, I.; Hong, J.W.; Tabuchi, T.; Motohashi, G.; Takemura, A.; Nakachi, T.; Kasuga, T.; Tabuchi, T. Prognostic significance of immunohistochemically detected blood and lymphatic vessel invasion in colorectal carcinoma: Its impact on prognosis. *Ann. Surg. Oncol.* **2007**, *14*, 470–477. [CrossRef]
19. Altunbay, D.; Cigir, C.; Sokmensuer, C.; Gunduz-Demir, C. Color Graphs for Automated Cancer Diagnosis and Grading. *IEEE Trans. Biomed. Eng.* **2010**, *57*, 665–674. [CrossRef]
20. Hou, L.; Samaras, D.; Kurc, T.M.; Gao, Y.; Davis, J.E.; Saltz, J.H. Patch-based Convolutional Neural Network for Whole Slide Tissue Image Classification. In Proceedings of the 2016 IEEE Conference on Computer Vision and Pattern Recognition (CVPR), Las Vegas, NV, USA, 27 June–30 June 2016; pp. 2424–2433. [CrossRef]
21. Pei, Y.; Mu, L.; Fu, Y.; He, K.; Li, H.; Gu, S.X.; Liu, X.M.; Li, M.Y.; Zhang, H.M.; Li, X.Y. Colorectal Tumor Segmentation of CT Scans Based on a Convolutional Neural Network With an Attention Mechanism. *IEEE Access* **2020**, *8*, 64131–64138. [CrossRef]
22. Zhou, Y.N.; Graham, S.; Koohbanani, N.A.; Shaban, M.; Heng, P.A.; Rajpoot, N. CGC-Net: Cell Graph Convolutional Network for Grading of Colorectal Cancer Histology Images. In Proceedings of the IEEE/CVF International Conference on Computer Vision Workshops, Seoul, Republic of Korea, 27 October–28 October 2019; pp. 388–398. [CrossRef]
23. Zhan, Z.W.; Liao, G.L.; Ren, X.; Xiong, G.S.; Zhou, W.L.; Jiang, W.C.; Xiao, H. RA-CNN: A Semantic-Enhanced Method in a Multi-Semantic Environment. *Int. J. Softw. Sci. Comput. Intell.* **2022**, *14*, 1–14. [CrossRef]
24. Shaban, M.; Awan, R.; Fraz, M.M.; Azam, A.; Tsang, Y.W.; Snead, D.; Rajpoot, N.M. Context-Aware Convolutional Neural Network for Grading of Colorectal Cancer Histology Images. *IEEE Trans. Med. Imaging* **2020**, *39*, 2395–2405. [CrossRef]
25. Vuong, T.L.T.; Lee, D.; Kwak, J.T.; Kim, K. Multi-task Deep Learning for Colon Cancer Grading. In Proceedings of the 2020 International Conference on Electronics, Information, and Communication (ICEIC), Barcelona, Spain, 19–22 January 2020. [CrossRef]
26. Sirinukunwattana, K.; Alham, N.K.; Verrill, C.; Rittscher, J. Improving Whole Slide Segmentation Through Visual Context—A Systematic Study. In *Medical Image Computing and Computer Assisted Intervention—MICCAI 2018, Pt II*; Springer: Cham, Switzerland, 2018; Volume 11071, pp. 192–200. [CrossRef]
27. Tummala, S.; Kadry, S.; Nadeem, A.; Rauf, H.T.; Gul, N. An Explainable Classification Method Based on Complex Scaling in Histopathology Images for Lung and Colon Cancer. *Diagnostics* **2023**, *13*, 1594. [CrossRef]
28. Bousis, D.; Verras, G.I.; Bouchagier, K.; Antzoulas, A.; Panagiotopoulos, I.; Katinioti, A.; Kehagias, D.; Kaplanis, C.; Kotis, K.; Anagnostopoulos, C.N.; et al. The role of deep learning in diagnosing colorectal cancer. *Prz. Gastroenterol.* **2023**, *18*, 266–273. [CrossRef]
29. Bokhorst, J.M.; Nagtegaal, I.D.; Fraggetta, F.; Vatrano, S.; Mesker, W.; Vieth, M.; van der Laak, J.; Ciompi, F. Deep learning for multi-class semantic segmentation enables colorectal cancer detection and classification in digital pathology images. *Sci. Rep.* **2023**, *13*, 8398. [CrossRef]
30. Reis, H.C.; Turk, V. Transfer Learning Approach and Nucleus Segmentation with MedCLNet Colon Cancer Database. *J. Digit. Imaging* **2023**, *36*, 306–325. [CrossRef] [PubMed]
31. Gertych, A.; Swiderska-Chadaj, Z.; Ma, Z.; Ing, N.; Markiewicz, T.; Cierniak, S.; Salemi, H.; Guzman, S.; Walts, A.E.; Knudsen, B.S. Convolutional neural networks can accurately distinguish four histologic growth patterns of lung adenocarcinoma in digital slides. *Sci. Rep.* **2019**, *9*, 1483. [CrossRef]
32. Chen, W.F.; Ou, H.Y.; Lin, H.Y.; Wei, C.P.; Liao, C.C.; Cheng, Y.F.; Pan, C.T. Development of Novel Residual-Dense-Attention (RDA) U-Net Network Architecture for Hepatocellular Carcinoma Segmentation. *Diagnostics* **2022**, *12*, 1916. [CrossRef]
33. Zhang, Z.; Liang, X.; Dong, X.; Xie, Y.; Cao, G. A Sparse-View CT Reconstruction Method Based on Combination of DenseNet and Deconvolution. *IEEE Trans. Med. Imaging* **2018**, *37*, 1407–1417. [CrossRef]
34. Eun, D.I.; Woo, I.; Park, B.; Kim, N.; Lee, A.S.; Seo, J.B. CT kernel conversions using convolutional neural net for super-resolution with simplified squeeze-and-excitation blocks and progressive learning among smooth and sharp kernels. *Comput. Methods Programs Biomed.* **2020**, *196*, 105615. [CrossRef] [PubMed]
35. Marques, G.; Ferreras, A.; de la Torre-Diez, I. An ensemble-based approach for automated medical diagnosis of malaria using EfficientNet. *Multimed. Tools Appl.* **2022**, *81*, 28061–28078. [CrossRef] [PubMed]

36. Sirinukunwattana, K.; Pluim, J.P.W.; Chen, H.; Qi, X.; Heng, P.A.; Guo, Y.B.; Wang, L.Y.; Matuszewski, B.J.; Bruni, E.; Sanchez, U.; et al. Gland segmentation in colon histology images: The glas challenge contest. *Med. Image Anal.* **2017**, *35*, 489–502. [CrossRef]
37. Shakeel, P.M.; Burhanuddin, M.A.; Desa, M.I. Automatic lung cancer detection from CT image using improved deep neural network and ensemble classifier. *Neural Comput. Appl.* **2022**, *34*, 9579–9592. [CrossRef]
38. Carcagnì, P.; Leo, M.; Cuna, A.; Mazzeo, P.L.; Spagnolo, P.; Celeste, G.; Distante, C. Classification of Skin Lesions by Combining Multilevel Learnings in a DenseNet Architecture. *Lect. Notes Comput. Sci.* **2019**, *11751*, 335–344. [CrossRef]
39. Montagnon, E.; Cerny, M.; Cadrin-Chenevert, A.; Hamilton, V.; Derennes, T.; Ilinca, A.; Vandenbroucke-Menu, F.; Turcotte, S.; Kadoury, S.; Tang, A. Deep learning workflow in radiology: A primer. *Insights Imaging* **2020**, *11*, 22. [CrossRef] [PubMed]
40. Ueno, H.; Kajiwara, Y.; Shimazaki, H.; Shinto, E.; Hashiguchi, Y.; Nakanishi, K.; Maekawa, K.; Katsurada, Y.; Nakamura, T.; Mochizuki, H.; et al. New criteria for histologic grading of colorectal cancer. *Am. J. Surg. Pathol.* **2012**, *36*, 193–201. [CrossRef] [PubMed]
41. Compton, C.C. Optimal pathologic staging: Defining stage II disease. *Clin. Cancer Res.* **2007**, *13*, 6862s–6870s. [CrossRef] [PubMed]
42. Chen, K.; Collins, G.; Wang, H.; Toh, J.W.T. Pathological Features and Prognostication in Colorectal Cancer. *Curr. Oncol.* **2021**, *28*, 5356–5383. [CrossRef]
43. Puppa, G.; Sonzogni, A.; Colombari, R.; Pelosi, G. TNM staging system of colorectal carcinoma: A critical appraisal of challenging issues. *Arch. Pathol. Lab. Med.* **2010**, *134*, 837–852. [CrossRef] [PubMed]
44. Klaver, C.E.L.; van Huijgevoort, N.C.M.; de Buck van Overstraeten, A.; Wolthuis, A.M.; Tanis, P.J.; van der Bilt, J.D.W.; Sagaert, X.; D'Hoore, A. Locally Advanced Colorectal Cancer: True Peritoneal Tumor Penetration is Associated with Peritoneal Metastases. *Ann. Surg. Oncol.* **2018**, *25*, 212–220. [CrossRef]
45. Maffeis, V.; Nicole, L.; Cappellesso, R. RAS, Cellular Plasticity, and Tumor Budding in Colorectal Cancer. *Front. Oncol.* **2019**, *9*, 1255. [CrossRef]
46. Maguire, A.; Sheahan, K. Controversies in the pathological assessment of colorectal cancer. *World J. Gastroenterol.* **2014**, *20*, 9850–9861. [CrossRef]
47. Harada, S.; Morlote, D. Molecular Pathology of Colorectal Cancer. *Adv. Anat. Pathol.* **2020**, *27*, 20–26. [CrossRef] [PubMed]
48. Nguyen, H.T.; Duong, H.Q. The molecular characteristics of colorectal cancer: Implications for diagnosis and therapy. *Oncol. Lett.* **2018**, *16*, 9–18. [CrossRef]
49. Vaswani, A.; Shazeer, N.; Parmar, N.; Uszkoreit, J.; Jones, L.; Gomez, A.N.; Kaiser, L.; Polosukhin, I. Attention Is All You Need. In Proceedings of the 31st Annual Conference on Neural Information Processing Systems (NIPS 2017), Long Beach, CA, USA, 4 December 2017; Volume 30. [CrossRef]
50. Awan, R.; Al-Maadeed, S.; Al-Saady, R.; Bouridane, A. Glandular structure-guided classification of microscopic colorectal images using deep learning. *Comput. Electr. Eng.* **2020**, *85*, 106450. [CrossRef]
51. Shi, Q.S.; Katuwal, R.; Suganthan, P.N.; Tanveer, M. Random vector functional link neural network based ensemble deep learning. *Pattern Recogn.* **2021**, *117*, 107978. [CrossRef]
52. Ho, C.; Zhao, Z.; Chen, X.F.; Sauer, J.; Saraf, S.A.; Jialdasani, R.; Taghipour, K.; Sathe, A.; Khor, L.Y.; Lim, K.H.; et al. A promising deep learning-assistive algorithm for histopathological screening of colorectal cancer. *Sci. Rep.* **2022**, *12*, 2222. [CrossRef] [PubMed]

Disclaimer/Publisher's Note: The statements, opinions and data contained in all publications are solely those of the individual author(s) and contributor(s) and not of MDPI and/or the editor(s). MDPI and/or the editor(s) disclaim responsibility for any injury to people or property resulting from any ideas, methods, instructions or products referred to in the content.

Article

New Convolutional Neural Network and Graph Convolutional Network-Based Architecture for AI Applications in Alzheimer's Disease and Dementia-Stage Classification

Md Easin Hasan [1,*] and Amy Wagler [2]

1 Department of Mathematical Sciences, The University of Texas at El Paso, 500 W. University Ave., El Paso, TX 79968, USA
2 Department of Public Health, The University of Texas at El Paso, 500 W. University Ave., El Paso, TX 79968, USA; awagler2@utep.edu
* Correspondence: mhasan8@miners.utep.edu; Tel.: +1-(915)-201-8521

Abstract: Neuroimaging experts in biotech industries can benefit from using cutting-edge artificial intelligence techniques for Alzheimer's disease (AD)- and dementia-stage prediction, even though it is difficult to anticipate the precise stage of dementia and AD. Therefore, we propose a cutting-edge, computer-assisted method based on an advanced deep learning algorithm to differentiate between people with varying degrees of dementia, including healthy, very mild dementia, mild dementia, and moderate dementia classes. In this paper, four separate models were developed for classifying different dementia stages: convolutional neural networks (CNNs) built from scratch, pre-trained VGG16 with additional convolutional layers, graph convolutional networks (GCNs), and CNN-GCN models. The CNNs were implemented, and then the flattened layer output was fed to the GCN classifier, resulting in the proposed CNN-GCN architecture. A total of 6400 whole-brain magnetic resonance imaging scans were obtained from the Alzheimer's Disease Neuroimaging Initiative database to train and evaluate the proposed methods. We applied the 5-fold cross-validation (CV) technique for all the models. We presented the results from the best fold out of the five folds in assessing the performance of the models developed in this study. Hence, for the best fold of the 5-fold CV, the above-mentioned models achieved an overall accuracy of 43.83%, 71.17%, 99.06%, and 100%, respectively. The CNN-GCN model, in particular, demonstrates excellent performance in classifying different stages of dementia. Understanding the stages of dementia can assist biotech industry researchers in uncovering molecular markers and pathways connected with each stage.

Keywords: Alzheimer's disease; image classification; transfer learning; convolutional neural networks; graph convolutional networks

1. Introduction

Dementia is a complex and debilitating condition that is not a single disease but a common term encompassing a range of specified medical conditions, characterized by abnormal brain changes. The cognitive abilities of a person experiencing dementia decline significantly, which is substantial enough to impair a person's daily life and ability to perform self-sustaining tasks. In addition to affecting cognitive abilities, dementia can significantly impact a person's behavior, feelings, and relationships. It can cause changes in a person's personality and emotional state and impact their ability to form and maintain social connections. The loss of cognitive functioning that is associated with dementia can manifest in a variety of ways, including difficulties with memory, language, problem-solving, and attention. As the condition progresses, these difficulties can become more pronounced and interfere with a person's ability to perform daily activities. Some people with dementia may also experience changes in their behavior, such as increased agitation or aggression, and struggle to control their emotions [1].

Dementia refers to numerous cognitive problems that all involve a loss in cognitive function. The levels of dementia vary and can include a healthy brain (no dementia), mild dementia, and severe dementia [2]. Because dementia is a progressive condition and its severity can range from very mild to severe, it is imperative to have models that can classify disease status and automate the process for classification for both treatment purposes and drug development. Early on in the condition's development, a person may only experience minor difficulties with cognitive functioning and may still be able to carry out many of their daily activities independently. However, as the condition progresses, these difficulties become more pronounced, and a person may require more assistance with tasks such as dressing, bathing, and feeding themselves. When dementia has advanced to later stages, people may become completely dependent on others for their basic needs and require round-the-clock care to maintain their health and well-being. Clinical medical professionals are not easily able to identify disease progression based on behavior and other outward manifestations of the disease. Hence, a tool for disease classification can advance early diagnoses and assist in drug development.

One pathway for developing models for assisting in dementia classification is to use image analysis of brain cells. This is a reasonable approach since dementia manifests due to harm caused to brain cells, leading to disruption in communication between them. As a result, this disruption can negatively impact an individual's behavior, emotions, and thought processes. Dementia is a prevalent condition that primarily affects older individuals, with a higher incidence rate among those over the age of 85 [3]. However, it is not considered a natural aspect of the aging process since many people can live well into their 90s without experiencing dementia symptoms. Alzheimer's disease (AD) is the most frequent type of dementia, though there are many other types [4].

A medical disorder, mild cognitive impairment (MCI) manifests as mild impairments in cognitive functioning such as memory or thinking. Although the symptoms are more severe than those typically expected for a healthy individual of the same age, they are not severe enough to impede daily life and, thus, are not classified as dementia. MCI is estimated to affect between 5% and 20% of individuals over the age of 65 [5]. While it is not a form of dementia, it may increase the likelihood of developing dementia in the future. MCI is a term for a condition that affects the brain. It does not have as severe symptoms as AD or dementia, and individuals with MCI can still perform their everyday tasks. It is considered to be in between regular age-related changes and dementia.

Symptoms of MCI include forgetfulness, trouble remembering appointments or events, difficulty finding words, and, in some cases, problems with movement and sense of smell. These symptoms do not significantly interfere with daily life but may indicate an increased risk of developing dementia. MCI does not have a singular cause, and the likelihood of developing it rises with age. Certain conditions like depression, diabetes, and stroke may also raise the risk of developing MCI [6].

A neurological disorder, AD progressively impairs memory and cognitive abilities, ultimately hindering an individual's ability to perform even basic tasks. Most people with Alzheimer's are diagnosed with the late-onset type, which typically manifests in their mid-60s. Beginning-onset AD, which is much less common, occurs between the ages of 30 and the mid-60s. Among older adults, the most common kind of dementia is caused by AD. Dr. Alois Alzheimer, for whom the illness is named, discovered changes in the brain tissue of a patient who died in 1906 from an uncommon mental ailment. She exhibited symptoms such as language problems, memory loss, and unpredictable behavior. After she passed away, Dr. Alzheimer investigated her brain and discovered numerous unusual clumps, now known as amyloid plaques, and tangled bundles of fibers known as tau tangles, which are still considered among the main features of AD [7].

Some of the main signs of AD that are still known today are the buildup of amyloid plaque and neurofibrillary tangles in the brain. Along with this, the disease also involves a decrease in the connections between neurons, which are responsible for sending signals between different parts of the brain and between the brain and other parts of the body.

Additionally, it is believed that various other intricate changes in the brain also contribute to the development and progression of Alzheimer's. Damage to certain kinds of brain cells in particular regions of the brain is linked to AD. Abnormally high levels of certain proteins inside and outside brain cells hinder the health of brain cells and disrupt communication between them. Memory loss is one of the early signs of AD because the hippocampus, which is responsible for learning and memory, is frequently the first area of the brain to experience damage. In the United States, AD is presently the seventh primary cause of death and the leading cause of dementia in elderly people [7].

Convolutional filters identify the image characteristics of a complex AD image. These characteristics are the edges, corners, or textures of an image. Each filter detects a feature and learns its values during training. CNNs detect numerous features concurrently using multiple convolutional filters. Each filter focuses on a unique element, helping the network learn hierarchical features from basic edges to complex patterns. Adding pooling layers after convolutional layers reduces the size of activation maps in space while keeping important data. After numerous layers, convolutional filters might identify attributes of the images for the classification of dementia stages [8]. Since convolution and pooling layers can learn the feature maps accurately, we will use a CNN for feature selection from the different types of dementia magnetic resonance imaging (MRI) scans.

The initial symptoms of AD differ among individuals. Scientists are investigating biomarkers, such as biological indicators of disease found in brain scans, cerebrospinal fluid, and blood, to identify changes in the brain at an earlier stage in those who suffer from MCI and those without cognitive impairment who may be at increased risk for AD. This study contributes to providing a mechanism for detecting changes in the brain consistent with dementia as a diagnostic and clinical tool. With this objective in mind, we developed CNNs, pre-trained VGG16 with additional convolutional layers, GCNs, and a fusion network of CNNs with GCNs for classifying different stages of dementia and AD. Knowing the stages of dementia helps healthcare professionals deliver the best treatments and medicines, since each stage of the disease has unique symptoms and patterns of progression. Hence, this paper introduces a CNN-GCN technique, which is a deep learning methodology, to predict various stages of dementia. The method combines a CNN for feature mapping and GCN layers for the final classification tasks. The deep learning approach we present may effectively integrate resilient feature selection and achieve accurate classification of various stages of dementia. The performance of the model is evaluated using a variety of criteria, including accuracy, precision, recall, and F1 score, on the test set when training is complete. With these measures, we can determine how well the CNN- and GCN-based methods can classify the distinct stages of dementia. We hope that by bringing CNN-GCN to the problem of dementia-stage classification, we will help improve the medical community's ability to diagnose the condition early and help practitioners provide better care for those who suffer from it.

2. Literature Review

Lim et al. [9] presented a prediction model based on deep learning to predict the progressive MCI to AD using structural MRI scans. The methodology of the paper involved training a 3D CNN model on MRI scans of patients with MCI, which aimed to predict whether a patient will progress to AD within a certain period. The authors evaluated the proposed model on a dataset of 352 patients with MCI and compared its performance with several baseline models. The results showed that the proposed deep learning model achieved a high accuracy of 89.5% in predicting the conversion from MCI to AD, outperforming several baseline models. However, one of the main drawbacks of the paper is the limited sample size of the dataset used for evaluation. Additionally, the study was conducted retrospectively, and the model was not validated on an external dataset, which could limit the generalizability of the results. Therefore, further studies with larger and more diverse datasets are needed to validate the effectiveness of their proposed model.

A deep-learning-based model was proposed by Basaia et al. for the automated classification of AD and MCI from a single MRI dataset [10]. The methodology of the paper involved training a deep neural network model on a dataset of MRI scans from patients with AD, MCI, and healthy controls. However, one of the main drawbacks of the paper is that the dataset used for evaluation was relatively small and homogeneous, which could limit the generalizability of the results to other populations. Additionally, the authors did not explore the interpretability of the model, which could be an important consideration for clinical applications. Therefore, further studies are needed to validate the effectiveness and interpretability of a deep learning model on larger and more diverse datasets.

Jiang et al. [11] presented a deep-learning-based approach for the diagnosis of MCI using structural MRI images. The methodology of the paper involved training a CNN model on a dataset of MRI scans from patients with MCI and healthy controls. The authors evaluated the proposed model on a separate dataset and compared its performance with several state-of-the-art methods for MCI diagnosis. Overall, 120 participants were tested using the publicly accessible Alzheimer's Disease Neuroimaging Initiative (ADNI) dataset. Using a relatively small dataset for model training and validation, they classified MCI versus healthy controls with 89.4% accuracy. Hence, there is a possibility to obtain higher accuracy by utilizing a comparatively larger dataset on an advanced graph-based deep learning model.

Aderghal et al. [12] presented a deep-learning-based approach for the categorization of different stages of AD using different MRI modalities. The methodology of the paper involved using transfer learning and fine-tuning a pre-trained CNN model on a dataset of MRI scans from patients with AD at different stages. The authors evaluated the proposed model on a dataset and compared its performance with several state-of-the-art deep learning methods for AD stage categorization.

In a related study, Basheera et al. [13] proposed a deep-learning-based approach for the classification of AD using a hybrid enhanced independent component analysis (ICA) on the segmented gray matter of MRI. The methodology of the paper involved using a CNN model trained on a dataset of MRI scans from patients with AD and healthy controls. The authors preprocessed the MRI images using a hybrid enhanced ICA method to segment the gray matter regions of interest.

Acharya et al. proposed a system that uses automated techniques to detect AD through brain MRI images [14]. The study emphasized the importance of the early detection of AD to improve treatment and patient care. Features were extracted from test images, and the dominant features were identified using the Student's t-test (ST). A KNN classifier was used to classify the test images based on their features. The ST + KNN technique provided better classification performance measures and outperformed the SVM (polynomial), RF, and Adaboost classifier methods. Hence, feature extraction plays a vital role in obtaining higher accuracy for classifying AD stages. So, we applied several feature selection techniques to our dataset before applying the proposed models.

Nagarathna et al. [15] proposed a method known as a multilayer feedforward neural network (MFNN) to categorize the stages of AD. The study used a dataset of MRI images obtained from the ADNI database. The images were preprocessed to remove noise and artifacts, and features were extracted. The extracted features were used to train and test the MFNN classifier. The feature extraction model consisted of five sets of convolutional blocks, and the classifier model used a multilayer feedforward network with three layers, including a hidden layer and an output layer. The results showed that the proposed model performed well on this dataset, even though the study had some limitations, such as a small dataset size and a lack of comparison with other classification techniques. In our study, we developed the CNN model for feature extraction, consisting of five blocks of convolutional layers.

Using medical imaging data, Kapadnis et al. [16] proposed an approach that explored the use of deep learning techniques for the detection of AD. The authors used CNNs for feature extraction and a support vector machine (SVM) for classification. The study first preprocessed the images and then extracted features using CNNs. The SVM was trained on these features to classify the images as either healthy or AD. The study highlights the potential of deep learning techniques for detecting AD, which can aid in early diagnosis and treatment. AI systems' capacity to learn intricate details through nonlinear transformations could produce promising results for the identification of AD. The study concludes by emphasizing the need for further research to improve the accuracy and efficiency of AD detection using AI techniques.

To distinguish between patients with MCI and AD by incorporating information about the thickness and geometry of the cortex, Wee et al. [17] proposed a method in which a neural network called a spectral graph CNN can be used. The suggested method used a spectral graph CNN framework to find the difference between AD and MCI and predict when MCI will turn into AD. The spectral graph CNN outperformed voxel-based CNN models and achieved balanced prediction for imbalanced sample sizes. The framework was also effective in predicting MCI-to-AD conversion. The authors suggested that the model could be applied to other brain imaging data and be integrated with other classification approaches on multi-modal brain image data for further improvement.

Guo et al. [18] described a way to use hierarchical GCNs on positron emission tomography (PET) imaging data to predict AD. They called it PETNet and used PET images from the ADNI 2 dataset for validation and evaluation. The ResNet-50 network was used for training the model with pre-trained weights. PETNet achieved similar performance to the pre-trained ResNet-50 for binary classification (MCI/NC) but outperformed ResNet-50 for MCI staging (EMCI/LMCI/NC). The limitations, including graph construction and inference, are still inconclusive issues in the fields of neuroimaging and medical image analysis. Additionally, there are difficulties in choosing the appropriate metrics and weight among different graph inference methods and in applying manifold learning.

Park et al. [19] used PET scans to create CNN-LSTM and 3D CNN models that can predict the difference between people with MCI and AD and those who do not have cognitive impairment (CU). The features were extracted using CNN layers, and then the flattened layer was passed as input into the LSTM. The area under the curve (AUC) for the classification of AD from the CU method was 0.964 using the CNN-LSTM. Since their proposed CNN-LSTM performed very well, we propose the CNN-GCN architecture to obtain higher accuracy for classifying different dementia stages.

Tajammal et al. [20] constructed a deep-learning-based ensembling technique that aimed to effectively extract features from input data and attain optimal performance. The experimental findings indicated that their method achieved an overall average accuracy of 98.8% for the classification task, including AD, MCI, and CN. They applied binary classification techniques for different classes. In our study, we performed multi-class classification for different dementia stages.

Liu et al. [21] came up with a new way to use a 3D deep CNN to predict the difference between people with mild Alzheimer's dementia, MCI, and CN by analyzing structural MRIs. The deep learning model demonstrated a high level of accuracy, achieving an AUC of 85.12 when differentiating between CN people and patients with either MCI or mild Alzheimer's dementia. Even though much research has been developed based on the CNN model for predicting AD dementia, there is active research ongoing to develop a more accurate prediction model by improving the CNN model. So, in our study, we developed an advanced CNN-GCN model for accurate dementia-stage prediction.

Building off the aforementioned work, our proposed method contributes to the literature in the following ways. First, Adeghal et al. [12] and Basheeraa et al. [13] used CNN-based approaches for their studies, but each study's purposes and methods differed. Adeghal et al. aimed to improve the categorization of AD stages through transfer learning using MRI data, while Basheeraa et al. focused on classifying AD using a hybrid enhanced ICA segmentation of gray matter in MRI images. In contrast, our study uses cutting-edge preprocessing methods and presents the pre-trained VGG16 model based on transfer learning with additional convolution layers to better identify the different stages of dementia. Moreover, we implement this advanced deep learning method on a more diverse multi-class dataset than in these previous studies. In a manner similar to [16,19], we utilize a CNN model for feature selection and GCNs for classifying the different AD stages, but anticipate that our proposed (CNN-GCN) method has higher accuracy in detecting AD compared to the CNNs-only model. Additionally, we work with a multi-class imbalanced dataset, as in [17], so GCNs could be a better classification technique for predicting different dementia stages. Finally, building upon [18], we use a highly accurate GCN model with appropriate graph construction techniques, metrics, and weights in this study to improve their proposed GCN model for dementia-stage classification.

3. Methodology

3.1. CNNs

CNNs are popular for image classification tasks due to their ability to automatically learn and extract features from images. CNNs have attained state-of-the-art performance in image classification tasks, often outperforming traditional machine learning algorithms. This is because CNNs can learn to identify complex features in images, such as edges, corners, and textures, without the need for explicit feature engineering. CNNs are designed to mimic the visual cortex of the brain and consist of several layers, including convolutional layers, pooling layers, and fully connected layers. Generally, convolutional layers apply a set of filters to the input image, which results in feature maps highlighting different aspects of the image. Pooling layers reduce the spatial dimensionality of the feature maps by selecting the most important features. Finally, the fully connected layers use the features to classify the image into different categories.

We applied a 5-fold cross-validation technique (a grid search on the validation set) to find the optimal layer size and network hyperparameters (learning rate, regularization, etc.). The original training set was divided into a new training set and a validation set with proportions of 80% and 20%, respectively. We used cross-validation to tune the hyperparameters and layer sizes on the following grid: 1×10^{-k} for $k = 1, \ldots, 5$ and 2^i for $i = 4, \ldots, 10$, respectively. Additionally, we tried different hyperparameters using the KerasTuner. This eliminates the difficulties associated with the hyperparameter search with its user-friendly and extensible optimization framework [22]. We utilized various search methods to discover the optimal values for our model's hyperparameters after configuring the search space using a define-by-run syntax.

The proposed CNN architecture consists of five convolutional layers, followed by ReLU activation, batch normalization (BN), and max pooling. The first two convolutional layers have 32 and 64 filters of size 4×4, respectively. The third convolutional layer has 128 filters of size 1×1. The fourth convolutional layer has 256 filters of size 1×1. The fifth convolutional layer has four filters of size 1×1, corresponding to the dataset's number of classes. The output of the fifth convolutional layer is flattened and passed to the final layer, which is a softmax layer that outputs the class probabilities. The L2 regularization loss of the weights is used to prevent overfitting.

3.2. VGG16 with Additional Convolutional Layers

A pre-trained neural network architecture for image classification is utilized in our work to develop a more advanced CNN model. The network architecture is made by following VGGNet, a popular neural network architecture for image classification.

VGGNet [23] is a CNN architecture that was introduced in 2014. VGGNet is known for its straightforward architecture, which consists of 16–19 convolutional layers and three fully connected layers. The convolutional layers are designed to extract features from the input image, while the fully connected layers are responsible for the classification task. VGGNet has been used in various computer vision applications, such as image classification, object detection, and semantic segmentation. One of the main benefits of VGGNet is its simplicity, which makes it easy to understand and implement. The uniform architecture of VGGNet also allows for easy experimentation with different layer configurations, which can be useful for fine-tuning the performance of the network. Additionally, VGGNet has achieved state-of-the-art results on several image classification benchmarks, such as the ImageNet Large Scale Visual Recognition Challenge. However, VGGNet's simplicity can also be a disadvantage in some cases. The large number of parameters in the network can make it difficult to train, especially with limited computational resources. VGGNet is also relatively slow compared to some other convolutional neural network architectures due to its large number of parameters and layers.

To further improve the performance of the pre-trained VGG16 architecture, we added five additional convolutional layers, a max pooling layer, a BN layer, and a ReLU activation layer. The number of layers, the sizes of the layers, and several other hyperparameters were modified in accordance with the cross-validation methods described earlier.

3.3. GCNs

In this part, we provide a comprehensive analysis of GCNs from distinct viewpoints. Additionally, we designed an upgrade to the current system by integrating CNNs with GCNs. This modification makes existing GCNs more suitable for the dementia and AD image classification problem.

At first, we cover some fundamentals of GCNs, such as the definitions and notation, as well as the formation of graphs. One-to-many relationships in non-Euclidean spaces can be explained through the use of graphs, which are highly nonlinear data structures. Here, an undirected graph is represented by $G = (V, E)$, where V and E stand for the sets of vertices and edges. The AD images serve as the vertex set, while the similarities between any pair of vertices (V_i and V_j) constitute the edge set. The connections between vertices are specified by the adjacency matrix, A. In our case, when two images are from the same class, we use the label 1, otherwise, we use the label 0 to generate the adjacency matrix. After obtaining A, the appropriate graph Laplacian matrix L is computed using the following equation: $L = D - A$ and the degrees of A are represented by the diagonal matrix D, where $D_{i,i} = \sum_j A_{i,j}$.

The symmetric normalized Laplacian matrix (L_{sym}) can be utilized to improve the graph's generalization, capitalizing on the decomposition $L_{sym} = D^{-1/2} L D^{-1/2}$. For example, the propagation rule for GCNs is

$$H^{l+1} = h(D^{-1/2} L D^{-1/2} H^l W^l + b^l)$$

The output of the lth layer is denoted by $H^{(l)}$, and the activation function ReLU is denoted by $h(\bullet)$, where $W^{(l)}$ and $b^{(l)}$ are the weights and biases of the layers that must be learned.

GCNs Architecture

The GCNs architecture is used to classify data represented as graphs, with each node representing a feature and each edge representing a relationship between nodes. The input layer receives the feature matrix of the graph as input. GCN layers use the graph's Laplacian matrix and learnable weights to perform a graph convolution operation on the input. Finally, the output layer produces the final classification output.

The GCNs architecture defines several helper functions for creating placeholders, initializing parameters, performing GCN operations, and optimizing the network. It also defines a function for training the network and returning it's accuracy. The training function takes in training and validation data, as well as the Laplacian matrix of the graph. It initializes the network's parameters, creates the placeholders for the input data, and defines the loss and optimization functions. We utilized the Xavier uniform initializer, then trained the network and returned the accuracy on the test set. We utilized the Proximal Adagrad Optimizer as an optimization function, although we tried other optimizers to determine the best performer. With $K = 5$, we used a KNN-based graph to calculate the adjacency matrix A. Before providing the features into the softmax layer, the GCNs implement a 128-unit graph convolutional hidden layer, similar to the CNN architecture described above.

3.4. CNN-GCN Architecture

Hong et al. [24] proposed the FuNet architectures that use a range of models and/or features to make it easier to predict the difference between features by training CNNs and GCNs at the same time to classify hyperspectral images. Additive (A), elementwise multiplicative (M), and concatenation (C) were the three fusion procedures by combining miniGCNs with the CNN model that were taken into consideration for their study. In this study, we proposed a novel fusion network by integrating CNNs with GCNs and considering the resulting features from CNNs before the final classifications of all the classes by GCNs. The proposed fusion network architecture (CNN-GCN) is an implementation of our previously mentioned CNN model for feature extraction and the GCN model to classify the graph nodes. So, in short, the features extracted from the CNN model are fed into the GCN classifier model to obtain the four nodes representing the class probabilities.

In Figure 1, the first convolution block to the fourth block consist of the convolution layer, BN layer, 2D max pooling layer, and the ReLU layer. We utilize three-dimensional input images with a height of 224 and a width of 224, and the number of channels is 3. Furthermore, it is worth noting that the receptive fields throughout the spatial and spectral domains for every single convolutional layer are expressed as follows: $4 \times 4 \times 32$, $4 \times 4 \times 64$, $1 \times 1 \times 128$, and $1 \times 1 \times 256$, respectively. We kept the number of filters in the early levels relatively low, and then, progressively increased the number as we moved deeper into the layers. The final block consists only of the convolution before flattening the features. Hence, we obtained the future maps by utilizing these five convolution blocks. After obtaining the feature maps by training the CNNs, we determined the adjacency matrix, training, validation, and test data to classify the four dementia stages. In GCNs, V represents vertexes, W indicates hidden features in the GCN layer, R denotes hidden features through the ReLU layer, Z represents hidden features in the softmax layer, and Y represents outcomes, respectively. The model has a single hidden layer with 128 nodes, and the output layer has 4 nodes representing the class probabilities. The input data consists of two parts: a feature vector and an adjacency matrix representing the graph structure. The feature vector is passed through a GCN layer to produce the hidden representation. The hidden layer is concatenated with a convolutional layer to process the feature vector representation of the graph and pass it through graph convolutional layers before being flattened to a vector. The final output is obtained by passing the flattened vector through a fully connected layer with four nodes. We trained the CNN-GCN model twice since, at first, the CNNs layers were trained to obtain robust feature maps and GCN layers were trained to classify the dementia stages.

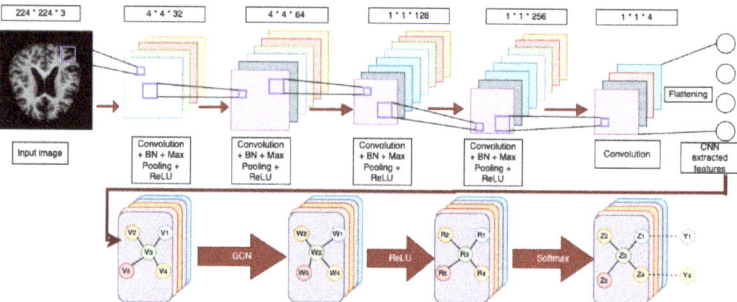

Figure 1. The architecture of the proposed CNN-GCN model.

Gradient-weighted class activation mapping (Grad-CAM) [25] is a technique used to precisely determine the specific features of input images that a model must capture. It achieves this by analyzing the gradients of a target concept which flow into the final convolutional layer. Grad-CAM then generates a coarse localization map that highlights the significant regions in the image that are crucial for improving the prediction accuracy. In Figure 2, we visualized how the Grad-CAM method makes the CNN-GCN model's outputs clearer for the input images so that the proposed CNN-GCN model can predict the stages of dementia perfectly. Hence, Grad-CAM uses targeted processing and captures the key image features to maintain the CNN-GCN model's accuracy and robustness.

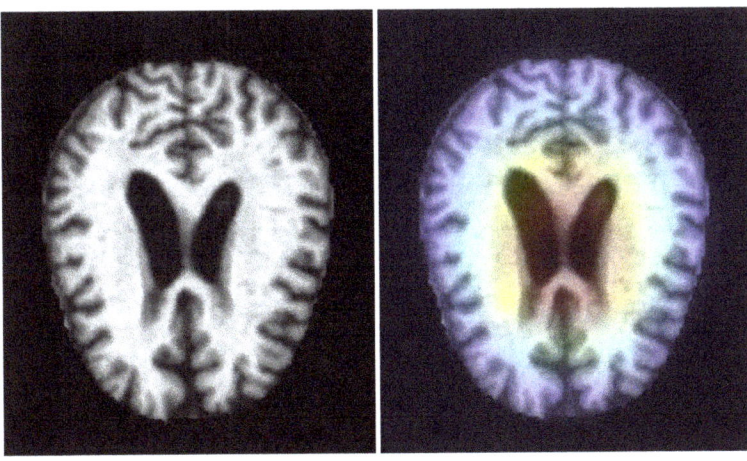

(a) Original image   (b) Grad-CAM image

Figure 2. Moderate dementia image: (**a**) original and (**b**) Grad-CAM image.

4. Results

There are several performance indicators that we assess, such as overall accuracy, F1 score, recall, and precision, for determining the model's performance in classifying different dementia stages. The F1 score is a metric that calculates the weighted average of recall and precision, whereas accuracy measures the proportion of properly classified individuals. Following the development of the models, several metrics were utilized in order to adjust parameters. The 5-fold cross-validation method is utilized to determine the performance of each model. Performance assessments are conducted using a multi-class approach and are represented by the confusion matrix. In the results section, we display the figures of loss, accuracy, confusion matrix, and the table of classification scores based on the best fold outputs from the 5-fold cross-validation for all models. Instead of displaying the loss, accuracy, and confusion matrix obtained from all folds of the 5-fold cross-validation, displaying the best fold outputs is better since it is not messy for following the outputs of this study. Moreover, AD- and dementia-stage prediction is crucial, since having knowledge about the stage enables physicians to have a more comprehensive understanding of the impact of the disease on the patient.

4.1. Data Description

The ADNI dataset is the most widely used structural and functional brain imaging scan in AD research to accelerate understanding and treatment development. We collected 6400 raw images from the ADNI database. There are four different categories, including healthy people, very mild, mild, and moderate dementia patients.

In Figure 3, we can see that we have 3200 healthy cases, 2240 very mild cases, 896 mild cases, and 64 moderate cases for training and testing the models.

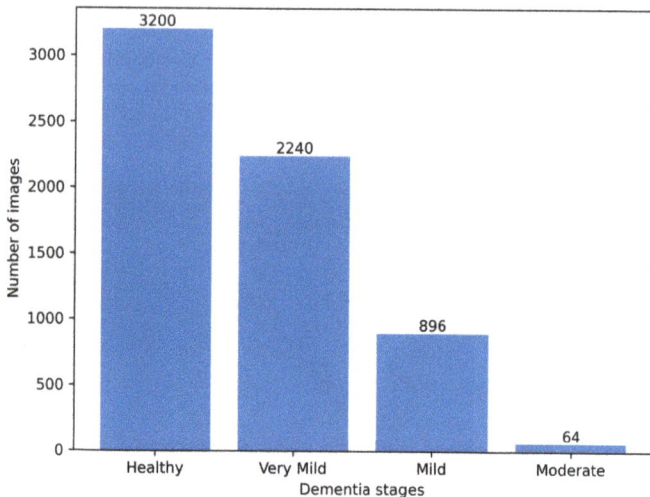

Figure 3. Total number of images by each category.

4.2. Preprocessing

The dataset used for dementia and AD analysis primarily consisted of MRI image data; however, the available data were imbalanced. So, there is an overwhelming dominance of samples from a single class over those from any other class. Data preprocessing techniques were employed to augment the dataset to address this issue. Two distinct augmentation methods, namely, Gaussian noise addition and rotation, were applied. The purpose of data augmentation was to increase the quantity of data in the dataset, thereby preventing overfitting of the model. The Gaussian noise addition process involves adding noise to a set of input images to augment the dataset by introducing variations to the images. Gaussian noise, with a specified standard deviation, is generated randomly and added to each image. This process creates noisy versions of the original images, allowing for a larger and more diverse dataset and, ultimately, more accurate predictions. By increasing the amount of data and introducing randomness, the model trained on this augmented dataset is less likely to overfit the available data, leading to potentially improved performance and generalization. Rotation is another way image augmentation is performed by applying random rotations to the image dataset. A random rotation angle within the specified range is generated, and the image is rotated accordingly. Random rotation of each image creates variations in their orientation. This process ensures that the augmented images are saved in a structured manner, replicating the directory structure of the original dataset. The implementation applies image augmentation to a collection of images. This process enhances the dataset by generating diverse versions of the images, which can be beneficial for subsequent analysis or training purposes.

4.3. Network Implementation

The TensorFlow platform is utilized to build the CNN and GCN networks, and the Adagrad optimizer [26] is employed to optimize the networks. The "exponential" learning rate strategy allows for the dynamic updating of the current learning rate by multiplying a base learning rate (such as 0.001) by every epoch. The maximum number of epochs allowed during network training is 100. The 0.8 momenta are used with BN [27], and the training phase's batch size is 32. Additionally, the weights are subject to a 2-norm regularization with a 0.001 setting to stabilize network training and minimize overfitting.

4.4. Evaluation Metrics

For each class of the dataset that was provided per model, we calculated the F1 score (4), precision (2), recall (3), and accuracy (1) to evaluate the performance of the proposed techniques. True positive (TP) is the number of images that are correctly classified as being in a particular class. False positive (FP) is the number of images that should belong to another class but are mistakenly assigned to that class. False negative (FN) is the number of images that are part of a class but are mistakenly assigned to another class. The number of images that are accurately classified as belonging to a different class are considered to be true negatives (TNs).

$$\text{accuracy} = \frac{TP + TN}{TP + FP + FN + TN} \times 100 \tag{1}$$

$$\text{precision} = \frac{TP}{TP + FP} \tag{2}$$

$$\text{recall} = \frac{TP}{TP + FN} \tag{3}$$

$$\text{F1-score} = 2 \times \frac{\text{precision} \times \text{recall}}{\text{precision} + \text{recall}} \tag{4}$$

In Figure 4, the value of the loss function is plotted against the number of completed iterations. Both the training and testing losses decreased for the first fifty iterations, even though the testing losses became stable. So, there is a deviation between the training and testing phases after approximately 50 iterations because of the complexity of the model. The CNN model has a high capacity to fit enough parameters of the training data that obstructs the model's capacity to generalize on testing data.

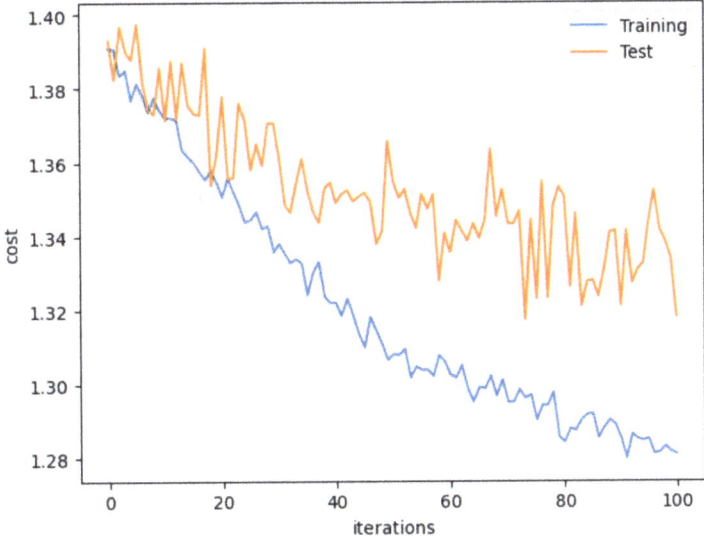

Figure 4. Epoch versus cost for the CNN model.

The accuracy vs. iterations curve provides us with the information we need to validate the performance of the CNN model. In Figure 5, we can see that both the training and testing accuracy are increasing. This indicates that the learning progress of this model is rising to the point of 100 iterations, beyond which point it stays constant when we run it for a greater number of iterations. So, in the case of accuracy, there was not a huge deviation between the training and testing phases.

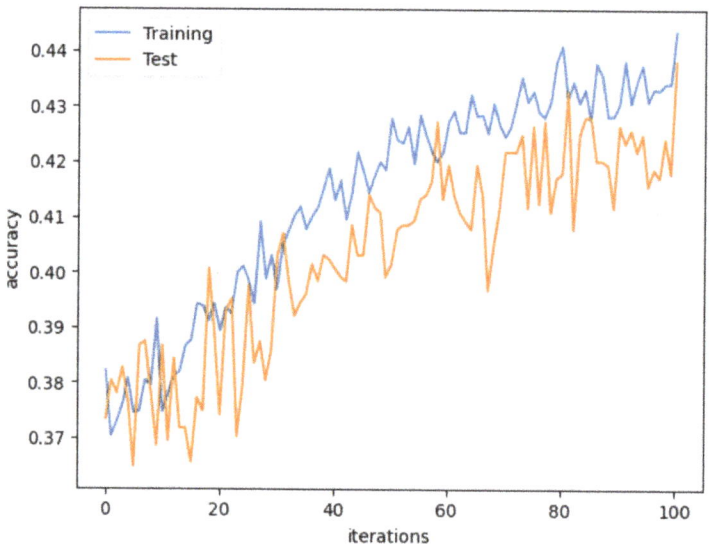

Figure 5. Epoch versus accuracy for the CNN model.

The confusion matrix that was produced for the CNN model is shown in Figure 6 for the classification of the healthy, very mild, mild, and moderate classes. Even though there is no correct prediction of the moderate class, the number of correctly predicted healthy class cases is 445; the number of correctly predicted very mild class cases is 100; and the number of correctly predicted mild class cases is 16. Due to the fact that there are only 64 images of the moderate class, it is difficult to make a precise prediction of the moderate class.

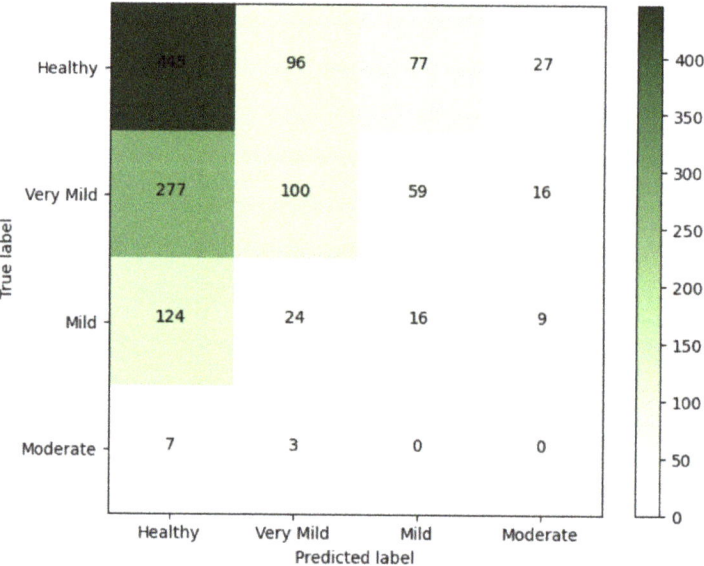

Figure 6. Confusion matrix for the CNN model.

The F1 score, precision, and recall of each of the classes that comprise the CNN model are detailed in Table 1. The overall accuracy of this model is calculated to be 43.83%. The

F1 score for the healthy, very mild, mild, and moderate classes are 0.59, 0.30, 0.10, and 0. The CNN algorithm properly predicted 561 out of 1280 test images. According to Table 1, the category that was predicted with the greatest degree of precision was healthy, while the category that was predicted with the least degree of precision was moderate dementia.

Table 1. Classification scores for the CNN model.

Class	n (Classified)	n (Truth)	F1 Score	Recall	Precision
Healthy	853	645	0.59	0.69	0.52
Very Mild	223	452	0.30	0.22	0.45
Mild	152	173	0.10	0.09	0.11
Moderate	52	10	0	0	0

In Figure 7, the value of the loss function is plotted against the number of completed iterations. Initially, the loss was high due to random parameters, but it started decreasing when the number of iterations increased. After iteration 40, both the training and testing losses were stable for the VGG16 with additional convolution layers.

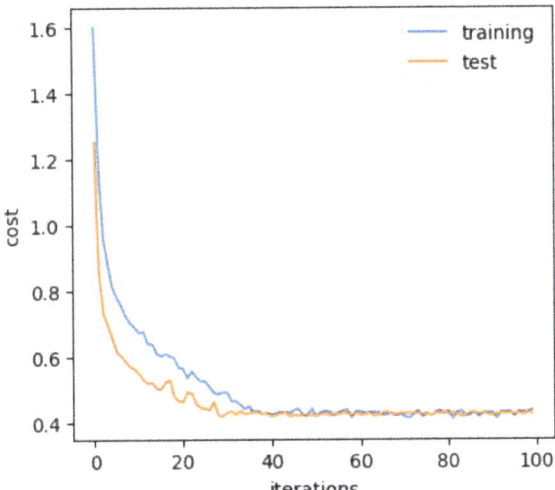

Figure 7. Epoch vs. cost for the VGG16 with additional convolutional layers model.

We can verify the VGG16 with additional convolutional layers model's performance from the accuracy versus iteration curve. In Figure 8, we can see that the training and testing accuracy is around 80% which shows that the learning progress of this model is increasing until 40 iterations and remains fixed after that.

In Figure 9, the confusion matrix for the VGG16 with additional convolutional layers model for the classes healthy, very mild, mild, and moderate is shown. The number of correctly predicted healthy classes is 505, the very mild class is 383, and the mild class is 23, even though there is no correct prediction of the moderate class out of 13 moderate class test images. Since there are only 64 moderate class images, there is very little chance for a correct prediction of the moderate class.

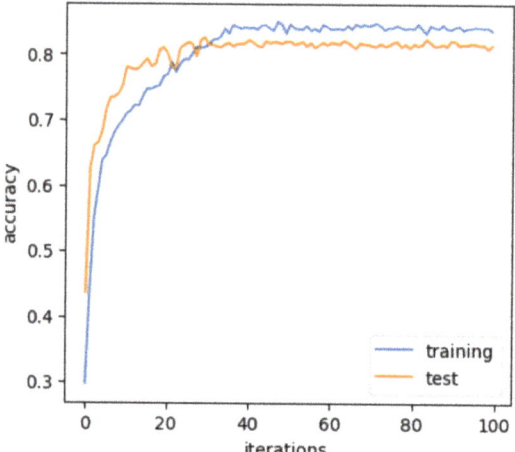

Figure 8. Epoch vs. accuracy for the VGG16 with additional convolutional layers model.

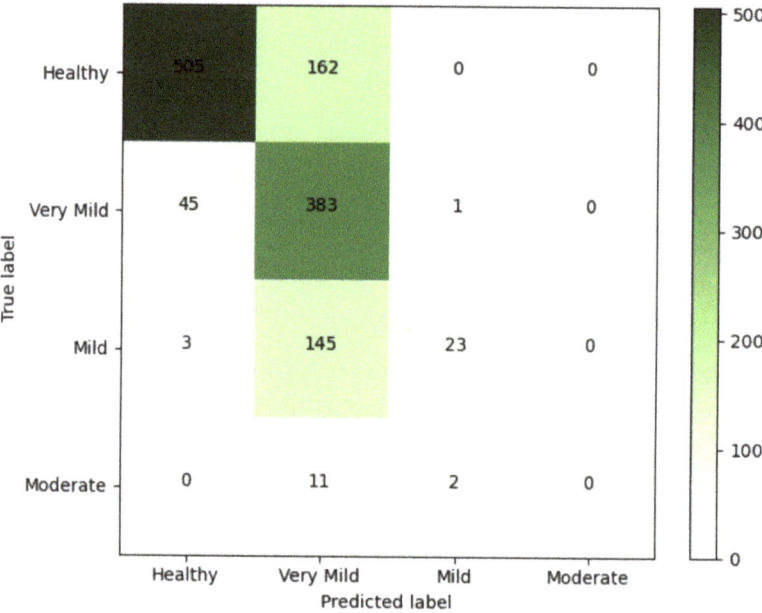

Figure 9. Confusion matrix for the VGG16 with additional convolutional layers model.

Table 2 describes the F1 score, precision, and recall of all the classes for the VGG16 with additional convolutional layers. The overall accuracy is 71.17% for this model. The F1 scores for the healthy, very mild, mild, and moderate classes are 0.83, 0.68, 0.23, and 0. Out of 1280 test images, our model correctly predicts 911. Table 2 shows that the class most accurately predicted is healthy, while the class least accurately predicted is moderate dementia. Since there are a very small number of moderate class images, the model performance for this class is very low.

Table 2. Classification scores for the VGG16 with additional convolutional layers model.

Class	n (Classified)	n (Truth)	F1 Score	Recall	Precision
Healthy	553	667	0.83	0.76	0.91
Very Mild	701	429	0.68	0.87	0.55
Mild	26	171	0.23	0.13	0.88
Moderate	0	13	0	0	0

The loss function's value versus the number of iterations is shown in Figure 10. The GCN model's loss decreased for the training and testing images, even though the loss was very high initially. After iteration 18, the cost was fixed at around zero for both the training and testing images.

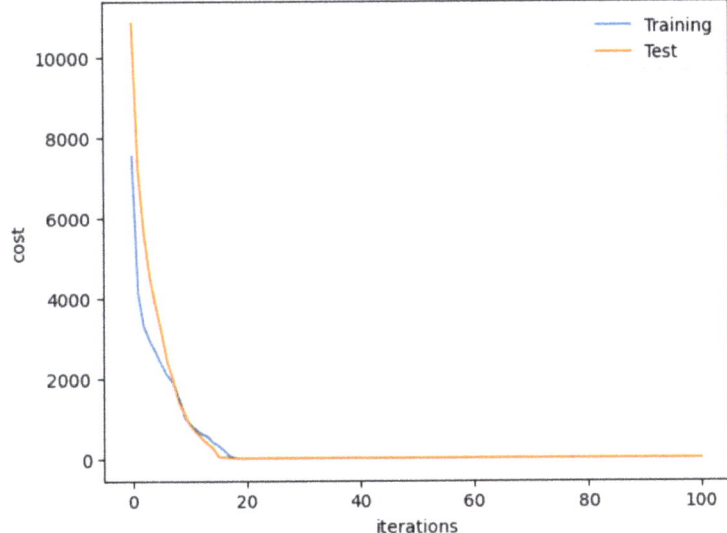

Figure 10. Epoch versus cost for the GCN model.

The accuracy versus iteration curve gives us the evidence we need to verify the GCN model's efficacy. Figure 11 shows a rise in accuracy throughout both training and testing until it becomes fixed close to 1. This shows that the model's learning rate increases up to about 20 iterations, after which it levels off and remains constant.

For the categorization of healthy, very mild, mild, and moderate, the GCN model's resulting confusion matrices are shown in Figure 12. The total number of correctly predicted healthy cases is 640; for very mild cases, this is 448; and for mild class cases, this is 180, although no moderate cases were identified in any of the 12 test images. Even though the GCN model was able to predict all of the other category images accurately, it was unable to predict the moderate dementia cases.

Table 3 shows the F1 score, precision, and recall of the GCN model for each class. This model is estimated to have a global accuracy of 99.06 percent. The F1 scores for the healthy, very mild, mild, and moderate classes are 1, 0.99, 1, and 0. Out of a total of 1280 test images, the GCN algorithm successfully predicted 1268. The most accurate prediction was made for the healthy and mild categories, while the least accurate prediction was made for the moderate dementia category.

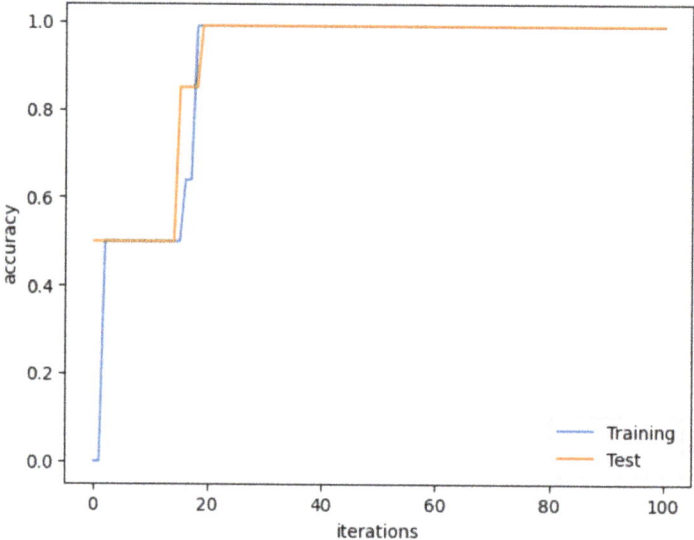

Figure 11. Epoch versus accuracy for the GCN model.

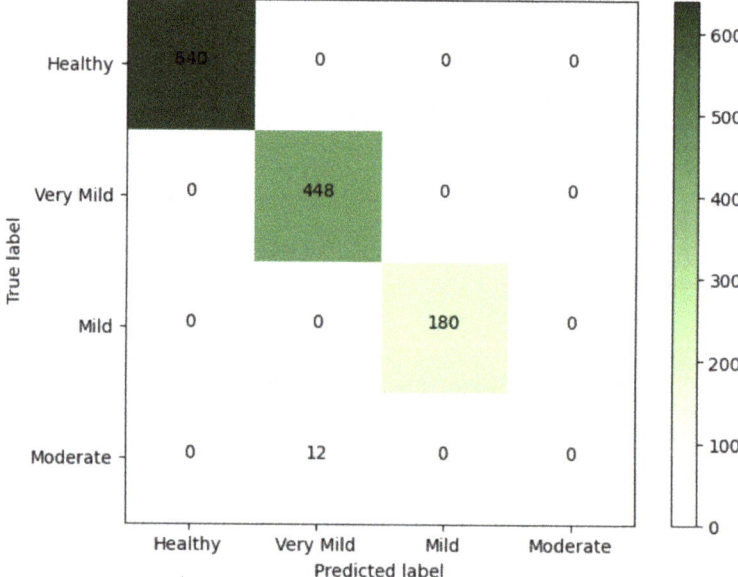

Figure 12. Confusion matrix for the GCN model.

Table 3. Classification scores for the GCN model.

Class	n (Classified)	n (Truth)	F1 Score	Recall	Precision
Healthy	640	640	1	1	1
Very Mild	460	448	0.99	1	0.97
Mild	180	180	1	1	1
Moderate	0	12	0	0	0

Figure 13 depicts the loss function's value versus the number of iterations. Even though the loss was initially quite high for the test images, the CNN-GCN model's loss decreased abruptly for the test images. After the first couple of iterations, the cost for both training and testing images became fixed at approximately zero.

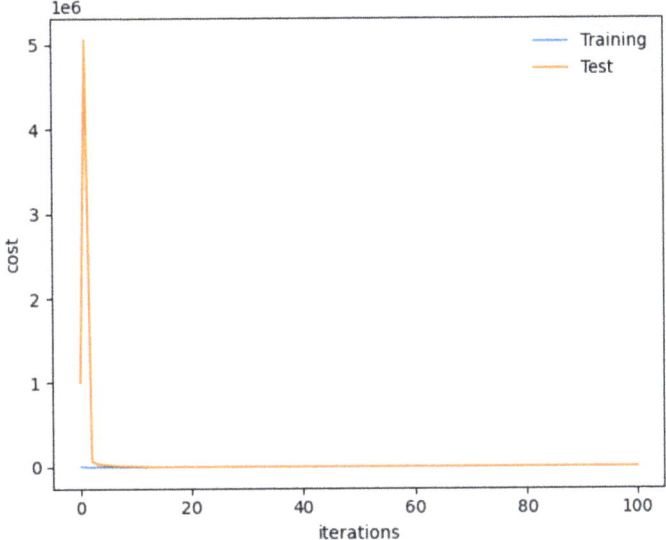

Figure 13. Epoch versus cost for the CNN-GCN model.

The accuracy versus iteration curve provides the evidence necessary to confirm the efficacy of the CNN-GCN model. Figure 14 depicts a rise in accuracy during both training and testing until it approaches 1 and stabilizes. This demonstrates that the model's learning rate increases after a couple of iterations before leveling off and remaining constant.

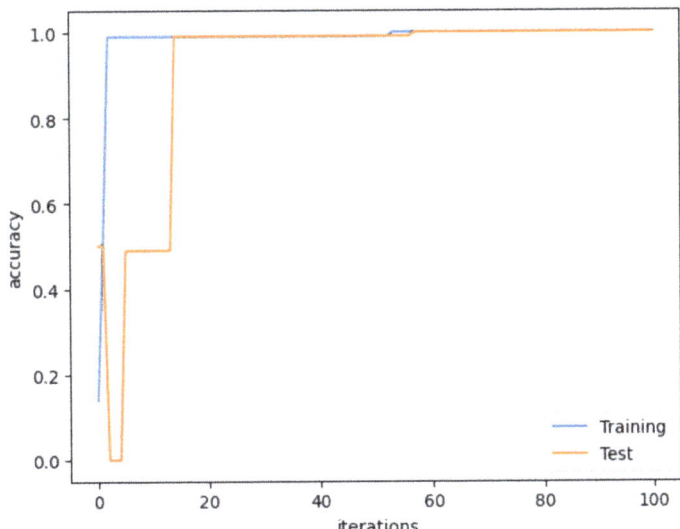

Figure 14. Epoch versus accuracy for the CNN-GCN model.

Figure 15 displays the confusion matrices produced by the CNN-GCN model for the categorization of the healthy, very mild, mild, and moderate classes. The number of correctly predicted healthy cases is 641, the number of very mild cases is 448, the number of mild cases is 179, and the number of moderate cases is 12. All category images are predicted correctly using the CNN-GCN model.

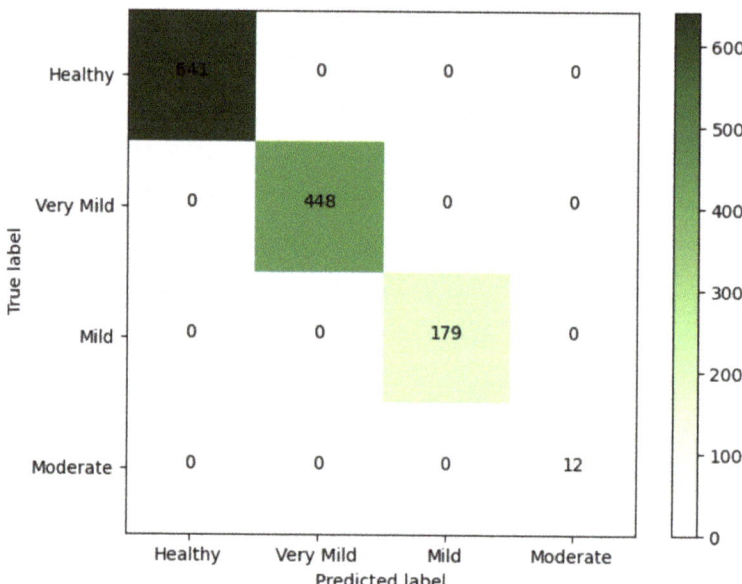

Figure 15. Confusion matrix for the CNN-GCN model.

Table 4 shows the F1 score, precision, and recall of the CNN-GCN model for each class. We obtained an overall accuracy of 100% from the CNN-GCN model. The F1 scores for the healthy, very mild, mild, and moderate classes are 1, 1, 1, and 1, respectively. The CNN-GCN algorithm successfully predicts all of the 1280 images.

Table 4. Classification scores for the CNN-GCN model.

Class	n (Classified)	n (Truth)	F1 Score	Precision	Recall
Healthy	641	641	1	1	1
Very Mild	448	448	1	1	1
Mild	179	179	1	1	1
Moderate	12	12	1	1	1

Our proposed CNN-GCN model achieves 100% accuracy on both the training and test data and may overfit the training data by capturing even irrelevant and abnormal patterns, such as noise and outliers. Consequently, the model may exhibit sub-par performance when presented with novel, unfamiliar data. The high accuracy may indicate a lack of generalizability of the model to novel contexts or datasets. This is particularly crucial when dealing with health-related data since it might exhibit significant variability. Hence, it is important to verify the accuracy of the CNN-GCN model by using distinct test datasets and ensuring its efficacy in real-world scenarios rather than just relying on controlled experimental settings. So, we collected a separate dataset for implementing our proposed CNN-GCN model. Neeraj [28] provided a dataset to Kaggle, which consists of 2D images collected from the ADNI baseline dataset that were originally Nifti images. The dataset has three distinct classes: AD, MCI, and CN. After implementing our proposed CNN-GCN model, we presented the confusion matrix in Figure 16 to categorize the AD, MCI, and CN classes. There are 8 accurately predicted instances of AD, 21 cases of MCI, and 15 cases of CN. The CNN-GCN model accurately predicted all of the category images. This illustrates the potential for its use with novel and unfamiliar data.

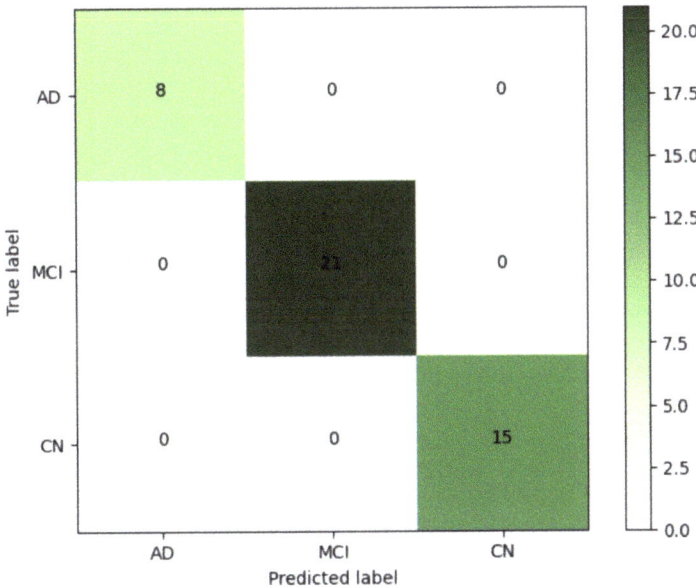

Figure 16. Confusion matrix for the CNN-GCN model for classifying AD, MCI, and CN.

5. Discussion

Dementia includes the very mild, mild, and moderate cognitive impairment phases that may or may not evolve into AD. The most common kind of dementia is AD. AD and other cognitive impairments fall under the general category of dementia. Because the cognitive impairment stages are the time during which AD may or may not develop, it is of the utmost importance to appropriately identify individuals during this stage [29]. Identifying and diagnosing the illness at its various phases helps doctors come up with more effective therapy and management solutions.

So, in this study, we developed a CNN model, a transfer-learning-based CNN model, a GCN model, and the proposed fusion network model (CNN-GCN) for identifying AD and dementia stages.

In Table 5, HC, CN, MCI, EMCI, and AD represent healthy control, normal control, mild cognitive impairment, early mild cognitive impairment, and Alzheimer's disease, respectively. We can see that the above works are based on different datasets and different methods. Some authors considered multi-class classification, and others considered binary classification. Since our approach, CNN-GCN, is a new approach for classifying the healthy, very mild dementia, mild dementia, and moderate dementia classes, no one has utilized this technique for classification tasks. We present each method's accuracy, which is defined as the percentage of accurate predictions on the test set.

In Table 6, we presented the GPU times in seconds for the four methods. We can see that the CNN, pre-trained VGG16 with additional convolutional layers, GCN, and CNN-GCN models took 411, 2364, 64, and 95 seconds, respectively, by using the NVIDIA T4 Tensor Core GPU for completing 100 epochs. The CNN-based methods are more computationally expensive compared to the GCN model. Our proposed CNN-GCN model is less computationally expensive and provides better accuracy.

Table 5. Review of selected existing works for the classification of AD and MCI.

Paper	No. of Classes	CNNs	Pre-Trained VGG	GCNs	CNN-GCN	ResNet-50	VGG16-SVM
Our work	Multi-class (4 way)	43.83%	71.17%	99.06%	100%	59.69%	
Lim et al. [9]	Multi-class (3 way: CN vs. MCI vs. AD)	72.70%	78.57%			75.71%	
Jiang et al. [11]	Binary (EMCI vs. NC)						89.4%
Payan et al. [30]	Binary (AD vs. HC, MCI vs. HC, AD vs. MCI)	95.39%, 92.13%, 86.84%					
Khvostikov et al. [31]	Binary (AD vs. HC, MCI vs. HC, AD vs. MCI)	93.3%, 73.3%, 86.7%					
Valliani et al. [32]	Multi-class (3 way: AD vs. MCI vs. CN)	49.2%				50.8%	
Helaly et al. [33]	Multi-class (4 way: AD vs. EMCI vs. LMCI vs. NC)	93%					

Table 6. Numerical comparison of the GPU times for all the models.

Model	CNNs	VGG16 with Additional Convolutional Layers	GCNs	CNN-GCN
GPU time (s)	411	2364	64	95

The performance of the models differed significantly. The performance of the CNN model was very poor compared to other models. By performing hyperparameter tuning, we found Adagrad to be the best optimizer. Additionally, we tried several optimizers, like gradient descent, Adam, RMSprop, and the proximal Adagrad optimizer. Since the AD MRI dataset is imbalanced, the performance of the CNN model was not sufficiently accurate in all cases.

We incorporated the VGG16 transfer learning model with the five additional convolutional layers to improve the performance of the CNN model. By utilizing the VGG16 model with additional convolutional layers, we obtained better accuracy compared to our developed CNN model. To determine the best transfer learning model, we also implemented the DenseNet, MobileNet, InceptionNet, and ResNet transfer learning models and received an overall accuracy of 70.70%, 70.37%, 65%, and 59.69%, respectively. We found that VGG16 is the best transfer learning model in our case. Although the VGG16 with additional convolutional layers model's performance seems to be behind that of competing approaches, our findings are on par with other CNN models developed so far for biomedical imaging.

Even though CNN-based models are very popular for analyzing image datasets, we developed the GCN model for AD- and dementia-stage prediction. This is due to the fact that GCNs give a strong and flexible representation of the connections between the many components in a complex AD image. Often, the AD MRI images include complicated structures, patterns, and interactions, all of which are amenable to being comprehended and examined to a greater degree by using graph-based methods. The graph-based methods were helpful in the prediction since they take into account the global context and linkages, which assists in mitigating the impacts of class imbalance. For the GCN and CNN-GCN models, we applied hyperparameter tuning and the above-mentioned optimizers. We received almost perfect accuracy in each case. The GCN model's overall accuracy was 99.06% and correctly predicted healthy, very mild, and mild dementia classes, but could not correctly predict any of the moderate dementia class test images. We then utilized our proposed CNN-GCN fusion network to classify the AD and dementia stages. We developed the same GCN model but utilized the features from the CNN model as input data for the CNN-GCN model. So, we obtained an overall accuracy of 100% by using the CNN-GCN model, which is supplied with features that have been extracted from CNNs. Only the CNN-GCN model was able to predict the moderate class test images accurately, whereas all the other previously mentioned models could not predict them correctly. This study provides evidence that a CNN-GCN modeling approach can work well and obtain high accuracy for applications involving imbalanced data.

6. Conclusions

To sum up, we created four models for identifying healthy, very mild, mild, and moderate dementia patients by utilizing both CNN- and GCN-based algorithms. When compared to the CNN model, the performance of the pre-trained VGG16 with additional convolutional layers model is superior. Moreover, when measured against different works in the literature, its performance is regarded as satisfactory. Even though we achieved an overall accuracy of 99.06% by utilizing the GCN model, it could not accurately predict any of the 12 test images from the moderate stage of dementia. The CNN-GCN model demonstrated the highest F1 score, precision, and recall, as well as an overall accuracy of 100%, out of all the algorithms that we examined. The CNN-GCN model was able to predict all the classes accurately, including the 12 test images from the moderate class. The major limitation of this project is the imbalanced dataset. Although it is common to have low accuracy for an imbalanced dataset in the field of biomedical imaging, our proposed GCNs and CNN-GCN models worked excellently with the imbalanced dataset. This model's performance may not be helpful for clinical diagnosis, but it marks a significant development in the classification of AD and different stages of dementia.

Author Contributions: Data curation, M.E.H.; methodology, M.E.H.; writing: M.E.H. and A.W. All authors have read and agreed to the published version of the manuscript.

Funding: This research did not receive any specific grant from funding agencies in the public, commercial, or not-for-profit sectors.

Institutional Review Board Statement: The data for this article were collected from ADNI. The ADNI study was conducted according to Good Clinical Practice guidelines, the Declaration of Helsinki, US 21CFR Part 50—Protection of Human Subjects, and Part 56—Institutional Review Boards, and pursuant to state and federal HIPAA regulations. Each participating site obtained ethical approval from their Institutional Review Board before commencing subject enrollment. So, the Institutional Review Board approval does not apply to this manuscript.

Informed Consent Statement: Informed consent was obtained from all subjects involved in the study. The human data were acquired from the publicly available ADNI database, which meets the ethics requirements.

Data Availability Statement: The subject data used in this study were obtained from the Alzheimer's Disease Neuroimaging Initiative (ADNI) database (adni.loni.usc.edu, accessed on 10 August 2023). Meanwhile, data supporting the findings of this study are available from the corresponding authors upon reasonable request.

Acknowledgments: The authors express their gratitude to the anonymous reviewers who contributed to raising the paper's standard.

Conflicts of Interest: The authors declare that this study was conducted without any commercial or financial relationship that could be considered a potential conflict of interest.

References

1. WHO. *Dementia*; WHO: Geneva, Switzerland, 2023.
2. Javeed, A.; Dallora, A.; Berglund, J.; Ali, A.; Ali, L.; Anderberg, P. Machine Learning for Dementia Prediction: A Systematic Review and Future Research Directions. *J. Med. Syst.* **2023**, *47*, 17. [CrossRef] [PubMed]
3. NIH. *What Is Dementia*; NIH: Bethesda, MD, USA, 2022.
4. Alzheimer's Society. *What Is the Difference between Dementia and Alzheimer's Disease?* Alzheimer's Society: London, UK, 2023.
5. NIH. *Mild Cognitive Impairment* ; NIH: Bethesda, MD, USA, 2022.
6. NIH. *Mild Cognitive Impairment*; NIH: Bethesda, MD, USA, 2021.
7. NIH. *What Is Alzheimers*; NIH: Bethesda, MD, USA, 2021.
8. Krizhevsky, A.; Sutskever, I.; Hinton, G. Imagenet classification with deep convolutional neural networks. In Proceedings of the Advances in Neural Information Processing Systems, Lake Tahoe, NV, USA, 3–6 December 2012; Volume 25.
9. Lim, B.Y.; Lai, K.W.; Haiskin, K.; Kulathilake, K.; Ong, Z.C.; Hum, Y.C.; Dhanalakshmi, S.; Wu, X.; Zuo, X. Deep learning model for prediction of progressive mild cognitive impairment to Alzheimer's disease using structural MRI. *Front. Aging Neurosci.* **2022**, *14*, 560. [CrossRef] [PubMed]

10. Basaia, S.; Agosta, F.; Wagner, L.; Canu, E.; Magnani, G.; Santangelo, R.; Filippi, M.; Alzheimer's Disease Neuroimaging Initiative. Automated classification of Alzheimer's disease and mild cognitive impairment using a single MRI and deep neural networks. *Neuroimage Clin.* **2019**, *21*, 101645. [CrossRef] [PubMed]
11. Jiang, J.; Kang, L.; Huang, J.; Zhang, T. Deep learning based mild cognitive impairment diagnosis using structure MR images. *Neurosci. Lett.* **2020**, *730*, 134971. [CrossRef] [PubMed]
12. Aderghal, K.; Afdel, K.; Benois-Pineau, J.; Catheline, G. Improving Alzheimer's stage categorization with Convolutional Neural Network using transfer learning and different magnetic resonance imaging modalities. *Heliyon* **2020**, *6*, e05652. [CrossRef] [PubMed]
13. Basheera, S.; Ram, M.S.S. A novel CNN based Alzheimer's disease classification using hybrid enhanced ICA segmented gray matter of MRI. *Comput. Med Imaging Graph.* **2020**, *81*, 101713. [CrossRef] [PubMed]
14. Acharya, U.R.; Fernandes, S.L.; WeiKoh, J.E.; Ciaccio, E.J.; Fabell, M.K.M.; Tanik, U.J.; Rajinikanth, V.; Yeong, C.H. Automated detection of Alzheimer's disease using brain MRI images—A study with various feature extraction techniques. *J. Med Syst.* **2019**, *43*, 1–14. [CrossRef] [PubMed]
15. Nagarathna, C.; Kusuma, M.; Seemanthini, K. Classifying the stages of Alzheimer's disease by using multi layer feed forward neural network. *Procedia Comput. Sci.* **2023**, *218*, 1845–1856.
16. Kapadnis, M.N.; Bhattacharyya, A.; Subasi, A. Artificial intelligence based Alzheimer's disease detection using deep feature extraction. In *Applications of Artificial Intelligence in Medical Imaging*; Elsevier: Amsterdam, The Netherlands, 2023; pp. 333–355.
17. Wee, C.Y.; Liu, C.; Lee, A.; Poh, J.S.; Ji, H.; Qiu, A.; Alzheimers Disease Neuroimage Initiative. Cortical graph neural network for AD and MCI diagnosis and transfer learning across populations. *Neuroimage Clin.* **2019**, *23*, 101929. [CrossRef] [PubMed]
18. Guo, J.; Qiu, W.; Li, X.; Zhao, X.; Guo, N.; Li, Q. Predicting Alzheimer's disease by hierarchical graph convolution from positron emission tomography imaging. In Proceedings of the 2019 IEEE International Conference on Big Data (Big Data), Los Angeles, CA, USA, 9–12 December 2019; IEEE: Piscataway, NJ, USA, 2019; pp. 5359–5363.
19. Park, S.; Yeo, N.; Kim, Y.; Byeon, G.; Jang, J. Deep learning application for the classification of Alzheimer's disease using 18F-flortaucipir (AV-1451) tau positron emission tomography. *Sci. Rep.* **2023**, *13*, 8096. [CrossRef] [PubMed]
20. Tajammal, T.; Khurshid, S.; Jaleel, A.; Wahla, S.Q.; Ziar, R.A. Deep Learning-Based Ensembling Technique to Classify Alzheimer's Disease Stages Using Functional MRI. *J. Healthc. Eng.* **2023**, *2023*, 6961346 [CrossRef] [PubMed]
21. Liu, S.; Masurkar, A.; Rusinek, H.; Chen, J.; Zhang, B.; Zhu, W.; Fernandez-Granda, C.; Razavian, N. Generalizable deep learning model for early Alzheimer's disease detection from structural MRIs. *Sci. Rep.* **2022**, *12*, 17106. [CrossRef] [PubMed]
22. O'Malley, T.; Bursztein, E.; Long, J.; Chollet, F.; Jin, H.; Invernizzi, L. KerasTuner. 2019. Available online: https://github.com/keras-team/keras-tuner (accessed on 1 August 2023).
23. Simonyan, K.; Zisserman, A. Very deep convolutional networks for large-scale image recognition. *arXiv* **2014**, arXiv:1409.1556.
24. Hong, D.; Gao, L.; Yao, J.; Zhang, B.; Plaza, A.; Chanussot, J. Graph convolutional networks for hyperspectral image classification. *IEEE Trans. Geosci. Remote. Sens.* **2020**, *59*, 5966–5978. [CrossRef]
25. Selvaraju, R.R.; Cogswell, M.; Das, A.; Vedantam, R.; Parikh, D.; Batra, D. Grad-cam: Visual explanations from deep networks via gradient-based localization. In Proceedings of the IEEE International Conference On Computer Vision, Venice, Italy, 22–29 October 2017; pp. 618–626.
26. Duchi, J.; Hazan, E.; Singer, Y. Adaptive subgradient methods for online learning and stochastic optimization. *J. Mach. Learn. Res.* **2011**, *12*, 2121–2159.
27. Ioffe, S.; Szegedy, C. Batch normalization: Accelerating deep network training by reducing internal covariate shift. In Proceedings of the International Conference on Machine Learning, PMLR, Lille, France, 6–11 July 2015; pp. 448–456.
28. Kumar, N. ADNI-Extracted-Axial. 2021. Available online: https://www.kaggle.com/ds/1830702 (accessed on 10 August 2023).
29. Gupta, Y.; Lama, R.K.; Kwon, G.R.; Initiative, A.D.N. Prediction and classification of Alzheimer's disease based on combined features from apolipoprotein-E genotype, cerebrospinal fluid, MR, and FDG-PET imaging biomarkers. *Front. Comput. Neurosci.* **2019**, *13*, 72. [CrossRef] [PubMed]
30. Payan, A.; Montana, G. Predicting Alzheimer's disease: A neuroimaging study with 3D convolutional neural networks. *arXiv* **2015**, arXiv:1502.02506.
31. Khvostikov, A.; Aderghal, K.; Benois-Pineau, J.; Krylov, A.; Catheline, G. 3D CNN-based classification using sMRI and MD-DTI images for Alzheimer disease studies. *arXiv* **2018**, arXiv:1801.05968.
32. Valliani, A.; Soni, A. Deep residual nets for improved Alzheimer's diagnosis. In Proceedings of the 8th ACM International Conference on Bioinformatics, Computational Biology, and Health Informatics, Boston, MA, USA, 20–23 August 2017; p. 615.
33. Helaly, H.; Badawy, M.; Haikal, A. Deep learning approach for early detection of Alzheimer's disease. *Cogn. Comput.* **2021**, *14*, 1711–1727. [CrossRef] [PubMed]

Disclaimer/Publisher's Note: The statements, opinions and data contained in all publications are solely those of the individual author(s) and contributor(s) and not of MDPI and/or the editor(s). MDPI and/or the editor(s) disclaim responsibility for any injury to people or property resulting from any ideas, methods, instructions or products referred to in the content.

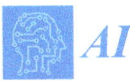

Review

AI and Face-Driven Orthodontics: A Scoping Review of Digital Advances in Diagnosis and Treatment Planning

Juraj Tomášik [1,*], Márton Zsoldos [2], Ľubica Oravcová [1], Michaela Lifková [3], Gabriela Pavleová [1], Martin Strunga [1] and Andrej Thurzo [1,*]

1 Department of Orthodontics, Regenerative and Forensic Dentistry, Faculty of Medicine, Comenius University in Bratislava, 81102 Bratislava, Slovakia; gabriela.pavleova@fmed.uniba.sk (G.P.); martin.strunga@fmed.uniba.sk (M.S.)
2 Department of Orthodontics and Pediatric Dentistry, Faculty of Dentistry, University of Szeged, H-6720 Szeged, Hungary; zsoldos.marton@stoma.szote.u-szeged.hu
3 Department of Stomatology and Maxillofacial Surgery, Faculty of Medicine, Comenius University in Bratislava, 81250 Bratislava, Slovakia
* Correspondence: juraj.tomasik@fmed.uniba.sk (J.T.); andrej.thurzo@uniba.sk (A.T.)

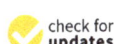

Citation: Tomášik, J.; Zsoldos, M.; Oravcová, Ľ.; Lifková, M.; Pavleová, G.; Strunga, M.; Thurzo, A. AI and Face-Driven Orthodontics: A Scoping Review of Digital Advances in Diagnosis and Treatment Planning. AI 2024, 5, 158–176. https://doi.org/10.3390/ai5010009

Academic Editor: Tim Hulsen

Received: 26 November 2023
Revised: 29 December 2023
Accepted: 3 January 2024
Published: 5 January 2024

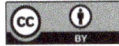

Copyright: © 2024 by the authors. Licensee MDPI, Basel, Switzerland. This article is an open access article distributed under the terms and conditions of the Creative Commons Attribution (CC BY) license (https://creativecommons.org/licenses/by/4.0/).

Abstract: In the age of artificial intelligence (AI), technological progress is changing established workflows and enabling some basic routines to be updated. In dentistry, the patient's face is a crucial part of treatment planning, although it has always been difficult to grasp in an analytical way. This review highlights the current digital advances that, thanks to AI tools, allow us to implement facial features beyond symmetry and proportionality and incorporate facial analysis into diagnosis and treatment planning in orthodontics. A Scopus literature search was conducted to identify the topics with the greatest research potential within digital orthodontics over the last five years. The most researched and cited topic was artificial intelligence and its applications in orthodontics. Apart from automated 2D or 3D cephalometric analysis, AI finds its application in facial analysis, decision-making algorithms as well as in the evaluation of treatment progress and retention. Together with AI, other digital advances are shaping the face of today's orthodontics. Without any doubts, the era of "old" orthodontics is at its end, and modern, face-driven orthodontics is on the way to becoming a reality in modern orthodontic practices.

Keywords: artificial intelligence; 3D printing; face scan; CBCT; facial analysis; treatment evaluation; treatment planning

1. Introduction

Modern orthodontics (orthodontics of the 21st century) has been shifting from "occlusion-driven" to "face-driven". The term "soft tissues paradigm" emerged at the end of the 20th century and stressed the importance to approach each patient requiring any kind of orthodontic treatment as an individual with a specific appearance, a unique facial composition and, last, but not least, their own expectations, while putting the aesthetics in focus [1]. In contrast, the Angle paradigm considered the ideal dental occlusion as paramount. In so doing, the role of soft tissues was completely disregarded or, at best, understated. With ever-evolving digital technologies and artificial intelligence, as well as established aesthetic rules and guidelines based on the assessment of anatomy, physiognomy and natural aesthetic parameters, the advent of advanced diagnostic methods as well as novel treatment modalities is underway [2].

Traditionally, an orthodontic treatment plan was based purely on hard tissue relationships as diagnosed using dental cast models and 2D cephalometric X-ray analyses [3]. At the end of the 20th century, the cone-beam CT (CBCT), consisting of a cone-shaped beam of X-rays and a reciprocating detector rotating around the patient, was introduced, which enabled obtaining 3D images with lower radiation doses compared to conventional CT scans [4]. With the increasing availability of cameras (especially digital cameras), taking intraoral and extraoral pictures before and after treatment has become a part of orthodontic documentation to help assess the impact of treatment on patients' dental arches and—to some extent—on their facial appearance. However, there are some limitations to the two-dimensional "reality". Three- and four-dimensional imaging methods have been developed to compensate for the missing depth in standard pictures. Active stereophotogrammetry is based on the analysis of a detected image that is projected on the scanned object. Passive stereophotogrammetry merges multiple pictures from different angles and computes one 3D object [5]. Adding the element of time to diagnostics allows for more detailed analyses, e.g., in cases of patients suffering from a cleft lip and/or palate or with facial asymmetries, while age is also an important diagnostic factor [6,7].

Intraoral scanning, laser scanning, cone-beam CT (CBCT), stereophotogrammetry and 3D images form a crucial part of modern orthodontics. Despite the fact that these technologies have their limitations and drawbacks, 3D technologies are taking the lead, especially in more complex cases [8]. They provide detailed and realistic input data to diagnostic and treatment-planning software [9–11]. Data from intraoral and/or facial scanners can combine with CBCT scans in order to allow for a better understanding of underlying clinical conditions [12,13]. Artificial intelligence allows for automatic cephalometric tracing that is both precise and accurate, thus making treatment planning more time-efficient [14,15]. The analysis of 3D images obtained from facial 3D scanners can be automatised using curvature maps and sagittal profile analyses [16]. Furthermore, intraoral scanners feed data into specific software that allows for planning changes in teeth positions, the shape of dental arches and interdental relations. Linking such software to various manufacturers of dental aligners completes the circle of a fully digital workflow in orthodontic treatment planning [17,18]. Modern protocols using pre- and post-treatment intraoral scans and an initial pretreatment CBCT scan can accurately predict the final post-treatment position of roots, thus eliminating the need of repeated X-ray exposure [12]. Even though the radiation dose of modern CBCT scanners is lower nowadays compared to the use of cephalostat in the past, following the ALARA (as low as reasonably achievable) principle, each CBCT scan acquisition should be well justified, even more so in treating growing patients [12,19,20]. As an alternative, MRI scans can be used in some patients (e.g., with craniofacial disorders); however, these remain inferior for orthodontic cephalometric analysis [21]. In a similar manner, digital photography alone can be used, to some extent, for landmark identification and facial analysis to alleviate the need of more invasive investigations [22,23].

Information technology has been applied in orthodontics for many decades. Extracting distances and angles from standardised cephalography and/or taking measurements on dental plaster models leads to the quantification of data. These can be further processed, which allows for the objective diagnosis of malocclusions based on various indices and standards [24]. Artificial intelligence (AI) has received much attention over the last few years. The term refers to such intelligent behaviour of computers that mimics the performance of humans in tasks related to cognition [25]. AI can be divided into two categories when it comes to its application in medicine: virtual AI, which includes electronic health record systems or systems assisting in treatment decisions, including surgical interventions, and predictive models in the disease state; on the other hand, physical AI concerns various "smart" prostheses, smart biomedical implants for health monitoring or robot-assisted surgeries [17,26–29]. Regarding AI-assisted decision making, it is necessary to emphasise that, whereas evidence-based dentistry drives dental professionals' daily decisions, machine-learning models learn from human expertise, and thus AI can serve as a good advisor that absorbs all relevant information available [30]. This might be of added value for less-experienced clinicians; however, some authors stress the need for an individualised approach granted by the human factor [31,32].

It has become clear that AI algorithms and the future of evidence-based orthodontics are inextricably interwoven. With the huge amount of digital data available, AI is expected to be a key player in yielding novel findings, which will ultimately lead to a treatment planning and diagnosis revolution in the future [33]. The aim of this paper is to identify the most-cited articles on digital advances within the field of orthodontics as ranked by the field-weighted citation impact ratio provided by Scopus, and to discuss the most-cited technologies in the context of modern orthodontics and dentistry.

2. Materials and Methods

This scoping review investigates the scope of current research on the use of digital technologies in facially driven orthodontic treatment. A literature search was conducted using the Scopus search engine to identify existing relevant studies: articles, reviews, conference papers and short surveys. The search was limited to papers written in English and published in years 2018–2023. The keywords used for the search were "orthodontics", "digital technologies", "facial analysis", "treatment planning", "stereophotogrammetry", "CBCT", "3D", "4D", "intraoral scan", "facial scan", "soft tissue analysis", "artificial intelligence" and "AI". The search query was as follows:

((orthodontics) AND (digital AND technologies) AND (facial AND analysis) AND ((treatment) AND ((planning) OR (plan)))) AND ((stereophotogrammetry) OR (cbct) OR (3d) OR (4d) OR (intraoral AND scan) OR (facial AND scan) OR (soft AND tissue AND analysis) OR (artificial AND intelligence) OR (ai)) AND PUBYEAR > 2017 AND PUBYEAR < 2024 AND TITLE-ABS-KEY (orthodontics)

Since the objective of this scoping review was to assess the trends of using modern technologies in facially driven orthodontic diagnosis and treatment planning, the goal was to identify the most-cited research in the relevant field and to assess the technologies studied therein. The field-weighted citation impact (FWCI) ratio within the Scopus search engine was used to identify the most-cited articles within the field. Because the aim of this review was to identify novel digital methods, the search was modified to identify articles written from 2018 to 2023. To ensure the searched articles were directly linked to orthodontics, the term "Orthodontics" needed to be included within the title, abstract or keywords.

The titles and abstracts of the searched articles were screened and relevant articles were checked for their FWCI value to identify the top twenty articles. Based on the content of these articles, focus areas to be discussed were identified.

3. Results

The search was carried out on 31 October 2023 at 1:47 pm. The search query yielded 147 results. After selecting only articles, reviews, conference papers and short surveys written in English, the number of papers dropped to 133. Their distributions with regard to the year of publication, subject area and document type are depicted in Figures 1–3, respectively.

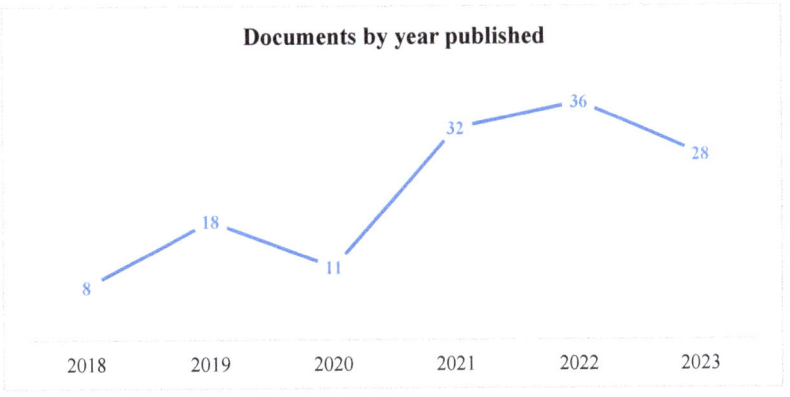

Figure 1. Number of searched documents per year from 2018 to 2023.

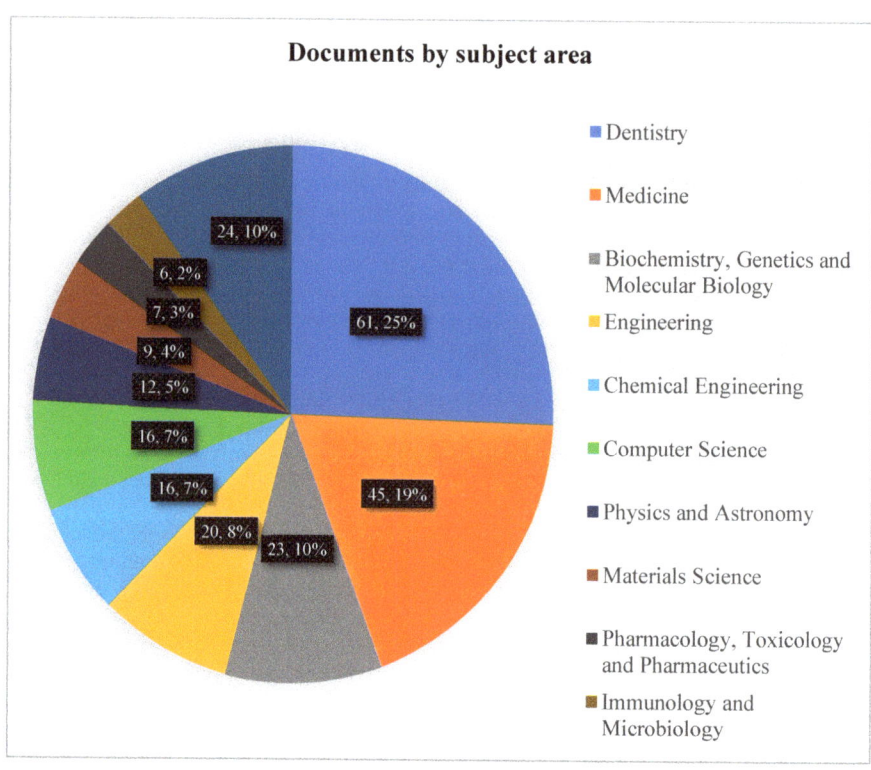

Figure 2. Distribution of searched documents within various subject areas.

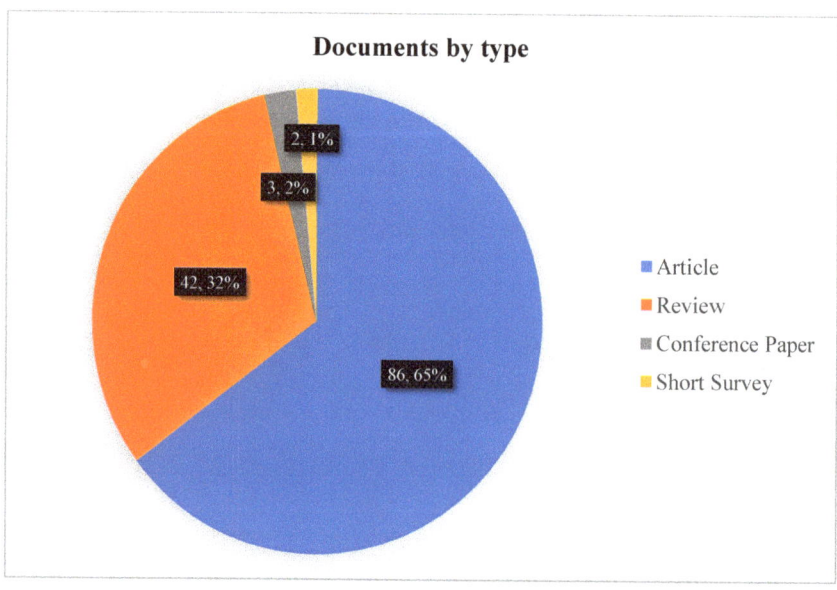

Figure 3. Proportion of various types of searched documents.

The greatest number of searched articles ($n = 36$) was published in 2022, whereas the smallest number ($n = 8$) was published in 2018. More than a quarter of all documents (25.5%) were published with a primary focus on dentistry, followed by medicine (18.8%), biochemistry, genetics and molecular biology (9.6%), engineering and chemical engineering (8.4% and 6.7%, respectively) and computer science (6.7%). The subject matter of the remaining fifty-eight documents varied from social sciences to material science. The largest proportion of searched documents (64.7%, $n = 86$) were articles, followed by reviews (31.6%, $n = 42$).

Based on the titles and abstracts, papers that were not relevant to the studied topic were excluded, which downsized the number from 133 to 101. Only sixty-nine articles had their FWCI value calculated. Table 1 lists twenty articles with the highest FWCI values.

Table 1. Top twenty most-cited articles relevant to the search query.

#	Title	Authors	Year	Main Focus	FWCI
1	A comparison between stereophotogrammetry and smartphone structured light technology for three-dimensional face scanning [34]	D'Ettorre, Giorgio; Farronato, Marco; Candida, Ettore; Quinzi, Vincenzo; Grippaudo, Cristina	2022	Face scanning	15.68
2	Deep convolutional neural network-based automated segmentation and classification of teeth with orthodontic brackets on cone-beam computed-Tomographic images: A validation study [35]	Ayidh Alqahtani, Khalid; Jacobs, Reinhilde; Smolders, Andreas; Van Gerven, Adriaan; Willems, Holger; Shujaat, Sohaib; Shaheen, Eman	2023	AI	13.2
3	Artificial intelligence in dentistry—A review [30]	Ding, Hao; Wu, Jiamin; Zhao, Wuyuan; Matinlinna, Jukka P.; Burrow, Michael F.; Tsoi, James K. H.	2023	AI	10.92
4	Artificial Intelligence: Applications in orthognathic surgery [36]	Bouletreau P.; Makaremi M.; Ibrahim B.; Louvrier A.; Sigaux N.	2019	AI	10.67
5	Where Is the Artificial Intelligence Applied in Dentistry? Systematic Review and Literature Analysis [37]	Thurzo, Andrej; Urbanová, Wanda; Novák, B.; Czako, Ladislav; Siebert, Tomáš; Stano; Mareková, Simona; Fountoulaki, Georgia; Kosnáčová, Helena; Varga, Ivan	2022	AI	5.83
6	Current concepts in orthognathic surgery [38]	Naran, Sanjay; Steinbacher, Derek M.; Taylor, Jesse A.	2018	Digital planning	5.62
7	Current state of the art in the use of augmented reality in dentistry: A systematic review of the literature [39]	Farronato, Marco; Maspero, Cinzia; Lanteri, Valentina; Fama, Andrea; Ferrati, Francesco; Pettenuzzo, Alessandro; Farronato, Davide	2019	Augmented reality	5.26
8	Machine learning in orthodontics: Automated facial analysis of vertical dimension for increased precision and efficiency [40]	Rousseau, Maxime; Retrouvey, Jean-Marc	2022	AI	5.22
9	Artificial Intelligence Systems Assisting in the Assessment of the Course and Retention of Orthodontic Treatment [41]	Strunga, Martin; Urban, Renáta; Surovková, Jana; Thurzo, Andrej	2023	AI	4.97
10	A Review of 3D Printing in Dentistry: Technologies, Affecting Factors, and Applications [42]	Tian, Yueyi; Chen, ChunXu; Xu, Xiaotong; Wang, Jiayin; Hou, Xingyu; Li, Kelun; Lu, Xinyue; Shi, HaoYu; Lee, Eui-Seok; Jiang, Heng Bo	2021	3D printing	4.51

Table 1. Cont.

#	Title	Authors	Year	Main Focus	FWCI
11	Scope and performance of artificial intelligence technology in orthodontic diagnosis, treatment planning, and clinical decision-making—A systematic review [43]	Khanagar, Sanjeev B.; Al-Ehaideb, Ali; Vishwanathaiah, Satish; Maganur, Prabhadevi C.; Patil, Shankargouda; Naik, Sachin; Baeshen, Hosam A.; Sarode, Sachin S.	2021	AI	4.47
12	Machine learning and orthodontics, current trends and the future opportunities: A scoping review [44]	Mohammad-Rahimi, Hossein; Nadimi, Mohadeseh; Rohban, Mohammad Hossein; Shamsoddin, Erfan; Lee, Victor Y.; Motamedian, Saeed Reza	2021	AI	4.02
13	The last decade in orthodontics: A scoping review of the hits, misses and the near misses! [45]	Gandedkar, Narayan H.; Vaid, Nikhilesh R.; Darendeliler, M. Ali; Premjani, Pratik; Ferguson, Donald J.	2019	3D printing	3.82
14	Advancements in Dentistry with Artificial Intelligence: Current Clinical Applications and Future Perspectives [46]	Fatima, Anum; Shafi, Imran; Afzal, Hammad; Díez, Isabel De La Torre; Lourdes, Del Rio-Solá M.; Breñosa, Jose; Espinosa, Julio César Martínez; Ashraf, Imran	2022	AI	3.59
15	Three-dimensional prediction of roots position through cone-beam computed tomography scans-digital model superimposition: A novel method [12]	Staderini, Edoardo,; Guglielmi, Federica; Cornelis, Marie A.; Cattaneo, Paolo M.	2019	CBCT, intraoral scanning	3.46
16	Augmented reality in dentistry: a current perspective [47]	Kwon, Ho-Beom; Park, Young-Seok; Han, Jung-Suk	2018	Augmented reality	2.83
17	Decoding Deep Learning applications for diagnosis and treatment planning [48]	Retrouvey, Jean-Marc; Conley, Richard Scott	2022	AI	2.35
18	Smartphone-Based Facial Scanning as a Viable Tool for Facially Driven Orthodontics? [49]	Thurzo, Andrej; Strunga, Martin; Havlínová, Romana; Reháková, Katarína; Urban, Renata; Surovková, Jana; Kurilová, Veronika	2022	Face scan	2.19
19	Effectiveness of a Novel 3D-Printed Nasoalveolar Molding Appliance (D-NAM) on Improving the Maxillary Arch Dimensions in Unilateral Cleft Lip and Palate Infants: A Randomized Controlled Trial [50]	Abd El-Ghafour, Mohamed; Aboulhassan, Mamdouh A.; Fayed, Mona M. Salah; El-Beialy, Amr Ragab; Eid, Faten Hussein Kamel; Hegab, Seif El-Din; El-Gendi, Mahmoud; Emara, Dawlat	2020	3D printing	2.18
20	Radiomics and Machine Learning in Oral Healthcare [51]	Leite, André Ferreira; Vasconcelos, Karla de Faria; Willems, Holger; Jacobs, Reinhilde	2020	AI	2.05

Figure 4 depicts the proportion of the primary areas of interest of the top twenty articles ranked by FWCI values. More than half ($n = 11$) of the selected articles focused on artificial intelligence, while three articles studied or reviewed 3D printing and its application in orthodontics, two articles researched facial scanning, two articles were devoted to augmented reality, one article focused on digital planning in orthodontics and one article was about merging CBCT with intraoral scans.

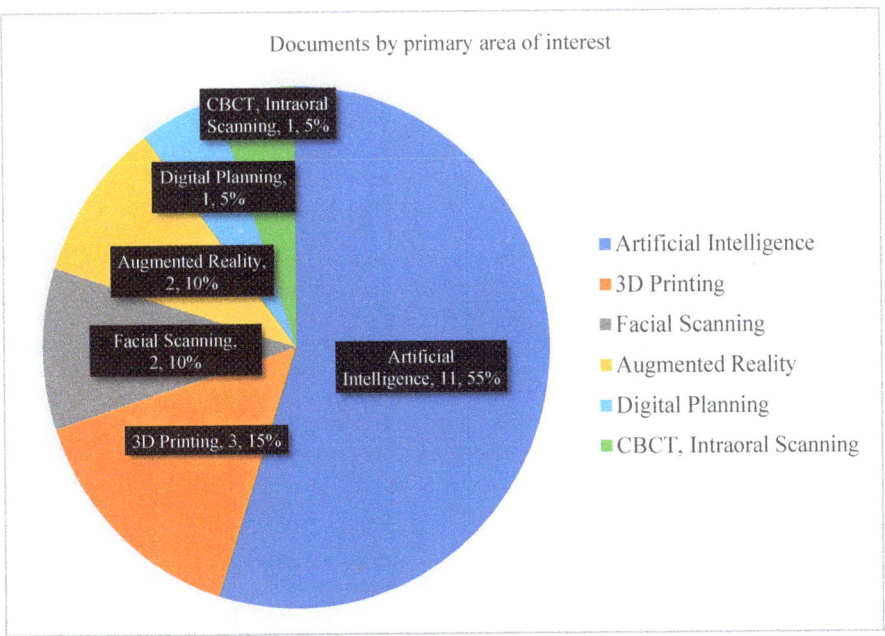

Figure 4. Number of most-cited documents by their primary area of interest.

The results of this scoping review of the recent literature (2018–2023) on the application of digital technologies in orthodontics identified the most relevant articles based on the field-weighted citation impact (FWCI) metric.

The top three digital technologies with the highest research potential were identified as: artificial intelligence (AI), 3D printing and facial scanning. AI has been used in a variety of applications in orthodontics, including cephalometric analysis, facial analysis, treatment planning and patient monitoring. Three-dimensional printing has been used to fabricate orthodontic appliances, surgical guides and aligners. Facial scanning has been used to collect the 3D data of patients' faces, which can be used for diagnosis, treatment planning and aesthetic evaluation.

4. Discussion

Artificial intelligence, 3D printing and facial scanning are the three digital technologies with the greatest research potential, as shown by the FWCI values of the researched articles. In the sections below, their use in orthodontics, as well as the limitations of this scoping review, are discussed.

4.1. Artificial Intelligence Tools and Datasets

Based on the literature search, it seems that radiology is the medical specialty that benefits the most from AI technologies now. A substantial amount of studies focused either on assessing the quality of obtained images or even on identifying CT, MRI scans and X-rays that showed no pathologies [52,53]. On the other hand, AI techniques can also detect pathological processes, e.g., dental caries on radiographs, with an increasing level of accuracy [54].

AI and machine learning—a part of AI that enables machines to expand their capabilities by self-adapting algorithms—find application in various fields within orthodontics [55]. Orthodontists, residents as well as general dentists could use artificial intelligence in diagnosis, decision making, treatment planning as well as patient monitoring. There is an AI functionality that determines the quality of 2D cephalometric X-rays, which could eliminate lower-quality X-rays from being further evaluated due to a possible distortion of the analysis [56]. On top of that, machine learning has found use in both lateral and 3D cephalogram analysis to provide ever-improving quality in landmark localisation [57,58].

Current studies on combining radiomics- and AI-based analysis with a radiologist's input in the field of dentomaxillofacial imaging seem very promising, and it seems that the paradigm shift will have a prominent impact on daily clinical practice as well as curricula in dental schools [51]. What is more, recent research showed that healthcare professionals would prefer if AI algorithms completely replaced manual and semiautomatic approaches in cephalometry—not only because it allows professionals to be more time-efficient, but also because it could increase the accuracy of obtained analysis results [59].

Nowadays, the question is not whether CBCT scans are accurate, but how automated processes can aid professionals in landmark detection, skeletal classification, scan analysis and CBCT data management [57,58,60,61]. Based on current research, it has been concluded that AI can be of great use in assessing mandibular shape asymmetry as well as in the screening of upper airways to measure multiple parameters [62,63].

Artificial intelligence has become an extensively researched field in the past decade [37]. Apart from CBCT analysis and automated teeth segmentation, AI aids professionals in treatment planning, including decisions on teeth extractions [35,43,44]. Even though recent research shows that the AI technology in the abovementioned areas, as well as in determining the degree of cervical vertebra maturation and the prediction of postoperative facial attractiveness, performs exceptionally well, and in its precision and accuracy is comparable to trained professionals, more studies are expected to elucidate and further discuss all the advantages and disadvantages of this novel technology [43,64,65]. It is highly probable that, in a few years, the advantages of AI applications (not only) in orthodontics will be indisputable. The professional opinion shifts depending on the data, experience and evidence. After all, it was only a few years ago that some authors claimed that a lateral cephalogram is more precise and accurate than a 3D CBCT scan [66]. Nobody argues for that now. One of the means of making AI more believable could be demystifying the AI algorithms ("the black box") and making them comprehensible to humans, which may become quite challenging—especially with the ever-increasing complexity of used algorithms [67]. Another way of ensuring trust towards an AI algorithm is its robustness, i.e., good practice in plentiful varied subject populations [68].

AI finds its application at all levels of decision-making processes in orthodontics and medicine (e.g., in such specialties as radiotherapy): data collection, storage, management, processing in-depth analysis, communication and education [69,70]. In-depth analysis also includes automated facial analysis and the use of AI in spotting craniofacial deformities and syndromes on facial scans, and even predicting diseases [27,36,40,48]. There has been some research on scoring facial attractiveness in relation to facial proportions and profiles [71,72]. It is likely that AI will soon enough enable automated aesthetic evaluation, smile design and treatment planning [2]. Based on machine-learning algorithms, given pretreatment variables, AI can successfully predict the duration of an orthodontic treatment [73]. Apart from that, dental monitoring software that uses AI has proven effective during the treatment phase to track progress, as well as during the retention phase to detect relapse and assess the stability of treatment outcomes, with the benefit of assessing the compliance of patients even without regular in-office visits [41]. After all, the goal of modern technologies is to make dental care high-quality, smooth, time-efficient and cost-effective, with improved treatment planning as well as risk management, and AI certainly adds up to that [46,74,75].

AI has found application in human genome sequencing and in analysing large volumes of data that provide priceless information on various biological processes. Information regarding genes that scientists are still gathering and figuring out will play a crucial role in the transition towards a truly personalised medicine. These so-called omics records will likely become an integral part of orthodontic medical records that will be routinely used in diagnosis and treatment planning. It is, therefore, crucial to update orthodontic residency programs, for one needs to adapt and evolve to provide orthodontic care of the highest quality [76].

AI algorithms are currently used for automatic landmark identification, cephalometric analysis, the staging of skeletal maturation, facial recognition and the detection of syndromes, the automatic segmentation of CBCT scans and predicting the need for orthognathic surgery or extractions, and more. The diapason of recent research demonstrates that the accuracy of the discussed technologies is clinically acceptable, rendering them extremely useful in orthodontic practice [77–86]. Recent developments in the area of automated 3D landmarking has led to accuracy improvements [87]. Despite that, some authors emphasise that human intervention is still needed to minimise errors in automatic cephalometric analysis [88]. To eliminate that, more research is needed to increase both the precision and accuracy of AI algorithms. Furthermore, demystifying and explaining how AI works would very much add to its believability.

The rapid advancement of AI has led to the development of numerous AI tools, each with its unique capabilities and applications in orthodontics. These tools can be broadly classified into three categories: supervised learning, unsupervised learning and reinforcement learning.

Supervised learning algorithms are trained on labelled data, where the correct output for each input is known. This type of learning is well-suited for tasks such as cephalometric analysis, where the goal is to identify landmarks and measure facial dimensions. Popular supervised learning algorithms in orthodontics include support vector machines, random forests and neural networks.

Unsupervised learning algorithms are trained on unlabelled data, where the goal is to uncover patterns or structure in the data without the guidance of labelled examples. This type of learning is useful for tasks such as facial recognition and the detection of syndromes, where the focus is on identifying patterns that distinguish between different facial features. Common unsupervised learning algorithms in orthodontics include k-means clustering, principal component analysis and autoencoders.

Reinforcement learning algorithms interact with an environment to maximise a reward signal. This type of learning is well-suited for tasks such as treatment planning, where the goal is to optimise the outcome of orthodontic treatment. Popular reinforcement learning algorithms in orthodontics include deep Q-learning and policy gradient methods.

The choice of AI tool depends on the specific task at hand and the available data. For instance, supervised learning algorithms are typically used for tasks where there is a large amount of labelled data, while unsupervised learning algorithms are more suitable for tasks where there is less labelled data or where the goal is to uncover patterns rather than make predictions. Reinforcement learning algorithms are particularly well-suited for tasks that involve sequential decision making, such as treatment planning.

The quality and quantity of data used to train AI algorithms play a crucial role in the accuracy and performance of those algorithms. In orthodontics, datasets can be obtained from various sources, including cephalometric X-rays, 3D CBCT scans, facial photographs and clinical records.

The evaluation of AI algorithms in orthodontics typically involves measuring their accuracy and precision on a held-out test dataset. Accuracy measures the proportion of predictions that are correct, while precision measures the proportion of positive predictions that are correct. Additional metrics that are often used to evaluate AI algorithms in orthodontics include:

F1-score: A weighted harmonic mean of the accuracy and precision.

ROC–AUC: The area under the receiver operating characteristic curve, which measures the ability of an algorithm to distinguish between positive and negative examples.

Sensitivity: The proportion of true positives that are correctly identified.

Specificity: The proportion of true negatives that are correctly identified.

By carefully selecting AI tools, training them on high-quality datasets and evaluating their performance on rigorous benchmarks, orthodontists can harness the power of AI to revolutionise the field of orthodontics.

A persisting issue when it comes to AI is data protection and safety.

4.2. Three-Dimensional Printing

In contrast to subtractive manufacturing (also called milling processes) that give rise to objects by removing excesses from a chunk of material, additive manufacturing (three-dimensional printing) is a process that creates objects by adding material layer-by-layer. In dentistry, 3D printing finds its application in maxillofacial surgery, implantology, prosthodontics and orthodontics. Metals (e.g., titanium), ceramics (e.g., zirconia), polymers (e.g., polylactic acid—PLA, polyetheretherketone—PEEK) and hydrogels (e.g., gelatine methacryloyl-based hydrogel, hyaluronic acid) are used for 3D-printing purposes. More recently, (bio)printing that uses cells, matrices and growth factors to produce tissues, such as tooth, jawbone and periodontal tissues, has achieved more and more attention. Various methods are used in 3D printing: stereolithography, laser-based techniques, electron beam melting, fused deposition modelling, laminated object manufacturing and inkjet printing [89]. Just like everything else, 3D-printing technologies have both advantages and disadvantages. The disadvantages include a high cost and rather time-demanding postprocessing. Undoubtedly, the advantages include the high yield of materials used, the possibility to fabricate complex structures and the high precision and accuracy of 3D-printed objects [42,90].

Orthodontics and orthognathic surgery have been transformed by 3D-printing methods. Additive manufacturing is used to fabricate study models, clear aligners (direct printing or using 3D-printed models), surgical guides of any kind (including guides for mini-implant insertions), components for fixed or removable appliances and occlusal splints [18]. It seems that having highly individualised lingual appliances have the added value of excellent outcomes [32,91]. In the same manner, there have been attempts to promote in-office custom-made brackets for vestibular appliances [92]. In patients with unilateral complete cleft lip and palate, a 3D-printed nasoalveolar moulding appliance was used prior to surgery to achieve better treatment results [50].

Considering all aspects of additive manufacturing, it seems reasonable to state that it will be used increasingly in individualised orthodontics, regenerative dentistry, implantology and maxillofacial surgery. Therefore, both the knowledge and skills necessary for mastering digital workflow in daily practice need to be cultivated in pre- and postgraduate students, residents as well as specialists. In order to provide patients with quality care, dental curricula and elective courses must respond to technological advances without any delay [93,94].

4.3. Facial Scanning

One of the most popular topics in the current research on digital technologies used in orthodontics is facial scanning. As with other novel diagnostic or therapeutic methods, one needs to first step out of their comfort zone to start considering them, then study the evidence behind them and decide to move on with current trends and technological developments in clinical settings. Proper theoretical background and some practical experience prior to approaching patients are essential to eliminate possible errors due to a total lack of expertise. This is where modernised formal education, lectures, study groups and various practical courses play an indispensable role [93].

The key prerequisite for digital transformation is the purpose of the change. It was noted that progress for the sake of progress is not wise. Reliability, accuracy and time-efficiency are some of the measures that might drive the change. Facial scans obtained using the 3D light scanner Artec Eva were compared to direct craniofacial measurements using a calliper. The study showed the excellent accuracy of the digital workflow. However, the digital method required twice as much time compared to the direct method [95].

Multiple studies have evaluated less-pricey devices in terms of the accuracy and reliability. Stereophotogrammetry seems to have great potential as an alternative to laser scanning in medical practice [96]. Based on a meta-analysis, professional 3D scanning systems are more precise than current facial scanning software in smart portable devices [8]. However, the differences seem to be clinically acceptable [97]. Kinect devices offer a low-cost 3D imaging technique that can be used in orthodontics and/or surgical planning [98]. The Bellus3D and Capture applications seem promising when compared to the method of stereophotogrammetry carried out by a 3dMD system; however, they require much more patience on the patient's side, as both the capturing and processing times are considerably greater [34]. Another study compared Bellus3D captures and facial surfaces segmented from CBCT scans. The authors concluded that there is some clinical applicability of Bellus3D in orthodontics; however, current technologies have their limitations when it comes to accuracy [49]. More studies are needed to showcase to what extent the differences between various face-scanning systems influence clinical outcomes and how they correlate with pre- and post-treatment CBCT scans. One such study did not show that acquisition technologies play a major role in measurement variations [99].

A question remains: Can we reconstruct faces using already-taken pictures? The process of creating 3D faces from 2D pictures is validated, as the acquired measurements are clinically acceptable. Nonetheless, this process is time- and labour-demanding [100].

With no doubts, the advantage of this radiation-free diagnostic tool needs to be emphasised, especially for growing subjects. Research shows that facial scans and subsequent soft tissue analyses can be used for the evaluation of extraction or orthognathic surgery outcomes with both sufficient reproducibility and reliability [101,102].

This paper highlighted the potential of AI to revolutionise the domains to which it is applied. The analysis demonstrates the versatility and adaptability of this technology. For example, in the case of bioelectronics, AI is helping to overcome the challenges associated with material development, fabrication processes and system integration. Similarly, in orthodontics, AI is enabling facial analysis to go beyond mere symmetry and proportionality, providing a more comprehensive understanding of facial structure and its impact on dental alignment. AI empowers the tailoring of treatment strategies to individual patient needs. AI can personalise device design and selection based on patient-specific characteristics in bioelectronics. In orthodontics, AI-driven facial analysis can identify unique facial features and optimise treatment plans accordingly. Data-driven decision making is fundamental for guiding AI-based decision-making processes. In bioelectronics, AI algorithms analyse vast amounts of data to identify patterns and optimise device performance. Similarly, facial analysis tools in orthodontics rely on patient data, such as 2D or 3D scans, to generate insights for treatment planning [103].

4.4. Limitations of the Paper

For this scoping review, only one search engine was used. Scopus was chosen because of the quality metrics it provides. The field-weighted citation impact (FWCI) of a paper is calculated as a ratio between received citations in a 3-year window after its publication and the expected average of paper citations in the subject field. Unfortunately, papers that may receive a high FWCI score in the coming months and/or years did not rank high in our search because their FWCI has not been calculated yet or was lower compared to older papers, only because of the time factor. To eliminate this, only articles older than 3 years could have been considered. However, had the search been carried out that way, the majority of articles would have been eliminated and our results would not have been valid, only because the point of finding the most researchable digital technologies in orthodontics would have been missed. There was a steep incline in the number of published articles corresponding to our search query from the year 2020 onwards, and so this trend should not be disregarded.

Despite the endeavour to propose the most suitable search query based on the current literature, it is possible that some novel digital technologies and applications of AI in orthodontics were not mentioned at all. As a consequence, some high-quality papers may have been potentially missed.

While reading the abstracts and titles of all searched articles, a human error needs to be accounted for. This is why there were two reviewers, each performing the literature search twice—one week apart.

Some searched papers, albeit interesting and seemingly relevant, did not have any relation to orthodontics and thus were excluded from the final list. In a similar manner, it might be possible that some relevant papers were not listed by the search engine in the original search and thus were not found.

Only papers written in English were studied. Papers written in other languages ($n = 10$) were additionally screened and some of them were considered as relevant and intriguing; however, none would have qualified for the top twenty FWCI articles, even if they had been included in the search.

In conclusion, this scoping review acknowledges the limitations of its scope and selection criteria. While the use of Scopus and the FWCI metric provided a valuable framework, the review's focus on English-language publications and the possibility of overlooking novel technologies and applications underscore the need for continued exploration and refinement. As AI continues to evolve in orthodontics, it is imperative to address the challenges and limitations identified in this study to ensure the responsible and effective integration of AI-powered tools into clinical practice. And while AI holds immense potential to revolutionise orthodontics, it is crucial to acknowledge the limitations, current challenges, and potential risks associated with its integration into clinical practice [37].

The current limitations are:

Data dependency: AI algorithms require vast amounts of high-quality data to train and develop their predictive capabilities. In orthodontics, acquiring comprehensive datasets with standardised measurements and clinical outcomes can be challenging due to ethical considerations and the variability of patient presentations.

Interpretability and explainability: The inner workings of complex AI algorithms can be opaque, making it difficult for clinicians to understand the rationale behind their recommendations. This lack of transparency can hinder the development of trust and acceptance among practitioners.

Bias and discrimination: AI algorithms can inherit biases from the data they are trained on. If the training data inadvertently reflect societal or systemic prejudices, these biases can be perpetuated in AI-generated predictions, leading to unfair treatment or misdiagnosis.

Human oversight and decision making: AI should not replace the expertise and judgment of qualified orthodontists. AI tools should serve as assistants, providing data-driven insights and recommendations that complement, not replace, human clinical decision making.

The current problems are:

Limited clinical validation: Many AI-powered orthodontic tools are still in their early stages of development and lack extensive clinical validation. Their effectiveness in real-world settings and their ability to translate into improved patient outcomes require rigorous testing and evaluation.

Interoperability and integration: Integrating AI tools into existing orthodontic workflows and software systems can be challenging. Compatibility issues and the lack of standardised data formats can hinder the seamless integration of AI into clinical practice.

Standardisation and regulatory oversight: Establishing standardised protocols for the development, validation and deployment of AI tools in orthodontics is essential to ensure their safety, efficacy and ethical use. Regulatory oversight and guidelines are needed to ensure compliance with professional standards and patient protection.

The potential risks are:

Overreliance on AI: Overconfidence in AI-generated predictions can lead to complacency and a decreased emphasis on clinical judgment and experience. Practitioners must maintain a critical approach, carefully evaluating AI suggestions and ensuring they align with patient-specific needs and clinical aspects.

Automation of decision making: While AI can assist in decision making, it should not entirely automate the process. Orthodontic treatment planning requires a comprehensive understanding of patient factors, clinical considerations and the nuances of treatment options. Overreliance on AI could diminish the patient-centred aspect of care and reduce the opportunity for shared decision making.

Privacy and data security: AI-powered orthodontic tools often handle sensitive patient data, including images, dental records and personal information. Ensuring the security and privacy of these data is paramount to protect patient confidentiality and prevent unauthorised access or misuse.

AI offers a transformative approach to orthodontics, providing greater accuracy, personalisation and efficiency. While AI should complement and augment human expertise, its integration holds the promise of revolutionising orthodontics and delivering the highest quality care for patients [41]. A comparison of the possibilities of AI with current orthodontic treatment concepts is shown in Table 2.

Table 2. Comparison of the possibilities of AI with current orthodontic treatment concepts.

Feature	Current Orthodontic Treatment Concepts	AI-Powered Orthodontics
Approach	Subjective interpretation and limited data analysis	Objective and data-driven
Diagnosis	Manual assessment of patient records and imaging	AI algorithms analysing digital scans and images
Treatment Planning	Generalised approaches	Personalised treatment plans tailored to individual patients
Monitoring	Periodic checkups	Real-time insights and the prediction of potential issues
Efficiency	Manual tasks and time-consuming assessments	Automation and streamlining of workflows
Outcomes	Potential for misdiagnoses and treatment errors	Improved patient outcomes, increased treatment efficiency and reduced diagnostic errors
Engagement	Limited patient involvement	Enhanced patient understanding and engagement

4.5. Attention-Based Models

Attention-based models and hybrid solutions are increasingly being employed in orthodontics to enhance diagnostic accuracy, treatment planning and patient management. These models leverage the power of deep learning to extract meaningful insights from complex dental data, including images, measurements and patient records.

Attention-based models, in particular, excel at capturing long-range dependencies and contextual relationships within these datasets. This ability is crucial for orthodontic applications, where the intricate relationships between various dental structures and their overall alignment play a critical role in diagnosis and treatment planning [104–108].

Here are some specific examples of how attention-based models and hybrid solutions are being used in orthodontics:

1. Dental image segmentation: Attention-based models can be used to accurately segment and identify specific dental structures in images, such as teeth, alveolar bones and soft tissues. This information can then be used for various purposes, such as measuring tooth positions, assessing periodontal health and predicting orthodontic treatment outcomes.
2. Predicting orthodontic treatment outcomes: Attention-based models can be trained on large datasets of patient records and treatment outcomes to identify patterns and correlations that predict the success of orthodontic treatment. This information can be used to personalise treatment plans and make informed decisions about the treatment duration and complexity.
3. Automated tooth segmentation: Attention-based models can be used to automate the segmentation of teeth in dental images, removing the need for manual segmentation

by orthodontists. This can save time and improve the efficiency of patient diagnosis and treatment planning.
4. Real-time patient monitoring: Attention-based models can be used to analyse real-time data from intraoral cameras or sensors to monitor patient progress and provide feedback to orthodontists. This can help ensure timely interventions and optimise treatment outcomes.
5. Virtual orthodontic simulations: Attention-based models can generate virtual simulations of orthodontic treatment outcomes, allowing orthodontists and patients to visualise the expected changes in tooth positions and facial aesthetics. This can enhance patient understanding and engagement in the treatment process.

The use of attention-based models and hybrid solutions in orthodontics is still in its early stages, but they hold immense promise for improving the accuracy, efficiency and personalisation of orthodontic care. As these technologies continue to evolve, they are expected to play an increasingly important role in the future of dentistry [104–108].

4.6. Current Trends and Future Directions

The digital transformation of orthodontics is rapidly progressing, with AI, 3D printing and facial scanning leading the way. These technologies are not only improving the accuracy and efficiency of diagnostics, treatment planning and patient monitoring, but they are also paving the way for personalised and patient-centric orthodontic care.

Current Trends

AI-powered cephalometry: AI algorithms are being developed to automate the analysis of cephalometric X-rays, 3D CBCT scans and facial photographs. This reduces the time and effort required for manual analysis, leading to more efficient diagnoses and treatment planning.

Real-time patient monitoring: AI-powered dental monitoring software is being used to track patient progress during treatment and detect the early signs of relapse. This is enabling orthodontists to intervene quickly and prevent the treatment from failing.

Three-dimensionally printed orthodontic appliances: Three-dimensional printing is being used to fabricate custom-made orthodontic appliances, such as aligners, retainers and surgical guides. This improves the fit and comfort of appliances, reducing the treatment time and reducing the need for adjustments.

Facial scanning for aesthetic evaluation: AI-powered facial-scanning software is being used to assess facial symmetry, proportion and attractiveness. This is helping orthodontists to create more aesthetically pleasing treatment plans.

Future Directions

AI-powered treatment optimisation: AI algorithms will be used to optimise the timing, sequencing and intensity of orthodontic treatment. This will result in more efficient and effective treatments.

Personalised orthodontic care: AI will be used to create personalised orthodontic treatment plans based on each patient's individual needs and goals. This will create a more patient-centric approach to orthodontic care.

Virtual reality and augmented reality: Virtual reality and augmented reality will be used to provide patients with a more immersive and interactive orthodontic experience. This will help patients to better understand their treatment and participate more actively in the decision-making process.

Data-driven orthodontic research: AI will be used to analyse large datasets of patient data to identify new insights and develop new treatment protocols. This will lead to a better understanding of the causes of malocclusions and more effective treatment methods.

5. Conclusions

The integration of AI, 3D printing and facial scanning into orthodontics is leading to a paradigm shift in the field. These technologies are transforming the way orthodontics is practiced, making it more accurate, efficient and patient-centred. As these technologies continue to develop, they will have an even greater impact on the future of orthodontics.

The integration of AI into orthodontics has opened a new world of possibilities and promises to revolutionise the field and transform patient care. While AI is still at an early stage of development, its potential to improve diagnosis, treatment planning and patient outcomes is undeniable. As AI continues to advance, it is imperative for orthodontists and dental students to keep up-to-date with the latest advancements and develop a solid foundation in digital technologies. This will ensure that orthodontics embraces the power of AI and paves the way for a new era of personalised data-driven care.

This scoping review shows that face-guided (facially driven) orthodontics is on the rise and is part of a complex AI revolution in the field, leading to an unprecedented paradigm shift. AI will make it possible to handle even difficult tasks, such as analysing complex facial features and simulations. We are currently at the beginning of incorporating AI into daily orthodontic practice.

Author Contributions: Conceptualisation, J.T. and A.T.; methodology, J.T. and A.T.; software, J.T.; validation, A.T., M.Z. and Ľ.O.; formal analysis, J.T. and M.Z.; investigation, J.T. and Ľ.O.; resources, J.T. and M.Z.; data curation, J.T. and Ľ.O.; writing—original draft preparation, J.T.; writing—review and editing, M.Z., Ľ.O., M.S., M.L., G.P. and A.T.; visualisation, J.T.; supervision, A.T.; project administration, J.T.; funding acquisition, A.T. All authors have read and agreed to the published version of the manuscript.

Funding: This work was supported by the Slovak Grant Agency for Science (KEGA)—grant no. 054UK-4/2023, and by Slovak Research and Development Agency—grant no. APVV-21-0173.

Institutional Review Board Statement: Not applicable.

Informed Consent Statement: Not applicable.

Data Availability Statement: Not applicable.

Conflicts of Interest: The authors declare no conflicts of interest.

References

1. Proffit, W.R. The Soft Tissue Paradigm in Orthodontic Diagnosis and Treatment Planning: A New View for a New Century. *J. Esthet. Dent.* **2000**, *12*, 46–49. [CrossRef]
2. Blatz, M.B.; Chiche, G.; Bahat, O.; Roblee, R.; Coachman, C.; Heymann, H.O. Evolution of Aesthetic Dentistry. *J. Dent. Res.* **2019**, *98*, 1294–1304. [CrossRef]
3. Sinha, A. Evolving Trends in Orthodontic Imaging for Advance Patient Care. *Indian J. Forensic Med. Toxicol.* **2019**, *13*, 1835–1841. [CrossRef]
4. Nasseh, I.; Al-Rawi, W. Cone Beam Computed Tomography. *Dent. Clin. N. Am.* **2018**, *62*, 361–391. [CrossRef]
5. Thurzo, A.; Jančovičová, V.; Hain, M.; Thurzo, M.; Novák, B.; Kosnáčová, H.; Lehotská, V.; Varga, I.; Kováč, P.; Moravanský, N. Human Remains Identification Using Micro-CT, Chemometric and AI Methods in Forensic Experimental Reconstruction of Dental Patterns after Concentrated Sulphuric Acid Significant Impact. *Molecules* **2022**, *27*, 4346. [CrossRef]
6. Hallac, R.R.; Feng, J.; Kane, A.A.; Seaward, J.R. Dynamic Facial Asymmetry in Patients with Repaired Cleft Lip Using 4D Imaging (Video Stereophotogrammetry). *J. Cranio-Maxillofac. Surg.* **2017**, *45*, 8–12. [CrossRef]
7. Xue, Z.; Wu, L.; Qiu, T.; Li, Z.; Wang, X.; Liu, X. Three-Dimensional Dynamic Analysis of the Facial Movement Symmetry of Skeletal Class III Patients with Facial Asymmetry. *J. Oral Maxillofac. Surg.* **2020**, *78*, 267–274. [CrossRef]
8. Carvalho, P.E.G.; Ortega, A.O.; Maeda, F.A.; da Silva, L.H.; Carvalho, V.G.G.; Torres, F.C. Digital Scanning in Modern Orthodontics. *Curr. Oral Health Rep.* **2019**, *6*, 269–276. [CrossRef]
9. Erten, O.; Yılmaz, B.N. Three-Dimensional Imaging in Orthodontics. *Turk. J. Orthod.* **2018**, *31*, 86–94. [CrossRef]
10. Anistoroaei, D.; Zegan, G.; Golovcencu, L.; Cernei, E.R.; Sodor-Botezatu, A.; Saveanu, I.C. Cone-Beam Computed Tomography-a Useful Tool in Orthodontic Diagnosis. In Proceedings of the 2019 E-Health and Bioengineering Conference (EHB), Iasi, Romania, 21–23 November 2019.
11. Kenkare, P.; Shetty, S.; Mangal, U.; Ashith, M.V.; Shetty, S. The Utilization of Three-Dimensional Technology for an Accurate Diagnosis and Precise Treatment Planning in the Field of Orthodontics. *Biomed. Pharmacol. J.* **2021**, *14*, 2101–2107. [CrossRef]

12. Staderini, E.; Guglielmi, F.; Cornelis, M.A.; Cattaneo, P.M. Three-Dimensional Prediction of Roots Position through Cone-Beam Computed Tomography Scans-Digital Model Superimposition: A Novel Method. *Orthod. Craniofac. Res.* **2019**, *22*, 16–23. [CrossRef]
13. Xiao, Z.; Liu, Z.; Gu, Y. Integration of Digital Maxillary Dental Casts with 3D Facial Images in Orthodontic Patients: A Three-Dimensional Validation Study. *Angle Orthod.* **2020**, *90*, 397–404. [CrossRef]
14. Ahn, J.; Nguyen, T.P.; Kim, Y.-J.; Kim, T.; Yoon, J. Automated Analysis of Three-Dimensional CBCT Images Taken in Natural Head Position That Combines Facial Profile Processing and Multiple Deep-Learning Models. *Comput. Methods Programs Biomed.* **2022**, *226*, 107123. [CrossRef]
15. Tsolakis, I.A.; Tsolakis, A.I.; Elshebiny, T.; Matthaios, S.; Palomo, J.M. Comparing a Fully Automated Cephalometric Tracing Method to a Manual Tracing Method for Orthodontic Diagnosis. *J. Clin. Med.* **2022**, *11*, 6854. [CrossRef]
16. Lippold, C.; Liu, X.; Wangdo, K.; Drerup, B.; Schreiber, K.; Kirschneck, C.; Moiseenko, T.; Danesh, G. Facial Landmark Localization by Curvature Maps and Profile Analysis. *Head Face Med.* **2014**, *10*, 54. [CrossRef]
17. Adel, S.; Zaher, A.; El Harouni, N.; Venugopal, A.; Premjani, P.; Vaid, N. Robotic Applications in Orthodontics: Changing the Face of Contemporary Clinical Care. *BioMed Res. Int.* **2021**, *2021*, 9954615. [CrossRef]
18. Khan, M.I.; Laxmikanth, S.M.; Gopal, T.; Neela, P.K. Artificial Intelligence and 3D Printing Technology in Orthodontics: Future and Scope. *AIMS Biophys.* **2022**, *9*, 182–197. [CrossRef]
19. Sahoo, R.; Sahoo, N.R. Advances in Cephalometry in Relation to the Shift in Soft Tissue Paradigm for Orthodontic Treatment Planning. *Indian J. Forensic Med. Toxicol.* **2020**, *14*, 8745–8757. [CrossRef]
20. Abdelkarim, A. Cone-Beam Computed Tomography in Orthodontics. *Dent. J.* **2019**, *7*, 89. [CrossRef]
21. Grandoch, A.; Nestmann, F.; Kreppel, M.; Buller, J.; Borggrefe, J.; Zirk, M.; Zöller, J.E. Comparison of MRI with Dedicated Head and Neck Signal Amplification Coil and Cone Beam Computed Tomography: MRI Is a Useful Tool in Diagnostics of Cranio-Facial Growth Disorders. *J. Cranio-Maxillofac. Surg.* **2019**, *47*, 1827–1833. [CrossRef] [PubMed]
22. Jaiswal, P.; Gandhi, A.; Gupta, A.; Malik, N.; Singh, S.; Ramesh, K. Reliability of Photogrammetric Landmarks to the Conventional Cephalogram for Analyzing Soft-Tissue Landmarks in Orthodontics. *J. Pharm. Bioallied Sci.* **2021**, *13*, S171–S175. [CrossRef] [PubMed]
23. Proffit, W.R.; Fields, H.W.; Larson, B.; Sarver, D.M. *Contemporary Orthodontics*, 6th ed.; Mosby: St. Louis, MO, USA, 2018.
24. Hans, M.G.; Palomo, J.M.; Valiathan, M. History of Imaging in Orthodontics from Broadbent to Cone-Beam Computed Tomography. *Am. J. Orthod. Dentofac. Orthop.* **2015**, *148*, 914–921. [CrossRef] [PubMed]
25. Mintz, Y.; Brodie, R. Introduction to Artificial Intelligence in Medicine. *Minim. Invasive Ther. Allied Technol.* **2019**, *28*, 73–81. [CrossRef] [PubMed]
26. Amisha; Malik, P.; Pathania, M.; Rathaur, V.K. Overview of Artificial Intelligence in Medicine. *J. Fam. Med. Prim. Care* **2019**, *8*, 2328–2331. [CrossRef] [PubMed]
27. El-Sherbini, A.H.; Hassan Virk, H.U.; Wang, Z.; Glicksberg, B.S.; Krittanawong, C. Machine-Learning-Based Prediction Modelling in Primary Care: State-of-the-Art Review. *AI* **2023**, *4*, 437–460. [CrossRef]
28. Wan, T.T.H.; Wan, H.S. Predictive Analytics with a Transdisciplinary Framework in Promoting Patient-Centric Care of Polychronic Conditions: Trends, Challenges, and Solutions. *AI* **2023**, *4*, 482–490. [CrossRef]
29. Zhu, Z.; Ng, D.W.H.; Park, H.S.; McAlpine, M.C. 3D-Printed Multifunctional Materials Enabled by Artificial-Intelligence-Assisted Fabrication Technologies. *Nat. Rev. Mater.* **2021**, *6*, 27–47. [CrossRef]
30. Ding, H.; Wu, J.; Zhao, W.; Matinlinna, J.P.; Burrow, M.F.; Tsoi, J.K.H. Artificial Intelligence in Dentistry—A Review. *Front. Dent. Med.* **2023**, *4*, 1085251. [CrossRef]
31. Fawaz, P.; Sayegh, P.E.; Vannet, B.V. What Is the Current State of Artificial Intelligence Applications in Dentistry and Orthodontics? *J. Stomatol. Oral Maxillofac. Surg.* **2023**, *124*, 101524. [CrossRef]
32. Grauer, D. Quality in Orthodontics: The Role of Customized Appliances. *J. Esthet. Restor. Dent.* **2021**, *33*, 253–258. [CrossRef]
33. Yamashiro, T.; Ko, C.-C. Artificial Intelligence and Machine Learning in Orthodontics. *Orthod. Craniofac. Res.* **2021**, *24*, 3–5. [CrossRef]
34. D'Ettorre, G.; Farronato, M.; Candida, E.; Quinzi, V.; Grippaudo, C. A Comparison between Stereophotogrammetry and Smartphone Structured Light Technology for Three-Dimensional Face Scanning. *Angle Orthod.* **2022**, *93*, 358–363. [CrossRef] [PubMed]
35. Ayidh Alqahtani, K.; Jacobs, R.; Smolders, A.; Van Gerven, A.; Willems, H.; Shujaat, S.; Shaheen, E. Deep Convolutional Neural Network-Based Automated Segmentation and Classification of Teeth with Orthodontic Brackets on Cone-Beam Computed-Tomographic Images: A Validation Study. *Eur. J. Orthod.* **2023**, *45*, 169–174. [CrossRef] [PubMed]
36. Bouletreau, P.; Makaremi, M.; Ibrahim, B.; Louvrier, A.; Sigaux, N. Artificial Intelligence: Applications in Orthognathic Surgery. *J. Stomatol. Oral Maxillofac. Surg.* **2019**, *120*, 347–354. [CrossRef] [PubMed]
37. Thurzo, A.; Urbanová, W.; Novák, B.; Czako, L.; Siebert, T.; Stano, P.; Mareková, S.; Fountoulaki, G.; Kosnáčová, H.; Varga, I. Where Is the Artificial Intelligence Applied in Dentistry? Systematic Review and Literature Analysis. *Healthcare* **2022**, *10*, 1269. [CrossRef] [PubMed]
38. Naran, S.; Steinbacher, D.M.; Taylor, J.A. Current Concepts in Orthognathic Surgery. *Plast. Reconstr. Surg.* **2018**, *141*, 925e–936e. [CrossRef] [PubMed]

39. Farronato, M.; Maspero, C.; Lanteri, V.; Fama, A.; Ferrati, F.; Pettenuzzo, A.; Farronato, D. Current State of the Art in the Use of Augmented Reality in Dentistry: A Systematic Review of the Literature. *BMC Oral Health* **2019**, *19*, 135. [CrossRef] [PubMed]
40. Rousseau, M.; Retrouvey, J.-M. Machine Learning in Orthodontics: Automated Facial Analysis of Vertical Dimension for Increased Precision and Efficiency. *Am. J. Orthod. Dentofac. Orthop.* **2022**, *161*, 445–450. [CrossRef]
41. Strunga, M.; Urban, R.; Surovková, J.; Thurzo, A. Artificial Intelligence Systems Assisting in the Assessment of the Course and Retention of Orthodontic Treatment. *Healthcare* **2023**, *11*, 683. [CrossRef]
42. Tian, Y.; Chen, C.; Xu, X.; Wang, J.; Hou, X.; Li, K.; Lu, X.; Shi, H.; Lee, E.-S.; Jiang, H.B. A Review of 3D Printing in Dentistry: Technologies, Affecting Factors, and Applications. *Scanning* **2021**, *2021*, 9950131. [CrossRef]
43. Khanagar, S.B.; Al-Ehaideb, A.; Vishwanathaiah, S.; Maganur, P.C.; Patil, S.; Naik, S.; Baeshen, H.A.; Sarode, S.S. Scope and Performance of Artificial Intelligence Technology in Orthodontic Diagnosis, Treatment Planning, and Clinical Decision-Making—A Systematic Review. *J. Dent. Sci.* **2021**, *16*, 482–492. [CrossRef]
44. Mohammad-Rahimi, H.; Nadimi, M.; Rohban, M.H.; Shamsoddin, E.; Lee, V.Y.; Motamedian, S.R. Machine Learning and Orthodontics, Current Trends and the Future Opportunities: A Scoping Review. *Am. J. Orthod. Dentofac. Orthop.* **2021**, *160*, 170–192.e4. [CrossRef] [PubMed]
45. Gandedkar, N.H.; Vaid, N.R.; Darendeliler, M.A.; Premjani, P.; Ferguson, D.J. The Last Decade in Orthodontics: A Scoping Review of the Hits, Misses and the near Misses! *Semin. Orthod.* **2019**, *25*, 339–355. [CrossRef]
46. Fatima, A.; Shafi, I.; Afzal, H.; Díez, I.D.L.T.; Lourdes, D.R.-S.M.; Breñosa, J.; Espinosa, J.C.M.; Ashraf, I. Advancements in Dentistry with Artificial Intelligence: Current Clinical Applications and Future Perspectives. *Healthcare* **2022**, *10*, 2188. [CrossRef] [PubMed]
47. Kwon, H.-B.; Park, Y.-S.; Han, J.-S. Augmented Reality in Dentistry: A Current Perspective. *Acta Odontol. Scand.* **2018**, *76*, 497–503. [CrossRef]
48. Retrouvey, J.-M.; Conley, R.S. Decoding Deep Learning Applications for Diagnosis and Treatment Planning. *Dent. Press J. Orthod.* **2022**, *27*, e22spe5. [CrossRef]
49. Thurzo, A.; Strunga, M.; Havlínová, R.; Reháková, K.; Urban, R.; Surovková, J.; Kurilová, V. Smartphone-Based Facial Scanning as a Viable Tool for Facially Driven Orthodontics? *Sensors* **2022**, *22*, 7752. [CrossRef]
50. Abd El-Ghafour, M.; Aboulhassan, M.A.; Fayed, M.M.S.; El-Beialy, A.R.; Eid, F.H.K.; Hegab, S.E.-D.; El-Gendi, M.; Emara, D. Effectiveness of a Novel 3D-Printed Nasoalveolar Molding Appliance (D-NAM) on Improving the Maxillary Arch Dimensions in Unilateral Cleft Lip and Palate Infants: A Randomized Controlled Trial. *Cleft Palate-Craniofac. J.* **2020**, *57*, 1370–1381. [CrossRef]
51. Leite, A.F.; Vasconcelos, K.D.F.; Willems, H.; Jacobs, R. Radiomics and Machine Learning in Oral Healthcare. *Proteom.-Clin. Appl.* **2020**, *14*, e1900040. [CrossRef]
52. Mayo, R.C.; Leung, J. Artificial Intelligence and Deep Learning—Radiology's next Frontier? *Clin. Imaging* **2018**, *49*, 87–88. [CrossRef]
53. Ren, R.; Luo, H.; Su, C.; Yao, Y.; Liao, W. Machine Learning in Dental, Oral and Craniofacial Imaging: A Review of Recent Progress. *PeerJ* **2021**, *9*, e11451. [CrossRef] [PubMed]
54. Alphonse, A.S.; Kumari, S.V.; Priyanga, P.T. Caries Detection from Dental Images Using Novel Maximum Directional Pattern (MDP) and Deep Learning. *Int. J. Electr. Electron. Res.* **2022**, *10*, 100–104. [CrossRef]
55. Kondody, R.T.; Patil, A.; Devika, G.; Jose, A.; Kumar, A.; Nair, S. Introduction to Artificial Intelligence and Machine Learning into Orthodontics: A Review. *APOS Trends Orthod.* **2022**, *12*, 214–220. [CrossRef]
56. Kolsanov, A.V.; Popov, N.V.; Ayupova, I.O.; Khamadeeva, A.M.; Tiunova, N.V.; Kramm, E.K.; Makhota, A.Y. Determination of the Usability of Teleroentgenographic Studies in Orthodontic Practice. *Biomed. Eng.* **2023**, *57*, 195–199. [CrossRef]
57. Alsubai, S. A Critical Review on the 3D Cephalometric Analysis Using Machine Learning. *Computers* **2022**, *11*, 154. [CrossRef]
58. Suhail, S.; Harris, K.; Sinha, G.; Schmidt, M.; Durgekar, S.; Mehta, S.; Upadhyay, M. Learning Cephalometric Landmarks for Diagnostic Features Using Regression Trees. *Bioengineering* **2022**, *9*, 617. [CrossRef]
59. Lin, L.; Tang, B.; Cao, L.; Yan, J.; Zhao, T.; Hua, F.; He, H. The Knowledge, Experience, and Attitude on Artificial Intelligence-Assisted Cephalometric Analysis: Survey of Orthodontists and Orthodontic Students. *Am. J. Orthod. Dentofac. Orthop.* **2023**, *164*, e97–e105. [CrossRef]
60. Albalawi, F.; Alamoud, K.A. Trends and Application of Artificial Intelligence Technology in Orthodontic Diagnosis and Treatment Planning—A Review. *Appl. Sci.* **2022**, *12*, 11864. [CrossRef]
61. Urban, R.; Haluzová, S.; Strunga, M.; Surovková, J.; Lifková, M.; Tomášik, J.; Thurzo, A. AI-Assisted CBCT Data Management in Modern Dental Practice: Benefits, Limitations and Innovations. *Electronics* **2023**, *12*, 1710. [CrossRef]
62. Fan, Y.; Zhang, Y.; Chen, G.; He, W.; Song, G.; Matthews, H.; Claes, P.; Pei, Y.; Zha, H.; Penington, A.; et al. Automated Assessment of Mandibular Shape Asymmetry in 3-Dimensions. *Am. J. Orthod. Dentofac. Orthop.* **2022**, *161*, 698–707. [CrossRef]
63. Balashova, M.; Khabadze, Z.; Popaduk, V.; Kulikova, A.; Bakaev, Y.; Abdulkerimova, S.; Generalova, Y.; Dashtieva, M.; Gadzhiev, F.; Umarov, A.; et al. Artificial Intelligence Application in Assessment of Upper Airway on Cone-Beam Computed Tomography Scans. *J. Int. Dent. Med. Res.* **2023**, *16*, 105–110.
64. Seo, H.; Hwang, J.; Jeong, T.; Shin, J. Comparison of Deep Learning Models for Cervical Vertebral Maturation Stage Classification on Lateral Cephalometric Radiographs. *J. Clin. Med.* **2021**, *10*, 3591. [CrossRef]
65. Liao, N.; Dai, J.; Tang, Y.; Zhong, Q.; Mo, S. iCVM: An Interpretable Deep Learning Model for CVM Assessment Under Label Uncertainty. *IEEE J. Biomed. Health Inform.* **2022**, *26*, 4325–4334. [CrossRef]

66. Kulikova, A.A.; Khabadze, Z.S.; Abdulkerimova, S.M.; Bakaev, Y.A.; El-Khalaf Ramiz, M.; Bagdasarova, I.V. Comparison of Accuracy of 2D- and 3D-Diagnostic Methods in Analysis of Maxillofacial Region for Cephalometry in Orthdontic Practice Based on Literature. *Russ. Electron. J. Radiol.* **2019**, *9*, 171–180. [CrossRef]
67. Hulsen, T. Explainable Artificial Intelligence (XAI): Concepts and Challenges in Healthcare. *AI* **2023**, *4*, 652–666. [CrossRef]
68. Marcus, G. The Next Decade in AI: Four Steps Towards Robust Artificial Intelligence. *arXiv* **2020**, arXiv:2002.06177. [CrossRef]
69. Al Turkestani, N.; Bianchi, J.; Deleat-Besson, R.; Le, C.; Tengfei, L.; Prieto, J.C.; Gurgel, M.; Ruellas, A.C.O.; Massaro, C.; Aliaga Del Castillo, A.; et al. Clinical Decision Support Systems in Orthodontics: A Narrative Review of Data Science Approaches. *Orthod. Craniofac. Res.* **2021**, *24*, 26–36. [CrossRef]
70. Chow, J.C.L.; Sanders, L.; Li, K. Design of an Educational Chatbot Using Artificial Intelligence in Radiotherapy. *AI* **2023**, *4*, 319–332. [CrossRef]
71. He, D.; Gu, Y.; Sun, Y. Correlations between Objective Measurements and Subjective Evaluations of Facial Profile after Orthodontic Treatment. *J. Int. Med. Res.* **2020**, *48*, 1–13. [CrossRef]
72. Putrino, A.; Abed, M.R.; Barbato, E.; Galluccio, G. A Current Tool in Facial Aesthetics Perception of Orthodontic Patient: The Digital Warping. *Dent. Cadmos* **2021**, *89*, 46–52. [CrossRef]
73. Volovic, J.; Badirli, S.; Ahmad, S.; Leavitt, L.; Mason, T.; Bhamidipalli, S.S.; Eckert, G.; Albright, D.; Turkkahraman, H. A Novel Machine Learning Model for Predicting Orthodontic Treatment Duration. *Diagnostics* **2023**, *13*, 2740. [CrossRef]
74. Ahmed, N.; Abbasi, M.S.; Zuberi, F.; Qamar, W.; Halim, M.S.B.; Maqsood, A.; Alam, M.K. Artificial Intelligence Techniques: Analysis, Application, and Outcome in Dentistry—A Systematic Review. *BioMed Res. Int.* **2021**, *2021*, 9751564. [CrossRef]
75. Akdeniz, B.S.; Tosun, M.E. A Review of the Use of Artificial Intelligence in Orthodontics. *J. Exp. Clin. Med.* **2021**, *38*, 157–162. [CrossRef]
76. Graber, L.W.; Vig, K.W.L.; Huang, G.J.; Fleming, P.S. *Orthodontics*, 7th ed.; Elsevier Health Sciences: Amsterdam, The Netherlands, 2022; ISBN 978-0-323-77859-6.
77. Bulatova, G.; Kusnoto, B.; Grace, V.; Tsay, T.P.; Avenetti, D.M.; Sanchez, F.J.C. Assessment of Automatic Cephalometric Landmark Identification Using Artificial Intelligence. *Orthod. Craniofac. Res.* **2021**, *24* (Suppl. S2), 37–42. [CrossRef]
78. Tanikawa, C.; Lee, C.; Lim, J.; Oka, A.; Yamashiro, T. Clinical Applicability of Automated Cephalometric Landmark Identification: Part I-Patient-Related Identification Errors. *Orthod. Craniofac. Res.* **2021**, *24* (Suppl. S2), 43–52. [CrossRef]
79. Kim, J.; Kim, I.; Kim, Y.-J.; Kim, M.; Cho, J.-H.; Hong, M.; Kang, K.-H.; Lim, S.-H.; Kim, S.-J.; Kim, Y.H.; et al. Accuracy of Automated Identification of Lateral Cephalometric Landmarks Using Cascade Convolutional Neural Networks on Lateral Cephalograms from Nationwide Multi-Centres. *Orthod. Craniofac. Res.* **2021**, *24* (Suppl. S2), 59–67. [CrossRef]
80. Kim, D.-W.; Kim, J.; Kim, T.; Kim, T.; Kim, Y.-J.; Song, I.-S.; Ahn, B.; Choo, J.; Lee, D.-Y. Prediction of Hand-Wrist Maturation Stages Based on Cervical Vertebrae Images Using Artificial Intelligence. *Orthod. Craniofac. Res.* **2021**, *24* (Suppl. S2), 68–75. [CrossRef]
81. Kök, H.; Izgi, M.S.; Acilar, A.M. Determination of Growth and Development Periods in Orthodontics with Artificial Neural Network. *Orthod. Craniofac. Res.* **2021**, *24* (Suppl. S2), 76–83. [CrossRef]
82. Yurdakurban, E.; Duran, G.S.; Görgülü, S. Evaluation of an Automated Approach for Facial Midline Detection and Asymmetry Assessment: A Preliminary Study. *Orthod. Craniofac. Res.* **2021**, *24* (Suppl. S2), 84–91. [CrossRef]
83. Rousseau, M.; Vargas, J.; Rauch, F.; Marulanda, J.; Retrouvey, J.-M. Members of the BBDC Facial Morphology Analysis in Osteogenesis Imperfecta Types I, III and IV Using Computer Vision. *Orthod. Craniofac. Res.* **2021**, *24*, 92–99. [CrossRef]
84. Lo Giudice, A.; Ronsivalle, V.; Spampinato, C.; Leonardi, R. Fully Automatic Segmentation of the Mandible Based on Convolutional Neural Networks (CNNs). *Orthod. Craniofac. Res.* **2021**, *24* (Suppl. S2), 100–107. [CrossRef]
85. Lim, J.; Tanikawa, C.; Kogo, M.; Yamashiro, T. Determination of Prognostic Factors for Orthognathic Surgery in Children with Cleft Lip and/or Palate. *Orthod. Craniofac. Res.* **2021**, *24* (Suppl. S2), 153–162. [CrossRef]
86. Auconi, P.; Ottaviani, E.; Barelli, F.; Giuntini, V.; McNamara, J.A.; Franchi, L. Prognostic Approach to Class III Malocclusion through Case-Based Reasoning. *Orthod. Craniofac. Res.* **2021**, *24* (Suppl. S2), 163–171. [CrossRef]
87. Serafin, M.; Baldini, B.; Cabitza, F.; Carrafiello, G.; Baselli, G.; Del Fabbro, M.; Sforza, C.; Caprioglio, A.; Tartaglia, G.M. Accuracy of Automated 3D Cephalometric Landmarks by Deep Learning Algorithms: Systematic Review and Meta-Analysis. *Radiol. Medica* **2023**, *128*, 544–555. [CrossRef]
88. Duran, G.S.; Gökmen, Ş.; Topsakal, K.G.; Görgülü, S. Evaluation of the Accuracy of Fully Automatic Cephalometric Analysis Software with Artificial Intelligence Algorithm. *Orthod. Craniofac. Res.* **2023**, *26*, 481–490. [CrossRef]
89. Huang, G.; Wu, L.; Hu, J.; Zhou, X.; He, F.; Wan, L.; Pan, S.-T. Main Applications and Recent Research Progresses of Additive Manufacturing in Dentistry. *BioMed Res. Int.* **2022**, *2022*, 5530188. [CrossRef]
90. Tang, Y.; Zhang, Y.; Meng, Z.; Sun, Q.; Peng, L.; Zhang, L.; Lu, W.; Liang, W.; Chen, G.; Wei, Y. Accuracy of Additive Manufacturing in Stomatology. *Front. Bioeng. Biotechnol.* **2022**, *10*, 964651. [CrossRef]
91. Michiko, A.; Shirahama, S.; Shimizu, A.; Romanec, C.; Anka, G. The Surgical Guides for TADs: The Rational and Laboratory Procedures. *Appl. Sci.* **2023**, *13*, 10332. [CrossRef]
92. Panayi, N.C. In-House Three-Dimensional Designing and Printing Customized Brackets. *J. World Fed. Orthod.* **2022**, *11*, 190–196. [CrossRef]

93. Nakornnoi, T.; Chantakao, C.; Luangaram, N.; Janbamrung, T.; Thitasomakul, T.; Sipiyaruk, K. Perceptions of Orthodontic Residents toward the Implementation of Dental Technologies in Postgraduate Curriculum. *BMC Oral Health* **2023**, *23*, 625. [CrossRef]
94. Oberoi, G.; Nitsch, S.; Edelmayer, M.; Janjic, K.; Müller, A.S.; Agis, H. 3D Printing-Encompassing the Facets of Dentistry. *Front. Bioeng. Biotechnol.* **2018**, *6*, 172. [CrossRef]
95. Franco de Sá Gomes, C.; Libdy, M.R.; Normando, D. Scan Time, Reliability and Accuracy of Craniofacial Measurements Using a 3D Light Scanner. *J. Oral Biol. Craniofac. Res.* **2019**, *9*, 331–335. [CrossRef]
96. Pojda, D.; Tomaka, A.A.; Luchowski, L.; Tarnawski, M. Integration and Application of Multimodal Measurement Techniques: Relevance of Photogrammetry to Orthodontics. *Sensors* **2021**, *21*, 8026. [CrossRef]
97. Mai, H.-N.; Lee, D.-H. Accuracy of Mobile Device–Compatible 3D Scanners for Facial Digitization: Systematic Review and Meta-Analysis. *J. Med. Internet Res.* **2020**, *22*, e22228. [CrossRef]
98. Badr, A.M.; Refai, W.M.M.; El-Shal, M.G.; Abdelhameed, A.N. Accuracy and Reliability of Kinect Motion Sensing Input Device's 3d Models: A Comparison to Direct Anthropometry and 2D Photogrammetry. *Open Access Maced. J. Med. Sci.* **2021**, *9*, 54–60. [CrossRef]
99. Eliasova, H.; Dostalova, T.; Urbanova, P. A Comparison of the Precision of 3D Images of Facial Tissues from the Forensic Point of View. *Forensic Imaging* **2022**, *28*, 200471. [CrossRef]
100. Mao, B.; Li, J.; Tian, Y.; Zhou, Y. The Accuracy of a Three-Dimensional Face Model Reconstructing Method Based on Conventional Clinical Two-Dimensional Photos. *BMC Oral Health* **2022**, *22*, 413. [CrossRef]
101. Rongo, R.; Nissen, L.; Leroy, C.; Michelotti, A.; Cattaneo, P.M.; Cornelis, M.A. Three-Dimensional Soft Tissue Changes in Orthodontic Extraction and Non-Extraction Patients: A Prospective Study. *Orthod. Craniofac. Res.* **2021**, *24* (Suppl. S2), 181–192. [CrossRef]
102. Perrotti, G.; Reda, R.; Rossi, O.; D'apolito, I.; Testori, T.; Testarelli, L. A Radiation Free Alternative to CBCT Volumetric Rendering for Soft Tissue Evaluation. *Braz. Dent. Sci.* **2023**, *26*, 1–7. [CrossRef]
103. Goh, G.D.; Lee, J.M.; Goh, G.L.; Huang, X.; Lee, S.; Yeong, W.Y. Machine Learning for Bioelectronics on Wearable and Implantable Devices: Challenges and Potential. *Tissue Eng. Part A* **2023**, *29*, 20–46. [CrossRef]
104. Mekruksavanich, S.; Phaphan, W.; Hnoohom, N.; Jitpattanakul, A. Attention-Based Hybrid Deep Learning Network for Human Activity Recognition Using WiFi Channel State Information. *Appl. Sci.* **2023**, *13*, 8884. [CrossRef]
105. Mengara Mengara, A.G.; Park, E.; Jang, J.; Yoo, Y. Attention-Based Distributed Deep Learning Model for Air Quality Forecasting. *Sustainability* **2022**, *14*, 3269. [CrossRef]
106. Lee, S.; Yang, Y.; Aiyanyo, I.; Keith, M.; Boussougou, M.; Park, D.-J. Attention-Based 1D CNN-BiLSTM Hybrid Model Enhanced with FastText Word Embedding for Korean Voice Phishing Detection. *Mathematics* **2023**, *11*, 3217. [CrossRef]
107. Singh, J.; Singh, N.; Fouda, M.M.; Saba, L.; Suri, J.S. Attention-Enabled Ensemble Deep Learning Models and Their Validation for Depression Detection: A Domain Adoption Paradigm. *Diagnostics* **2023**, *13*, 2092. [CrossRef]
108. Deng, J.; Zhang, S.; Ma, J.; Lu, J.; Deng, J.; Zhang, S.; Ma, J. Self-Attention-Based Deep Convolution LSTM Framework for Sensor-Based Badminton Activity Recognition. *Sensors* **2023**, *23*, 8373. [CrossRef]

Disclaimer/Publisher's Note: The statements, opinions and data contained in all publications are solely those of the individual author(s) and contributor(s) and not of MDPI and/or the editor(s). MDPI and/or the editor(s) disclaim responsibility for any injury to people or property resulting from any ideas, methods, instructions or products referred to in the content.

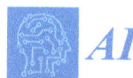

Article

A Flower Pollination Algorithm-Optimized Wavelet Transform and Deep CNN for Analyzing Binaural Beats and Anxiety

Devika Rankhambe [1], Bharati Sanjay Ainapure [1,*], Bhargav Appasani [2,*] and Amitkumar V. Jha [2]

1 Department of Computer Engineering, Vishwakarma University, Pune 411046, India; rankhambedevika@gmail.com
2 School of Electronics Engineering, Kalinga Institute of Industrial Technology, Bhubaneswar 751024, India; amit.jhafet@kiit.ac.in
* Correspondence: ainapuressa@gmail.com (B.S.A.); bhargav.appasanifet@kiit.ac.in (B.A.)

Abstract: Binaural beats are a low-frequency form of acoustic stimulation that may be heard between 200 and 900 Hz and can help reduce anxiety as well as alter other psychological situations and states by affecting mood and cognitive function. However, prior research has only looked at the impact of binaural beats on state and trait anxiety using the STA-I scale; the level of anxiety has not yet been evaluated, and for the removal of artifacts the improper selection of wavelet parameters reduced the original signal energy. Hence, in this research, the level of anxiety when hearing binaural beats has been analyzed using a novel optimized wavelet transform in which optimized wavelet parameters are extracted from the EEG signal using the flower pollination algorithm, whereby artifacts are removed effectively from the EEG signal. Thus, EEG signals have five types of brainwaves in the existing models, which have not been analyzed optimally for brainwaves other than delta waves nor has the level of anxiety yet been analyzed using binaural beats. To overcome this, deep convolutional neural network (CNN)-based signal processing has been proposed. In this, deep features are extracted from optimized EEG signal parameters, which are precisely selected and adjusted to their most efficient values using the flower pollination algorithm, ensuring minimal signal energy reduction and artifact removal to maintain the integrity of the original EEG signal during analysis. These features provide the accurate classification of various levels of anxiety, which provides more accurate results for the effects of binaural beats on anxiety from brainwaves. Finally, the proposed model is implemented in the Python platform, and the obtained results demonstrate its efficacy. The proposed optimized wavelet transform using deep CNN-based signal processing outperforms existing techniques such as KNN, SVM, LDA, and Narrow-ANN, with a high accuracy of 0.99%, precision of 0.99%, recall of 0.99%, F1-score of 0.99%, specificity of 0.999%, and error rate of 0.01%. Thus, the optimized wavelet transform with a deep CNN can perform an effective decomposition of EEG data and extract deep features related to anxiety to analyze the effect of binaural beats on anxiety levels.

Keywords: binaural beats; EEG signals; wavelet transform; flower pollination optimization algorithm; deep convolutional neural network

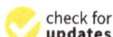

Citation: Rankhambe, D.; Ainapure, B.S.; Appasani, B.; Jha, A.V. A Flower Pollination Algorithm-Optimized Wavelet Transform and Deep CNN for Analyzing Binaural Beats and Anxiety. *AI* **2024**, *5*, 115–135. https://doi.org/10.3390/ai5010007

Academic Editor: Tim Hulsen

Received: 6 September 2023
Revised: 23 November 2023
Accepted: 24 November 2023
Published: 29 December 2023

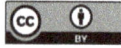

Copyright: © 2023 by the authors. Licensee MDPI, Basel, Switzerland. This article is an open access article distributed under the terms and conditions of the Creative Commons Attribution (CC BY) license (https://creativecommons.org/licenses/by/4.0/).

1. Introduction

Anxiety has progressively grown in incidence over the last 24 years, particularly among adolescents and young adults [1]. Individuals in the United States were three times more likely to screen positive for anxiety disorders in April/May 2020 than in April/May 2019, due to the COVID-19 pandemic lockdowns [2]. Brainwave entrainment, also known as brainwave synchronization [3,4], is a technique for reducing anxiety and stress. It is said to improve moods, aid in deep sleep, boost the immune system (delta frequency: 1–4 Hz) [5], improve memory, aid in deep relaxation, and meditation (theta frequency: 4–8 Hz), improve positive thinking (alpha frequency: 8–13 Hz), and improved alertness (beta frequency: 14–24 Hz).

A binaural beat is a form of acoustic stimulation that has been shown to help with anxiety reduction and the attenuation or augmentation of various psychological conditions and states [6,7]. The binaural beat is the brain impression of a low-frequency sound that occurs when a person is exposed to two slightly distinct wave frequencies, both between 200 and 900 Hz [8,9]. Recent studies seem to back up the idea that binaural beats can change the operational connectivity between brain regions [10–12] and cortical network connectivity [13–15].

Several experiments have concentrated on the measurement of the effect of binaural beats on anxiety reduction. However, researchers only focused on state anxiety and trait anxiety using the state-trait anxiety inventory (STA-I) [16–18]. Moreover, anxiety has been classified into four categories, minimal anxiety, mild anxiety, moderate anxiety, and severe anxiety, which have not yet been analyzed with binaural beats. To do this, the Beck Anxiety Inventory (BAI) can be utilized, which has a score of 0–63, where BAI scores < 7 represent minimal anxiety, 8–15 represent mild anxiety, 16–25 represent moderate anxiety, and 26–63 represent severe anxiety. Similar to the self-reported analysis through anxiety inventories, the effect of binaural beats is analyzed using electroencephalography (EEG) signals [19].

In the processing of EEG signals, artifact removal is one of the most important stages due to their contamination with other signals. Unwanted signals, called artifacts, are caused by noise in the environment, experimental errors, and physiological abnormalities. Extrinsic artifacts include environmental artifacts and experiment errors, which are caused by external causes, whereas intrinsic artifacts include physiological artifacts caused by the body itself (e.g., eye blink, muscle activity, heartbeat) [20,21]. Significant artifacts in EEG recordings are caused by ocular artifacts, recorded as electrooculogram (EOG) signals [22]. Eye movement and blinks cause ocular aberrations, which can spread over the scalp and be detected as EEG activity. The contamination of EEG data by muscle activity is a well-known and difficult challenge since it manifests as electromyogram (EMG) signals from various muscle groups [23,24]. When electrodes are put on or near a blood vessel [25], cardiac artifacts such as electrocardiogram (ECG) signals can be created, causing the heart to expand and contract. Thus, the objective of this work is to examine the effect of binaural beats on four levels of anxiety and their signal processing. However, the improper selection of the mother wavelet parameter will result in it performing poorly in artifact removal in EEG signals, which can reduce the original energy of the EEG signal. For feature extraction and classification, MLP was not optimal for brainwaves other than delta waves, which led to a reduction in the accuracy analysis of the binaural beats' effects. However, there is a need to improve this for effective and promising results for the effect of binaural beats on the level of anxiety experienced. The major contributions provided by this paper are as follows:

- In EEG signals, the improper selection of the wavelet parameter reduces the original signal energy, hence an optimized wavelet transform has been introduced using the flower pollination optimization algorithm to remove artifacts from the EEG signal.
- Consequently, the impact of the binaural beats on brainwaves is analyzed via deep-based signal processing which has the capability of extracting all the deep features belonging to anxiety from EEG signals while classifying various anxiety levels.

This paper is presented as follows: some articles related to binaural beats' effect on EEG signals are surveyed in Section 2. The mathematical derivations and the experimental analysis of the optimized wavelet transform with deep CNN-based signal processing are stated in Sections 3 and 4. Lastly, the conclusion to this paper is given in Section 5.

2. Literature Review

Yusim, et al. [26] found that a binaural beat meditation technique reduced self-reported anxiety measurements in psychiatric outpatients and non-patients. Gkolias, et al. [27] found that binaural beats at 5 Hz reduced pain intensity, anxiety, and analgesic usage in chronic pain sufferers compared to sham stimulation. Sekirin et al. [28] found that binaural beating techniques reduced reactive and personal anxiety in individuals scheduled to have hip joint endoprosthesis. Menziletoglu et al. [29] found that both binaural beats and music reduced preoperative dental anxiety, but did not assess which treatment was more successful. Mallik et al. [30] found that a combination of quiet music and theta auditory beat stimulation reduced anxiety measurements in people prescribed anxiolytics. Da Silva Junior et al. [31] found significant changes in high alpha and beta, as well as theta, brainwaves in participants who listened to a 5 Hz binaural beat for 20 min. Amarasinghe et al. [32] used self-organizing maps (SOM) to detect thinking patterns and identify two patterns in five users. El Houda et al. [33] investigated the effects of marijuana binaural beats on EEG signals but found no significant results. Pluck et al. [34] conducted a double-blind study and found no effect of theta-frequency binaural beats on cognitive fluency but found a significant induction of dread in the binaural beat condition compared to control. Lee et al. [35] proposed a combination of 6 Hz binaural beats and ASMR triggers to promote theta brainwaves and psychological stability for sleep induction.

Da Silva Junior et al. [31] examined the effects of binaural beats on brainwaves and found significant changes in higher alpha, high beta, and theta brainwaves using multi-layer perceptron (MLP) and LORETA methods. Chouhan et al. [31,36] used an entropy-based approach to assess a person's degree of attentiveness using EEG signals recorded from an Emotiv EPOC headset. Lee et al. [35] investigated the effects of different binaural beat frequencies on EEG signals and found that a combination of binaural beats and ASMR triggers induced sleep. Jayasinghe et al. [37,38] presented software that uses feedback from the Apple Health Kit and Google Fit to identify and minimize stress using machine learning classifiers, including k-nearest neighbors and Naive Bayes. Amarasinghe et al. [32] proposed an approach based on self-organizing maps (SOM) for detecting thinking patterns using EEG signals and a feed-forward ANN. That et al. [39,40] investigated the use of an ANN classifier to classify EEG data from stressed and non-stressed females women using energy spectral density (ESD) characteristics. Advanced et al. [41] presented a CRNN for simultaneous sound event detection. Cheah et al. [42] found that a CNN can categorize EEG signals without the need for manual features. Andrian et al. [43] used brainwave stimulators to enhance alpha brainwaves and alleviate stress, while El Houda et al. [33] examined the impact of marijuana binaural beats on the brain. Zaini et al. [44,45] monitored EEG data and evaluated the correlations between binaural beats' characteristics and mental states using a Bayesian Networks Processor. Jirakittayakorn et al. [46] investigated the impact of a 3 Hz binaural beat on snooze phases using EEG data and event-related potential analysis.

In addition, Loong et al. [47] conducted a prospective, randomized controlled study to examine the analgesic and anxiolytic benefits of binaural beat audio in cataract surgery patients. Abu-Taieh et al. [48] used an expanded TAM model to investigate the effect of parents' anxiety and depression on children's anxiety and depression when SNs were used. Lee et al. [49] investigated the brainwave entrainment impact of binaural beats as an adjunct treatment for insomnia symptoms. Yi et al. [50] studied the effects of audible and inaudible binaural beat stimuli on alpha brainwave elicitation, whereas Ignatius et al. [51] investigated the use of audiometric EEGs for identifying certain binaural hearing properties. These studies add to our understanding of the numerous applications and consequences of binaural beats in different neurological situations.

However, some studies did not consider artifacts due to eye blinking and muscle movements, while others used techniques that could reduce the original energy of the EEG signal. Thus, there is a need to improve the performance of these studies to provide an accurate analysis of binaural beats.

3. Optimized Wavelet Transform with Deep CNN-Based EEG Signal Processing

Binaural beats are produced when sine waves are transmitted to each ear separately and are near one another, which reduces anxiety by affecting mood and cognitive functions. The binaural beat is the brain perception of a low-frequency sound that occurs when a person is exposed to two wave frequencies that are very slightly different from one another (by a maximum of 30 Hz), both of which have frequencies between 200 and 900 Hz. To investigate the possible impacts of binaural beats on EEG signals, various transformation techniques have been used previously, but the selection of an incorrect mother wavelet reduces the system's accuracy and overlaps with the original signal, which can lower the EEG signal's initial energy. Hence, a novel resource-constrained model named the optimized wavelet transform has been proposed, in which optimized wavelet parameters are extracted from the EEG signal by integrating the flower pollination optimization algorithm with the wavelet transform for the selection of wavelet parameters. Thus, the proper wavelet parameters are selected to lessenthe reduction of the original signal's energy. Thus, an optimization that is based on the multi-objective function of a lower mean square error (MSE) and higher signal-to-noise ratio (SNR) removes the artifacts from the EEG signal to keep the valuable information, thus removing the artifact from the EEG is important to secure the quality of the EEG signal.

EEG signals have five types of brainwaves, which are delta, theta, alpha, beta, and gamma, but the existing models for binaural beats are not optimal for brainwaves other than delta waves. Furthermore, in this study, the level of anxiety has been categorized into minimal, mild, moderate, and severe anxiety, which has not yet been analyzed about binaural beats. Hence, novel, deep CNN-based signal processing has been integrated into EEG signal processing to analyze the effect of binaural beats on anxiety. The deep CNN model extracts all the deep features related to anxiety from EEG signals, which leads to more precise results for binaural beats' impacts on anxiety in terms of brainwaves, thereby achieving an effective and feasible result for the effect of binaural beats on minimal, mild, moderate, and severe of anxiety and accuracy for the analysis of binaural beats' effects.

Figure 1 shows a block diagram for proposed EEG signal processing based on a deep CNN with optimized wavelet transform, in which a raw EEG signal is transformed into a wavelet parameter and is analyzed in time–frequency space. Then, by integrating the flower pollination algorithm, the optimized wavelet parameters are obtained without artifacts in EEG signals, and the deep CNN is then used to extract features and classify the various levels of anxiety in the extracted signal.

3.1. BAI with Alpha Binaural Beats

The level of anxiety was determined by examining the effect of binaural beatsusing the Beck Anxiety Inventory (BAI), which meant in terms of determining the severity of the physical and cognitive symptoms of anxiety throughout the previous week, a four-point scale was considered that included more self-reported items. To accomplish this, some physically healthier subjects were selected and they filled in the BAI inventory. Based on their BAI scores, the subjects were divided into five groups, the minimal, mild, moderate, and severe anxiety groups, as well as a control group. The typical cut-offs are as follows: 0–9, minimal depression; 10–18, mild depression; 19–29, moderate depression; 30–63, severe depression. Multiple statements with the same score were noticed for some BAI items. For these statements, the four groups of subjects were listening to alpha binaural beats for a particular period, with ranges in a frequency of 7–13 Hz which may encourage relaxation. Although not quite meditation, alpha waves are connected to profound physical and mental calm. The consequences of stress are countered by the slight euphoria/excitement and tranquility brought on by alpha waves, which also lower cortisol levels and improve the immune system. Melatonin production is also increased by alpha waves, which significantly enhances the quality of sleep. The control group subjects, however, were not subjected to any music therapy. After the stimulation, all the subjects filled out the BAI inventory as a self-reported analysis of the effect of binaural beats on anxiety.

3.2. Optimized Wavelet Transform

The EEG signals acquired from all the subjects before and after stimulation are processed to technically analyze the effects of the binaural beats. Optimized wavelet transform (OWT) is applied to obtain information from non-stationary signals like EEGs in both the temporal and frequency domains. The contributions of the OWT towards extracting features from the source signal rely on the precise choice of wavelet parameters. Despite this, there is not a clear cutoff formula for choosing a wavelet basis function to effectively use this optimized wavelet, transform, in which artifacts are removed from the EEG signal using the concept of flower pollination optimization, which is integrated with the wavelet transform for the optimal selection of wavelet parameters to select the optimal parameter. A lower mean square error (MSE) and higher signal-to-noise ratio (SNR) are considered objective functions for solving optimization problems. The efficiency of noise reduction and unique feature extraction relies on the selection of optimized wavelet parameters. The optimized wavelet denoising process has two phases: first, the wavelet parameters are selected based on the decomposition level of the EEG signal, and second, the selection of appreciating parameters based on the flower pollination algorithm produces the denoised EEG signal.

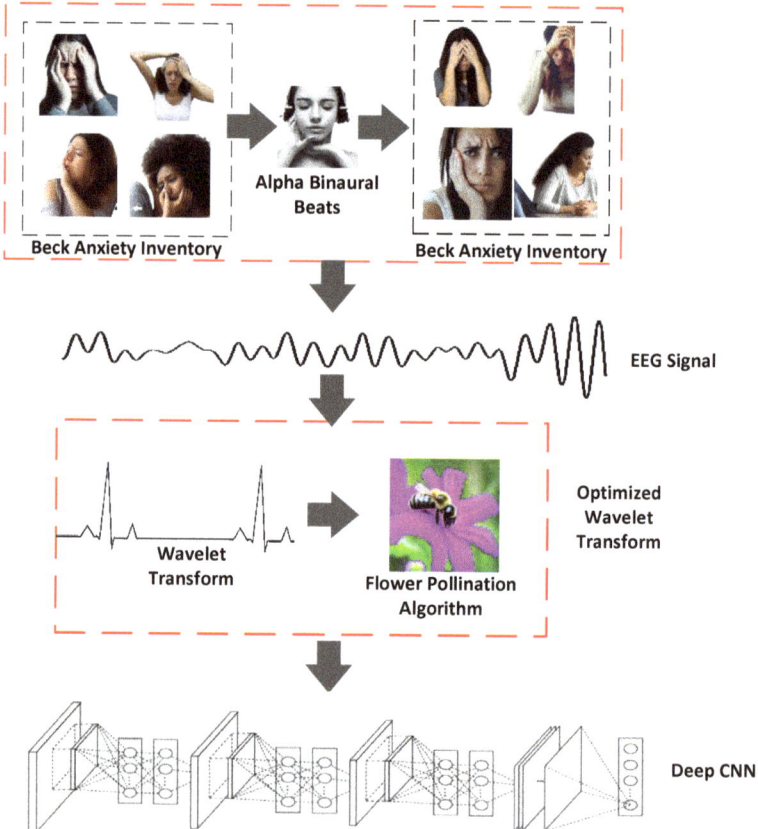

Figure 1. The architecture of the proposed EEG signal processing is based on a deep CNN with optimized wavelet transform.

The original (mother) wavelet $h_{m,k}(t)$ is often the source of the set of wavelet functions in the EEG signal. It is dilated by a value of $a = 2m$, translated by the constant $b = k\,2m$, and normalized so that it is given by Equation (1), as follows:

$$h_{m,k}(t) = 1\ \sqrt{a}h(\ t-b\,a\ ) = 1\ \sqrt{2m}h(2-m\,t-k) \tag{1}$$

According to the given integer values of m, k, and the initial wavelet, which is either determined analytically or by solving a dilation equation which is given in Equation (2) below.

$$x(n) = a_0 + \sum_{m=0}^{s-1} \sum_{k=0}^{2^{s-m}-1} a_{2^{s-m-1}+k} - h(2^{-m}n - k) \quad (2)$$

The $x(n)$, the dilation equation, is transformed to x_i^{t+1} due to the wavelet parameter initialization of the constant value, which is the global pollination operator, to determine the best suitable wavelet parameter. Thus, the modified form of the dilation equation is given by Equation (3).

$$x_i^{t+1} = x_i^t + L(X_i^t - g_*) \quad (3)$$

The levy distribution (L) is given in Equation (4), as follows:

$$L \sim \frac{\lambda \Gamma(\lambda) \sin(\pi \lambda / 2)}{\pi} \frac{1}{s^{1+\lambda}} (s \gg s0 > 0) \quad (4)$$

where λ is the wavelength parameter and s is the step vector, which is in the threshold limit of the transformed EEG signal for the distribution. Similarly, for local pollination, Equation (5) is used to update the x_i with the local parameter, k, of the decision factor, and ε is the switching probability. The local pollination operator x_i^{k+1} in the updation of the wavelet parameter is given by,

$$x_i^{k+1} = x_i^k + \varepsilon \left(x_i^k - x_t^k \right) \quad (5)$$

The proposed optimized wavelet transforms, via the flower pollination optimization algorithm, have two objective functions: $min\ (MSE)$ and $max\ (SNR)$ which are given in Equation (6), as thus the fitness function of the proposed system is given in Equation (6):

$$f = Min(Max(1 - SSIM(X\ N)) \quad (6)$$

The two objective functions, which are the mean squared error (MSE) and signal-to-noise ratio (SNR), are formulated in Equation (6). The fitness formulation makes use of the (1-SSIM), also known as the dissimilarity index, which is generated for each picture in the iteration and tends to further minimize its maximum value. Thus, the fitness function of the system is given by the minimum mean square error and the maximum signal-to-noise ratio in the optimized wave transform. The process takes place in an optimized wavelet transform using the flower pollination algorithm.

Figure 2 illustrates the conceptual diagram of an optimized wavelet transform using the flower pollination algorithm, in which the contaminated EEG signal is expanded using an optimized wavelet transform to obtain optimized wavelet coefficients, and then the wavelet transform is integrated with the flower pollination optimization algorithm to select the best wavelet parameters that remove the most artifacts from the EEG signal.

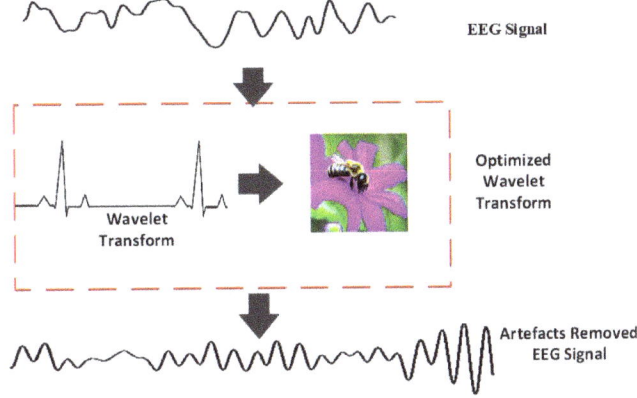

Figure 2. Conceptual diagram of optimized wavelet transform using flower pollination optimization.

The Algorithm 1 for the flower pollination optimization of the optimized wavelet parameter has been explained as follows:

Algorithm 1: Flower pollination optimization of the optimized wavelet parameter

---

Input: Wavelet parameter
Output: Best wavelet parameter without noise
Initialize: n parameters with random solution
Define a switch probability $p \in [0, 1]$
Calculate all f for n solutions
$t = 0$
while $(i \geq N)$ do
    for $i = 1, \ldots, N$ do
        if $rnd \leq p$ then
            Draw a (d-dimensional) step vector in the L which obeys a Levy distribution
            Perform $x_i^{t+1} = x_i^t + L(X_i^t - g_*)$
        else if
            Perform $x_i^{k+1} = x_i^k + \varepsilon\left(x_i^k - x_t^k\right)$
        Select $x_i^{t+1}(t) \leftarrow 1$;
        Else
         Draw from a uniform distribution $\in [0,1]$
        Select $x_i^{k+1} \leftarrow 0$;
        end if
        Calculate $f'(x)$ /*f' is the fitness function calculated at random distribution */
        if $f'(x^*) \leq f(x)$ then $x^* = x$
        end if
    end for
    Find the current best solution $g*$ among all x_i^k
    $t = t + 1$
end while

The flower pollination algorithm with optimized wavelet parameters shows the initialization of the n parameters with a random solution. The input is the wavelet transform parameter and the output obtained from the optimized wavelet parameter with the flower pollination algorithm is given as the best wavelet parameter with the solution to the input, thus, the uniform distribution of the parameters is taken into account to obtain the best solution g among all x_i^k of the probability switching function of the wavelet transform. The switching function determines the difference due to the high probability of the wavelet transform being in the best wavelet selection. It also generates a random function for the flower pollination optimization algorithm and the wavelet transform to obtain the step vector s from the levy distribution that provides the performance of global and local pollination, thus, the best solution is obtained by calculating the decision factors x_i^k of the current solution via the top solution discovered globally in a global pollination operator x_i^t. The improvement loop must be exchanged either locally or globally by the switch operator i, therefore, up until a point of stagnation, this procedure is repeated.

Figure 3 depicts the flow diagram of an optimal wavelet transform, which begins with the signal's initialization pattern for data collection. The input signal data is read first, then an efficient wavelet transform is performed for each signal to choose the best wavelet parameters. A greater signal-to-noise ratio (SNR) and a lower mean square error (MSE) are considered to be the objective functions for addressing optimization problems that remove artifacts from the EEG signal.

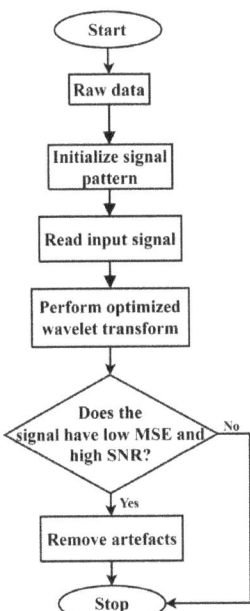

Figure 3. Flow chart of optimized wavelet transform.

3.3. Deep CNN-Based Signal Processing

Deep CNN-based signal processing extracts features and combines various classification elements, it also offers a good path for the precise detection of various brain states. Thus, several features were recovered from the denoised EEG signal to extract features such as the alpha, beta, theta, delta, and gamma brainwaves and both their time and frequency domains, including the mean, standard deviation, entropy, and energy, four widely used measurements of the signal. The electroencephalogram, with its mean value, provided the iteration varies from 1 to L, has a standard deviation with a different set of signal processing, thus, the energy of the system is given by the delta frequency domain, thus, the entropy of the electroencephalogram is also given by the DCNN-based signal processing. Therefore, to extract usable features from the EEG signal of each participant, the DCNN is trained individually. Each participant's number of channels that recorded high-quality data varied during the pre-processing stage, it was discovered. The EEG signal of each participant was left with a variable number of channels and some channels were eliminated based on the signal-to-noise ratio and low mean square error, therefore classification was accomplished via DCNN to extract useful features such as delta, theta, alpha, betta, and gamma brainwaves from the optimized wavelet coefficients. The DCNN predicts the associated class to which an independent variable belongs using a variety of independent variable values' features as input. For instance, for a specific feature x of a class y, the classifier is a function f that predicts the class $y = f(x)$. The DCNN's architecture has interconnected nodes that store and process data through connections formed between its nodes as a result of a learning process that recognizes patterns in the training data.

The input layer function based on time-frequency analysis is formalized as Equation (7):

$$I_t = \varphi(g_i * .(h_{t-1}, x_i^{t+1}) + x_i \tag{7}$$

The hidden layer function based on time-frequency analysis is formalized as Equation (8):

$$h_t = \varphi(g_f * .(h_{t-1}, x_i^{t+1}) + x_f \tag{8}$$

The output layer function based on time-frequency analysis is formalized as Equation (9):

$$O_t = \varphi(g_o *.(h_{t-1}, x_i^{t+1})+x_o \tag{9}$$

The output with the activation function of the deep CNN is formalized as Equation (10):

$$a = \varphi[\sum_j g * x_i^{k+1} + x] \tag{10}$$

where x_i^{k+1} are the unit inputs, b is the bias, φ is the nonlinear activation function, and a is the activation unit. As a result, a separate set of cases is used to test the classifier's performance, which gives the accurate classification of the anxiety level as mild, moderate, minimal, or severe. Thus the $g*$ is the output from the optimized wave parameters. Here, x_i is the unit of the input layer of the DCNN, x_f is the unit of the hidden layer function of the DCNN, and x_o is the unit of the output activation function of the DCNN. Thus, the activation unit of the deep convolution neural network is given by the summation of the EEG signal with the product of the best solution obtained from the wavelet parameter, thus, the activation unit stimulates the deep convolution neural network to classify the performance as a different level of anxiety. The architecture of the deep CNN-based signal processing's feature extraction and classification is shown in Figure 4.

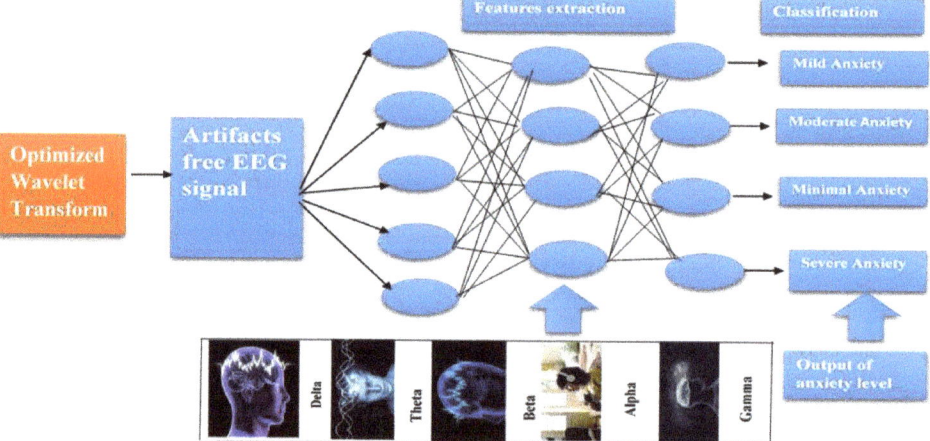

Figure 4. The architecture of deep CNN-based signal processing's feature extraction and classification.

Figure 4 shows the deep CNN-based signal processing's feature extraction and classification, in which five features were extracted from the artifacts-free EEG signal, which was the alpha, beta, theta, delta, and gamma time and frequency domains in brainwaves. Therefore, this model predicts the anxiety level of each feature by using a non-linear activation function in its classification.

Overall, the optimized wavelet transform removes artifacts from the EEG signal using the concept of flower pollination optimization, which is integrated with the wavelet transform for the optimal selection of wavelet parameters. Deep CNN-based signal processing has been integrated into the EEG signal's processing to analyze the effect of binaural beats on anxiety by extracting all the features belonging to anxiety from the EEG signal, providing more accurate results for the binaural beats' effects on anxiety in terms of brainwaves. The next section explains the results obtained from the proposed model in detail.

4. Results and Discussion

This section provides a detailed description of the implementation results as well as the performance of the proposed system and a comparison section to ensure that the proposed system works effectively.

4.1. Simulation Setup

This work has been implemented in the working platform of Python with the following system specifications, and its simulation results are discussed below.

- Platform: Python;
- OS: Windows;
- Processor: 64-bit Intel;
- RAM: 8 GB.

4.2. Dataset Description

The dataset used in this research was the EEG Brainwave Dataset: Feeling Emotions, in which data were gathered from two individuals, namely a man and a woman, for three minutes in each of the three states, namely positive, neutral, and negative. It also used Muse EEG headgear to capture the EEG locations at TP9, AF7, AF8, and TP10 using dry electrodes. The stimuli used to create the emotions were collected for six minutes along with the neutral data. The parameters used in the flower pollination algorithm are described in Table 1.

Table 1. Parameters of flower pollination algorithm.

Parameters	Value
Maximum generation	1000
Switch probability	0.8
Population size	25
Upper boundary	−10
Lower boundary	10
Model order	3
Number of parameters	6

4.3. Simulated Output of Proposed System

The simulated output of the proposed system in the analyses of anxiety levels after hearing alpha binaural beats is explained in this subsection.

Figure 5 shows the channel frequency by varying the time before the applying wavelet transform. The channel frequency ranges from −2000 to 2000 in the time range of 0.1 to 80,000 ns. From these channel frequencies, it is difficult to obtain the important parameters of the signal. Hence the wavelet transform has been applied to extract the signal parameters.

Figure 6 shows the channel frequency obtained by varying the time after applying the wavelet transform. The channel frequency ranges from −2000 to 2000 in the time range of 0.1 to 90,000 ns. The channel frequencies are optimized by selecting the best wavelet parameters by incorporating the flower pollination algorithm, and the level of anxiety is then analyzed via the DCNN based on the frequency range of the signal.

Figure 7 shows the classification results of the proposed system for the level of anxiety. The classification results show a mild level of anxiety in 20 cases, moderate anxiety in 30, minimal anxiety in 40, and severe anxiety in 10, based on the EEG signal processing of brainwaves.

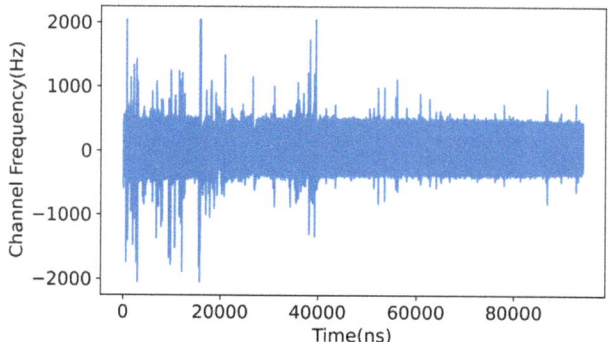

Figure 5. Channel frequency before wavelet transform.

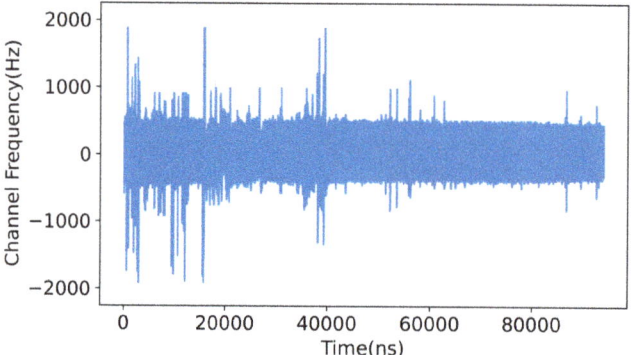

Figure 6. Channel frequency after wavelet transform.

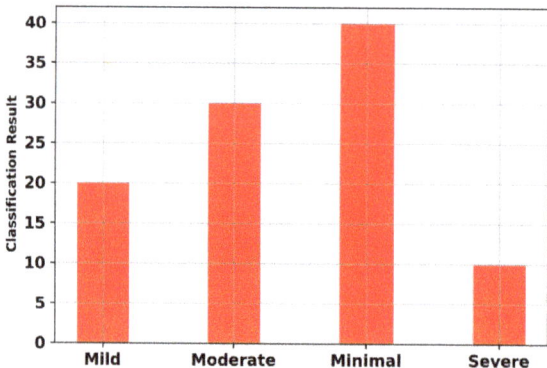

Figure 7. Classification results of the proposed system for determining anxiety levels.

4.4. Performance Metrics of the Proposed System

The performance of the proposed approach and the achieved outcomes are explained in detail in this section.

Figure 8 shows the accuracy of the proposed system with varying numbers of epochs. The accuracy attains a minimum value of 0.65 at the initial stage and attains a maximum value of 0.98 at 27 epochs. Thus, it was noticed that the accuracy increased with the increase in epochs. The accuracy of the proposed system was increased using deep CNN-based signal processing, which extracted all the features associated with anxiety from the brainwaves in the EEG signals.

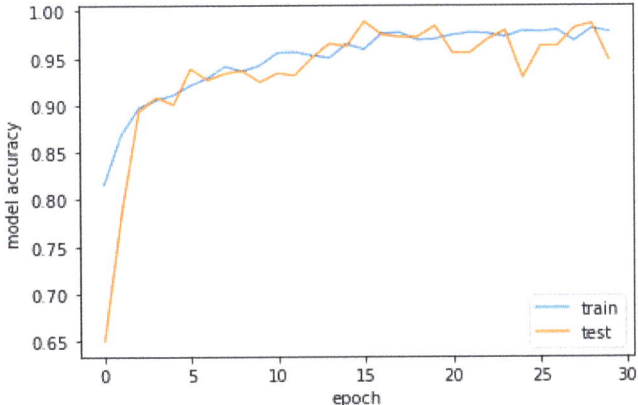

Figure 8. Accuracy of the proposed system with varying epochs.

Figure 9 shows the loss of the proposed system with varying numbers of epochs. The loss has a minimum value of 0.5 at one epoch. The loss of the proposed system has a maximum value of 2.5 at the initial stage. The loss of the proposed system is decreased by using deep CNN-based signal processing to extract all the characteristics linked to the anxiety of brainwaves in an EEG signal-optimized wavelet transform, in which artifacts are removed from the EEG signal, which does not reduce the original energy of the EEG signal.

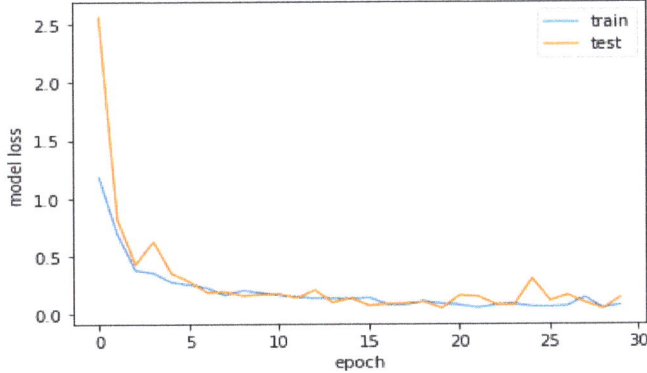

Figure 9. Loss of the proposed system with varying epochs.

Figure 10 shows the precision of the proposed system with varying numbers of epochs. The precision has a minimum value of 20 at one epoch and attains a maximum value of 100 at five epochs. The precision of the proposed system is increased using deep CNN-based signal processing, which extracts all the features belonging to anxiety from brainwaves in EEG signal, and classification is conducted after extracting all these features.

Figure 11 shows the recall of the proposed system with varying the numbers of epochs. The recall has a minimum value of 19.5 at one epoch and a maximum value of 99 at five epochs. The recall of the proposed system is increased using deep CNN-based signal processing, which extracts all features associated with anxiety from the brainwaves in an EEG signal.

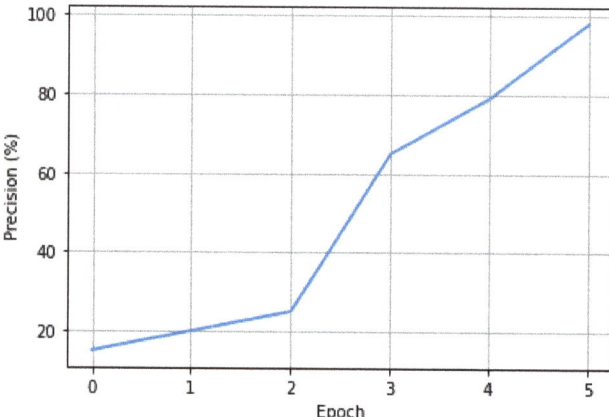

Figure 10. Precision of proposed system with varying epochs.

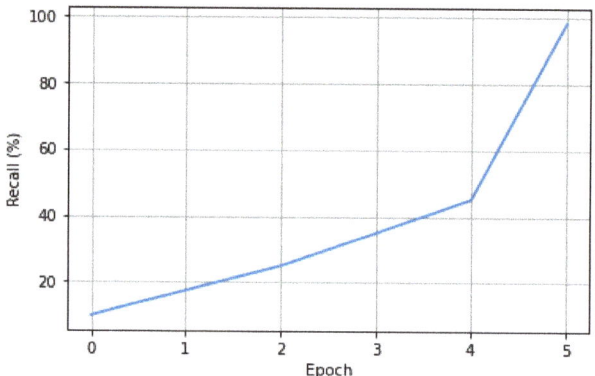

Figure 11. Recall the proposed system with varying epochs.

Figure 12 shows the F1-score of the proposed system with varying numbers of epochs. The F1 score has a minimum value of 17.5 at one epoch and a maximum value of 99.5 at five epochs. The F1-score of the proposed system is increased using deep CNN-based signal processing, which removes artifacts and extracts all the deep features belonging to anxiety from the brainwaves in the EEG signal.

Figure 13 shows the sensitivity of the proposed system with varying numbers of epochs. The sensitivity has a minimum value of 80 in epoch 25 and a maximum value of 99.8 in epoch 200. The sensitivity of the proposed system is increased using the optimized wavelet transform, which provides the process for artifact removal and examines the sensitivity of the brainwave EEG signal.

Figure 14 depicts the specificity of the proposed system with varying numbers of epochs. The specificity has a minimum value of about 85 in epoch 23 and a maximum value of about 98 at the specificity of about 200 epochs. The specificity of the proposed system is determined using the flower pollination optimization algorithm.

Figure 15 shows the sensitivity of the proposed system by varying the numbers of data counts. The sensitivity has a minimum value of about 94% with a data count of about 1000 and a maximum value of 98% in the realm of 6000 data counts. Thus, the sensitivity of the proposed system is increased using the optimized wavelet transform, in which the artifacts are removed and thus the sensitivity of the proposed system increases with the increasing data count.

Figure 16 shows the specificity of the proposed system with varying data counts. The specificity has a minimum value of about 96.75% at 2000 data counts and a maximum value of 99% at 6000 data counts. The specificity of the proposed system initially decreases suddenly with the increasing number of data counts and then it starts increasing with further increases in the number of data counts. Thus the specificity of the proposed system is at a maximum at the highest data counts due to the use the optimized wavelet transform.

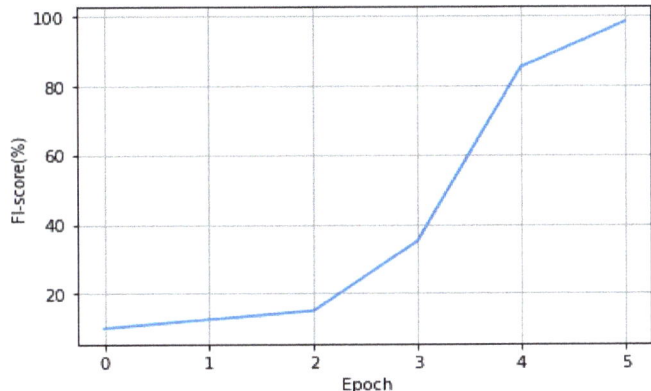

Figure 12. F1-score of the proposed system with varying epochs.

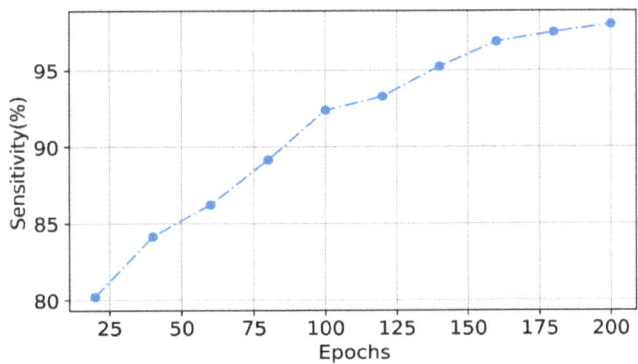

Figure 13. Sensitivity of the proposed system with varying epochs.

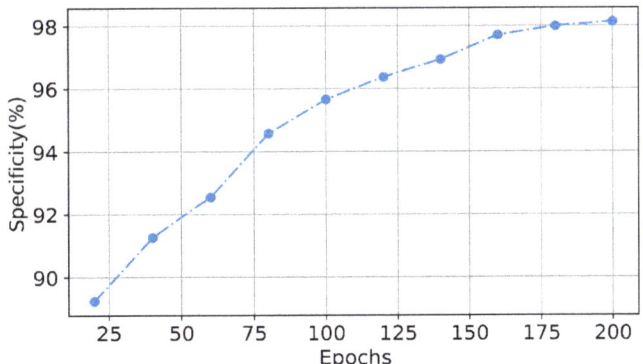

Figure 14. Specificity of the proposed system with varying epochs.

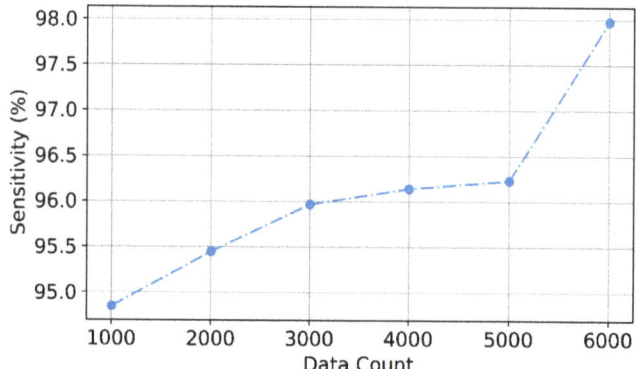

Figure 15. Sensitivity of the proposed system with varying data counts.

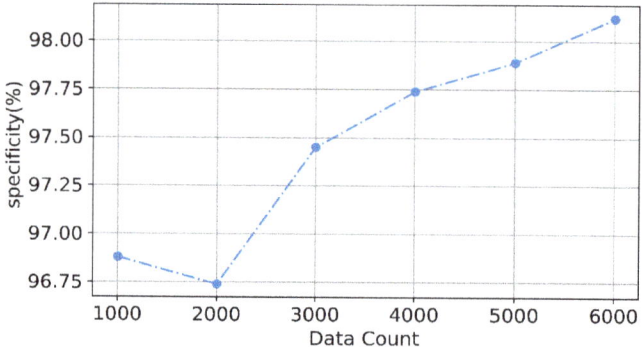

Figure 16. Specificity of the proposed system with varying data counts.

Figure 17 shows the accuracy of the proposed system with varying data counts. The accuracy has a minimum value of 96.3% at 1000 data counts and a maximum value of 98.0% at 6000 data counts. The accuracy of the proposed system is increased using the optimized wavelet transform of the EEG signal to remove artifacts via the concept of flower pollination optimization, which is integrated with the wavelet transform for choosing the best wavelet parameters to then choose the optimal parameter.

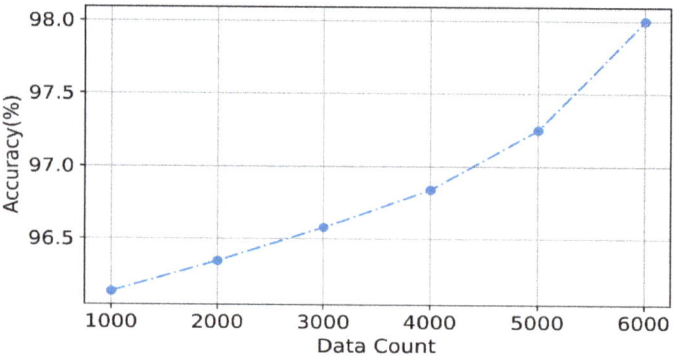

Figure 17. Accuracy of the proposed system with varying data counts.

Figure 18 shows the recall of the proposed system with varying data counts. The recall has a minimum value of 93.1% at 1000 data counts and a maximum value of 95.0% at 6000 data counts. The recall of the proposed system is increased via the optimized wavelet transform of the EEG signal, which removes artifacts using the flower pollination algorithm for choosing the best wavelet parameters to then choose the optimal parameter.

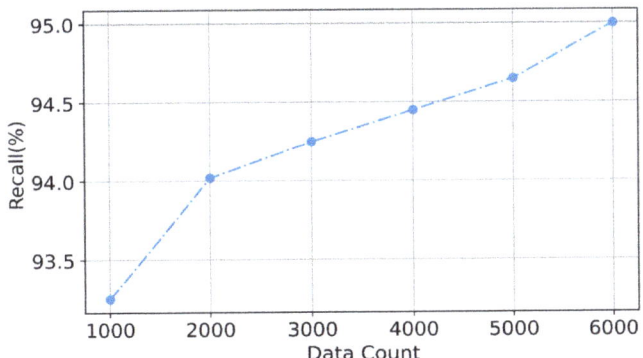

Figure 18. Recall the proposed system for varying data counts.

Figure 19 shows the F1-score of the proposed system with varying data counts. The F1-score has a minimum value of 94.2% at 1000 data counts and a maximum value of 95% at 6000 data counts. The recall of the proposed system is increased using the optimized wavelet transform of the EEG signal, in which the main objective of this WT approach is to identify an effective decomposition of the input EEG data that produces distinctive features from each sub-band using the flower pollination optimization algorithm, which is used to select optimal wavelet parameters to remove artifacts from EEG signals.

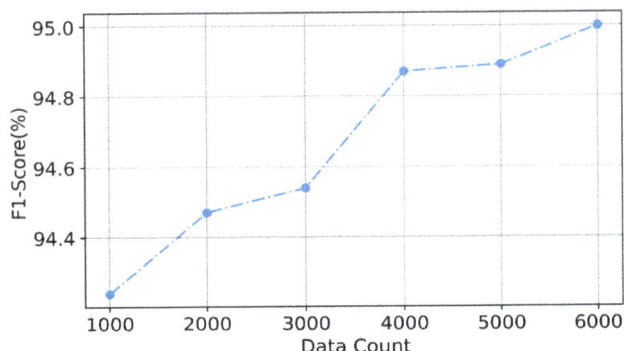

Figure 19. F1-score of the proposed system with varying aata counts.

Figure 20 shows the precision of the proposed system with varying data counts. The precision has a minimum value of 92.14% at 1000 data counts and a maximum value of 95% at 6000 data counts. The precision of the proposed system is increased by selecting the optimum wavelet parameters using the optimized wavelet transform of an EEG signal with a flower pollination algorithm.

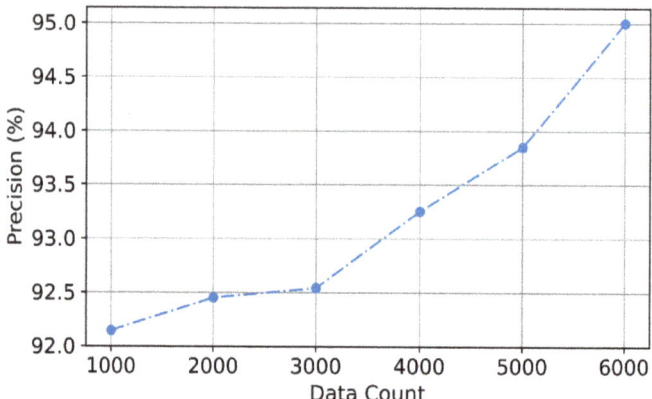

Figure 20. The precision of the proposed system for varying data counts.

4.5. Comparison of the Results of the Proposed Method

This section highlights the proposed system performance by comparing it to the outcomes of existing approaches and showing their results based on various metrics.

Below, Table 2 shows the comparison of the proposed model with the existing models such as KNN, SVM, LDA, and Narrow-ANN [38–42]. Compared with the existing models, the proposed deep CNN achieves a high accuracy of 0.99%, a precision value of 0.99%, and a specificity of 0.999%. The F1-score and recall of the proposed system have the maximum values of 0.99% and 0.99%, whereas the existing models KNN, SVM, LDA, and Narrow-ANN, have F1-scores of 0.90%, 0.98%, 0.921%, and 0.983%, respectively, and recalls of 0.90%, 0.98%, 0.92%, and 0.985%, respectively. Also, the proposed model attains a low error of 0.01. This shows that the proposed model achieved a better performance than the existing models.

Table 2. Comparison table.

Specification	KNN	SVM	LDA	Narrow-ANN	Proposed
Accuracy (%)	0.90	0.98	0.92	0.985	0.99
Recall (%)	0.90	0.98	0.92	0.985	0.99
Precision (%)	0.90	0.98	0.93	0.985	0.99
F1-Score (%)	0.90	0.98	0.921	0.983	0.99
Specificity (%)	0.975	0.995	0.980	0.9951	0.999
Error (%)	0.01	0.02	0.08	0.01	0.01

Table 3 depicts the cumulative survey on binaural beats processing and, from this table, it is understood that the accuracy can be further improved. The existing research that uses machine learning techniques such as KNN, MLP, and SVM, has accuracy values in the range of 60 to 75%, whereas the existing techniques that use some advanced deep learning techniques such as CNNs and ANNs have accuracy values in the range of 80 to 97%. However, these existing techniques have error and generalization issues while achieving high accuracy. Hence, the proposed model used an optimization algorithm along with a deep learning model to achieve a high accuracy of 99% without any error.

Table 3. Cumulative survey on binaural beats processing.

Ref.	Technique Used	Benefits	Limitations	Result Obtained
[31]	e-LORETA	Visual depiction of the impact of binaural beats	MLP shows better performance only on delta waves	Accuracy: 64.77%
[36]	Modified sample entropy feature	The interface system takes only 3 sec to determine the effect of stimuli	Attention-related movements can reduce accuracy	Takes only 3 seconds to determine the effect of audio and visual stimuli.
[35]	ASMR	Can lessen the annoyance of binaural beats while improving brainwave entrainment	N/A	CS could cause 6 Hz activity for inducing NREM sleep stage 1
[38]	Artificial neural network	Can identify and eliminate stress based on user preferences and treatment records	K-nearest neighbor shows better performance on some brainwaves only	Accuracy: 90%
[32]	DFT-SOM-ANN	Mental pattern recognition with high accuracy	Artifacts introduced in older adults cannot be removed via DFT	Accuracy: 98.68%
[40]	ESD-ANN	Excellent accuracy in identifying woman with and without stress, using the entire brain	Optimal channel selection difficult with ANN	Accuracy: 89.19%
[41]	C3RNN	Better performance than baseline CRNN with the same weights and high training speed	The error can be generated due to backpropagation	Accuracy: 84.1%
[42]	CNN	Accurately distinguishes EEGs of individuals listening to music from those of subjects without auditory input	May not consider the generalization issue	Accuracy: 97.68%
[43]	Brainwave stimulator	Promotes the production of alpha brainwaves to decrease stress	Artifacts due to eye blinking and muscle movements are not considered	A significant increase in the number of alpha brainwave PSD observed
[33]	Bi-spectral analysis	Extracts features providing information about the distribution and dispersion of signals	The usage of discrete Fourier transform for filtering could reduce the original energy of the EEG signal	The degree of synchronization ranged from 52.1% to 83.4%
[45]	Semantic-based Bayesian network engine	Records and analyzes correlations between binaural beats, EEG, and perceived mental states	Implementation outcomes are not provided in a detailed manner	Performance: 72.25%
[46]	Fast Fourier transform	Shows entrainments after the perception of binaural beats based on an associated EEG rhythm	The technique should be time-fixed for assessing the brain's reaction to quick shifts in auditory intensity	Absolute power value ranges between 5 and 15 μV^2
Proposed model	Deep CNN-based signal processing	Extraction of deep features from EEG signals, enabling precise identification of the impacts of binaural beats on various types of brainwaves and anxiety levels. This provides more accurate and detailed insights into the effects of binaural beats on different levels of anxiety, leading to a more effective and feasible outcome.	N/A	Accuracy: 99%

Overall, the optimized wavelet transform using deep CNN-based signal processing outperforms existing techniques such as KNN, SVM, LDA, and Narrow-ANN (andvarious forms of ANNs with a high accuracy of 0.99%, precision of 0.99%, recall of 0.99%, F1-score of 0.99%, specificity of 0.999%, and error rate of 0.01% in identifying an effective decomposition of the input EEG data and extracting all deep features belonging to anxiety and analyzing the effect of binaural beats on the level of anxiety.

5. Conclusions

An optimized wavelet transform with the flower pollination optimization algorithm has been proposed to remove artifacts from EEG signals without reducing the original signal's energy, in which the flower pollination optimization algorithm is integrated with the wavelet transform for the optimal selection of wavelet parameters, the result of which are that the artifacts are removed from the EEG signal with aminimum loss value of 0.4 and a high accuracy of 99%. Then, EEG signals have five types of brainwaves, delta, theta, beta, alpha, and gamma, which are optimally analyzed via deep CNN-based signal processing that is integrated into EEG signal processing and helps with analyzing the effect of binaural beats on the four levels of anxiety (minimal, mild, moderate, and severe). This model can extract all the deep features belonging to anxiety from EEG signals, which provide more accurate results for establishing binaural beats' effects on anxiety via brainwaves. Thus, the results obtained from the proposed method outperform existing techniques with a high accuracy of 99%, precision of 96%, recall of 97%, and F1-score of 96%. As a result, the novel methodology provides effective and promising results for determining the effect of binaural beats on four levels of anxiety.

While the deep CNN model extracts deep features from EEG signals, the complexity of interpreting brainwave patterns, especially in the context of anxiety, can pose challenges. There may be inherent difficulties in accurately quantifying the relationship between binaural beats and specific brainwave activities related to anxiety. Future studies might concentrate on developing real-time monitoring systems that use the proposed methodologies to offer instant feedback on the efficacy of binaural beats in controlling anxiety levels, allowing for immediate treatment.

Author Contributions: Conceptualization, B.S.A. and D.R.; methodology, D.R.; software, D.R.; validation, B.S.A. and B.A.; formal analysis, B.S.A. and D.R.; investigation, B.A. and A.V.J.; resources, B.A.; data curation, A.V.J.; writing—original draft preparation, D.R. and B.S.A.; writing—review and editing, B.A. and B.S.A.; visualization, B.A. and A.V.J.; supervision, B.A.; funding acquisition, B.A. All authors have read and agreed to the published version of the manuscript.

Funding: This research received no external funding.

Institutional Review Board Statement: Not applicable.

Informed Consent Statement: Not applicable.

Data Availability Statement: Data are contained within the article.

Conflicts of Interest: The authors declare no conflicts of interest.

References

1. Phillips, S.P.; Yu, J. Is anxiety/depression increasing among 5–25 year-olds? A cross-sectional prevalence study in Ontario, Canada, 1997–2017. *J. Affect. Disord.* **2021**, *282*, 141–146. [CrossRef] [PubMed]
2. Twenge, J.M.; Joiner, T.E. U.S. Census Bureau-assessed prevalence of anxiety and depressive symptoms in 2019 and during the 2020 COVID-19 pandemic. *Depress. Anxiety* **2020**, *37*, 954–956. [CrossRef] [PubMed]
3. Goodin, P.; Ciorciari, J.; Baker, K.; Carrey, A.M.; Harper, M.; Kaufman, J. A high-density EEG investigation into steady state binaural beat stimulation. *PLoS ONE* **2012**, *7*, e34789. [CrossRef]
4. Ossebaard, H.C. Stress reduction by technology? An experimental study into the effects of brainmachines on burnout and state anxiety. *Appl. Psychophysiol. Biofeedback* **2000**, *25*, 93–101. [CrossRef] [PubMed]
5. Huang, T.L.; Charyton, C. A comprehensive review of the psychological effects of brainwave entrainment. Database of Abstracts of Reviews of Effects (DARE): Quality-assessed Reviews [Internet]. *Altern. Ther. Health Med.* **2008**, *14*, 38–50.

6. Padmanabhan, R.; Hildreth, A.J.; Laws, D. A prospective, randomised, controlled study examining binaural beat audio and pre-operative anxiety in patients undergoing general anaesthesia for day case surgery. *Anaesthesia* **2005**, *60*, 874–877. [CrossRef]
7. Au, T.Y.; Assavarittirong, C. The overview of utilizing complementary therapy to relieve stress or anxiety in emergency department patients: Animal-assisted therapy, art therapy, and music therapy. *MHGC Proceeding* **2021**, *4*, 2. [CrossRef]
8. Wahbeh, H.; Calabrese, C.; Zwickey, H. Binaural beat technology in humans: A pilot study to assess psychologic and physiologic effects. *J. Altern. Complement. Med.* **2007**, *13*, 25–32. [CrossRef]
9. Chaieb, L.; Wilpert, E.C.; Reber, T.P.; Fell, J. Auditory beat stimulation and its effects on cognition and mood states. *Front. Psychiatry* **2015**, *6*, 70. [CrossRef]
10. Gao, X.; Cao, H.; Ming, D.; Qi, H.; Wang, X.; Wang, X.; Chen, R.; Zhou, P. Analysis of EEG activity in response to binaural beats with different frequencies. *Int. J. Psychophysiol.* **2014**, *94*, 399–406. [CrossRef]
11. Karino, S.; Yumoto, M.; Itoh, K.; Uno, A.; Yamakawa, K.; Sekimoto, S.; Kaga, K. Neuromagnetic responses to binaural beat in human cerebral cortex. *J. Neurophysiol.* **2006**, *96*, 1927–1938. [CrossRef] [PubMed]
12. Karino, S.; Yumoto, M.; Itoh, K.; Uno, A.; Matsuda, M.; Yamakawa, K.; Sekimoto, S.; Kaneko, Y.; Kaga, K. Magnetoencephalographic study of human auditory steady-state responses to binaural beat. *Int. Congr. Ser.* **2004**, *1270*, 169–172. [CrossRef]
13. Beauchene, C.; Abaid, N.; Moran, R.; Diana, R.A.; Leonessa, A. The effect of binaural beats on visuospatial working memory and cortical connectivity. *PLoS ONE* **2016**, *11*, e0166630. [CrossRef] [PubMed]
14. Beauchene, C.; Abaid, N.; Moran, R.; A Diana, R.; Leonessa, A. The effect of binaural beats on verbal working memory and cortical connectivity. *J. Neural Eng.* **2017**, *14*, 026014. [CrossRef] [PubMed]
15. Ioannou, C.I.; Pereda, E.; Lindsen, J.P.; Bhattacharya, J. Electrical brain responses to an auditory illusion and the impact of musical expertise. *PLoS ONE* **2015**, *10*, e0129486. [CrossRef] [PubMed]
16. Weiland, T.J.; A Jelinek, G.; E Macarow, K.; Samartzis, P.; Brown, D.M.; Grierson, E.M.; Winter, C. Original sound compositions reduce anxiety in emergency department patients: A randomised controlled trial. *Med. J. Aust.* **2011**, *195*, 694–698. [CrossRef] [PubMed]
17. Siminenco, A. The perspective of using binaural beat auditory stimulation in the treatment of pain. In *MedEspera: The 6th International Medical Congress for Students and Young Doctors: Abstract Book*; MedEspera: Chisinau, Moldova, 2016.
18. Alipoor, A.; Oraki, M.; Sabet, M.Y. Efficiency of brainwave entrainment by binaural beats in reducing anxiety. *J. Kermanshah Univ. Med. Sci.* **2014**, *18*, e74271.
19. Fougère, M.; Greco-Vuilloud, J.; Arnous, C.; Lowe, C. Sensory stimulations potentializing digital therapeutics pain control. *Front. Pain Res.* **2023**, *4*, 1168377. [CrossRef]
20. Urigüen, J.A.; Garcia-Zapirain, B. EEG artifact removal—State-of-the-art and guidelines. *J. Neural Eng.* **2015**, *12*, 031001. [CrossRef]
21. Huppert, T.J.; Diamond, S.G.; Franceschini, M.A.; Boas, D.A. HomER: A review of time-series analysis methods for near-infrared spectroscopy of the brain. *Appl. Opt.* **2009**, *48*, D280–D298. [CrossRef]
22. Islam, K.; Rastegarnia, A.; Yang, Z. Methods for artifact detection and removal from scalp EEG: A review. *Neurophysiol. Clin.* **2016**, *46*, 287–305. [CrossRef] [PubMed]
23. Wallstrom, G.L.; Kass, R.E.; Miller, A.; Cohn, J.F.; Fox, N. Automatic correction of ocular artifacts in the EEG: A comparison of regression-based and component-based methods. *Int. J. Psychophysiol.* **2004**, *53*, 105–119. [CrossRef]
24. Hamal, A.Q.; Rehman, A.W.b.A. Artifact processing of epileptic EEG signals: An overview of different types of artifacts. In Proceedings of the 2013 International Conference on Advanced Computer Science Applications and Technologies, Kuching, Malaysia, 23–24 December 2013; IEEE: New York, NY, USA, 2013.
25. Goncharova, I.; McFarland, D.; Vaughan, T.; Wolpaw, J. EMG contamination of EEG: Spectral and topographical characteristics. *Clin. Neurophysiol.* **2003**, *114*, 1580–1593. [CrossRef] [PubMed]
26. Yusim, A.; Grigaitis, J. Efficacy of Binaural Beat Meditation Technology for Treating Anxiety Symptoms: A Pilot Study. *J. Nerv. Ment. Dis.* **2020**, *208*, 155–160. [CrossRef] [PubMed]
27. Gkolias, V.; Amaniti, A.; Triantafyllou, A.; Papakonstantinou, P.; Kartsidis, P.; Paraskevopoulos, E.; Bamidis, P.D.; Hadjileontiadis, L.; Kouvelas, D. Reduced pain and analgesic use after acoustic binaural beats therapy in chronic pain-A double-blind randomized control cross-over trial. *Eur. J. Pain* **2020**, *24*, 1716–1729. [CrossRef] [PubMed]
28. Sekirin, A.B.; Prikuls, V.F.; Maybrodskaya, A.E. Assessment of clinical efficacy of the acoustic binaural beating method in the complex preparation of patients for hip replacement. *N. N. Priorov J. Traumatol. Orthop.* **2020**, *27*, 60–65. [CrossRef]
29. Menziletoglu, D.; Guler, A.; Cayır, T.; Isik, B. Binaural beats or 432 Hz music? Which method is more effective for reducing preoperative dental anxiety? *Med. Oral Patol. Oral Y Cirugía Bucal* **2021**, *26*, e97–e101. [CrossRef]
30. Mallik, A.; Russo, F.A. The Effect of Music & Auditory Beat Stimulation on Anxiety. *PLoS ONE* **2021**, *17*, e0259312.
31. da Silva Junior, M.; de Freitas, R.C.; dos Santos, W.P.; da Silva, W.W.A.; Rodrigues, M.C.A.; Conde, E.F.Q. Exploratory study of the effect of binaural stimulation on the EEG activity pattern in resting state using artificial neural networks. *Cogn. Syst. Res.* **2019**, *54*, 1–20. [CrossRef]
32. Amarasinghe, K.; Wijayasekara, D.; Manic, M. EEG based brain activity monitoring using Artificial Neural Networks. In Proceedings of the 2014 7th International Conference on Human System Interactions (HSI), Costa da Caparica, Portugal, 16–18 June 2014; IEEE: New York, NY, USA, 2014.
33. El Houda, B.Y.N.; El Amine, D.S.M. Effect of the Marijuana Binaural Beats on the Brain. *Ann. Clin. Cases* **2020**, *1*, 1022.

34. Pluck, G.; López-Águila, M.A. Induction of fear but no effects on cognitive fluency by theta frequency auditory binaural beat stimulation. *Psychol. Neurosci.* **2019**, *12*, 53–64. [CrossRef]
35. Lee, M.; Song, C.-B.; Shin, G.-H.; Lee, S.-W. Possible effect of binaural beat combined with autonomous sensory meridian response for inducing sleep. *Front. Hum. Neurosci.* **2019**, *13*, 425. [CrossRef] [PubMed]
36. Chouhan, T.; Panse, A.; Smitha, K.; Vinod, A. A comparative study on the effect of audio and visual stimuli for enhancing attention and memory in brain computer interface system. In Proceedings of the 2015 IEEE International Conference on Systems, Man, and Cybernetics, Hong Kong, China, 9–10 October 2015; IEEE: New York, NY, USA, 2015.
37. Sakurai, N.; Nagasaka, K.; Takahashi, S.; Kasai, S.; Onishi, H.; Kodama, N. Brain function effects of autonomous sensory meridian response (ASMR) video viewing. *Front. Neurosci.* **2023**, *17*, 1025745. [CrossRef] [PubMed]
38. Jayasinghe, T. Element Mindfulness Approach from Binaural Beats Using Mobile Application. Ph.D. Thesis, Informatics Institute of Technology, Colombo, Sri Lanka, 2019.
39. Rui, Z.; Gu, Z. A review of EEG and fMRI measuring aesthetic processing in visual user experience research. *Comput. Intell. Neurosci.* **2021**, *2021*, 2070209. [CrossRef] [PubMed]
40. Thafa'i, N.A.; Ghani, S.A.; Zaini, N. Classification of Normal and Stress Groups Among Females Based on Electroencephalography Signals Using Artificial Neural Network. *Adv. Sci. Lett.* **2017**, *23*, 5277–5281. [CrossRef]
41. Adavanne, S.; Politis, A.; Virtanen, T. Multichannel sound event detection using 3D convolutional neural networks for learning inter-channel features. In Proceedings of the 2018 International Joint Conference on Neural Networks (IJCNN), Rio de Janeiro, Brazil, 8–13 July 2018; IEEE: New York, NY, USA, 2018.
42. Cheah, K.H.; Nisar, H.; Yap, V.V.; Lee, C.-Y. Convolutional neural networks for classification of music-listening EEG: Comparing 1D convolutional kernels with 2D kernels and cerebral laterality of musical influence. *Neural Comput. Appl.* **2020**, *32*, 8867–8891. [CrossRef]
43. Andrian, Y.F.; Widiyanti, P.; Arisgraha, F.C.S. Alpha brainwave stimulator using light and binaural beats stimulation. *AIP Conf. Proc.* **2020**, *2314*, 1.
44. El Houda Baakek, Y.N.; El Amine Debbal, S.M. Digital drugs (binaural beats): How can it affect the brain/their impact on the brain. *J. Med. Eng. Technol.* **2021**, *45*, 546–551. [CrossRef]
45. Zaini, N.; Omar, H.L.; Latip, M.F.A. Semantic-based Bayesian Network to determine correlation between binaural-beats features and entrainment effects. In Proceedings of the 2011 IEEE International Conference on Computer Applications and Industrial Electronics (ICCAIE), Penang, Malaysia, 4–7 December 2011; IEEE: New York, NY, USA, 2011.
46. Jirakittayakorn, N.; Wongsawat, Y. A novel insight of effects of a 3-Hz binaural beat on sleep stages during sleep. *Front. Hum. Neurosci.* **2018**, *12*, 387. [CrossRef]
47. Loong, L.J.; Ling, K.K.; Tai, E.L.M.; Kueh, Y.C.; Kuan, G.; Hussein, A. The effect of binaural beat audio on operative pain and anxiety in cataract surgery under topical anaesthesia: A randomized controlled trial. *Int. J. Environ. Res. Public Health* **2022**, *19*, 10194. [CrossRef]
48. Abu-Taieh, E.M.; AlHadid, I.; Masa'deh, R.; Alkhawaldeh, R.S.; Khwaldeh, S.; Alrowwad, A. Factors affecting the use of social networks and its effect on anxiety and depression among parents and their children: Predictors using ml, sem and extended TAM. *Int. J. Environ. Res. Public Health* **2022**, *19*, 13764. [CrossRef] [PubMed]
49. Lee, E.; Bang, Y.; Yoon, I.-Y.; Choi, H.-Y. Entrapment of binaural auditory beats in subjects with symptoms of insomnia. *Brain Sci.* **2022**, *12*, 339. [CrossRef] [PubMed]
50. Yi, J.-H.; Kim, K.-B.; Kim, Y.-J.; Kim, J.-S.; Kim, H.-S.; Choi, M.-H.; Chung, S.-C. A Comparison of the Effects of Binaural Beats of Audible and Inaudible Frequencies on Brainwaves. *Appl. Sci.* **2022**, *12*, 13004. [CrossRef]
51. Ignatious, E.; Azam, S.; Jonkman, M.; De Boer, F. Frequency and time domain analysis of EEG based auditory evoked potentials to detect binaural hearing in noise. *J. Clin. Med.* **2023**, *12*, 4487. [CrossRef]

Disclaimer/Publisher's Note: The statements, opinions and data contained in all publications are solely those of the individual author(s) and contributor(s) and not of MDPI and/or the editor(s). MDPI and/or the editor(s) disclaim responsibility for any injury to people or property resulting from any ideas, methods, instructions or products referred to in the content.

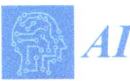

Review

Explainable Artificial Intelligence (XAI): Concepts and Challenges in Healthcare

Tim Hulsen

Department of Hospital Services & Informatics, Philips Research, 5656 AE Eindhoven, The Netherlands; tim.hulsen@philips.com

Abstract: Artificial Intelligence (AI) describes computer systems able to perform tasks that normally require human intelligence, such as visual perception, speech recognition, decision-making, and language translation. Examples of AI techniques are machine learning, neural networks, and deep learning. AI can be applied in many different areas, such as econometrics, biometry, e-commerce, and the automotive industry. In recent years, AI has found its way into healthcare as well, helping doctors make better decisions ("clinical decision support"), localizing tumors in magnetic resonance images, reading and analyzing reports written by radiologists and pathologists, and much more. However, AI has one big risk: it can be perceived as a "black box", limiting trust in its reliability, which is a very big issue in an area in which a decision can mean life or death. As a result, the term Explainable Artificial Intelligence (XAI) has been gaining momentum. XAI tries to ensure that AI algorithms (and the resulting decisions) can be understood by humans. In this narrative review, we will have a look at some central concepts in XAI, describe several challenges around XAI in healthcare, and discuss whether it can really help healthcare to advance, for example, by increasing understanding and trust. Finally, alternatives to increase trust in AI are discussed, as well as future research possibilities in the area of XAI.

Keywords: XAI; AI; artificial intelligence; explainable; explainability; machine learning; deep learning; data science; big data; healthcare; medicine

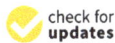

Citation: Hulsen, T. Explainable Artificial Intelligence (XAI): Concepts and Challenges in Healthcare. *AI* 2023, *4*, 652–666. https://doi.org/10.3390/ai4030034

Academic Editor: Kenji Suzuki

Received: 31 May 2023
Revised: 11 July 2023
Accepted: 9 August 2023
Published: 10 August 2023

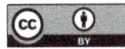

Copyright: © 2023 by the author. Licensee MDPI, Basel, Switzerland. This article is an open access article distributed under the terms and conditions of the Creative Commons Attribution (CC BY) license (https:// creativecommons.org/licenses/by/ 4.0/).

1. Introduction

Artificial Intelligence (AI) is "the theory and development of computer systems able to perform tasks that normally require human intelligence, such as visual perception, speech recognition, decision-making, and translation between languages" [1]. Examples of AI techniques are machine learning (ML), neural networks (NN), and deep learning (DL). AI can be applied to many different areas, such as econometrics (stock market predictions), biometry (facial recognition), e-commerce (recommendation systems), and the automotive industry (self-driving cars). In recent years, AI has found its way into the domain of biomedicine [2] and healthcare [3] as well. It is used to help researchers analyze big data to enable precision medicine [4] and to help clinicians to improve patient outcomes [5]. AI algorithms can help doctors to make better decisions ("clinical decision support", CDS), localize tumors in magnetic resonance (MR) images, read and analyze reports written by radiologists and pathologists, and much more. In the near future, generative AI and natural language processing (NLP) technology, such as Chat Generative Pre-trained Transformer (ChatGPT), could also help to create human-readable reports [6].

However, there are some barriers to the effective use of AI in healthcare. The first one is "small" data, resulting in bias [7]. When studies are carried out on a patient cohort with limited diversity in race, ethnicity, gender, age, etc., the results from these studies might be difficult to be applied to patients with different characteristics. An obvious solution for this bias is to create datasets using larger, more diverse patient cohorts and to keep bias in mind when designing experiments. A second barrier exists in privacy and security issues. Strict regulations (such as the European GDPR, the American HIPAA, and the Chinese PIPL) exist, limiting the use of personal data and imposing large fines for the leakage of such data. These issues can be solved in different ways, for example, by using federated or distributed learning. In this way, the algorithm travels to the data and sends results back to a central repository. The data do not need to be transferred to another party, avoiding privacy and security issues as much as possible [8]. Another solution is the use of synthetic data, artificial data, which might either be generated from scratch or based on real data, usually generated using AI algorithms such as Generative Adversarial Networks (GANs) [9]. A third barrier is the limited trust that clinicians and patients might have in AI algorithms. They can be perceived as a "black box": something goes in, and something comes out, with no understanding of what happens inside. This distrust in AI algorithms, their accuracy, and reliability is a very big issue in an area in which a decision could mean the life or death of the patient. As a result of this distrust, the term Explainable Artificial Intelligence (XAI) [10] has been gaining momentum as a possible solution. XAI tries to make sure that algorithms (and the resulting decisions) can be understood by humans.

XAI is being mentioned more and more in scientific publications, as can be seen in Figure 1. Its first mention in a PubMed title, abstract, or keywords was in 2018, in a paper about machine learning in neuroscience [11]. Since then, it has been mentioned a total of 488 times, of which more than 63% (311) in papers from 2022 or from the first months of 2023. The results for the Embase database show a similar trend. A full list of the publications can be found in Supplementary Tables S1 (PubMed) and S2 (Embase). This trend shows the growing importance of XAI in (bio)medicine and healthcare. Taking this growth into consideration, the number of manuscripts that discuss the concepts and challenges of XAI in the context of healthcare remains small. In this narrative review, we will have a look at several concepts around XAI and what their importance might be for the implementation and acceptance of AI in healthcare. This review will also provide some future directions. It will not attempt to give a full overview of the current literature on this topic or explain in detail which methods exist to explain AI algorithms, as several excellent reviews on this topic already exist [12–15]. First, we will go through some central concepts of XAI. We will explain the terminologies "black box" and "glass box". Then, we will look at two approaches to explainability, transparency, and post-hoc explanations, followed by a discussion on the collaboration between humans (e.g., clinicians) and AI. The subsequent two sections introduce scientific XAI and discuss the explanation methods of granular computing and fuzzy modeling. Second, we will discuss some challenges of XAI in healthcare. The first section is about legal and regulatory compliance, which is of particular importance in healthcare, dealing with sensitive personal data. The next sections discuss the effects of XAI on privacy and security and the question of whether the explanations always raise trust. Another section discusses the balance between explainability and accuracy/performance, followed by an overview of methods to measure explainability and a contemplation on the future increasing complexity of AI algorithms. The penultimate section shows some examples of XAI applied in a healthcare setting. Finally, the discussion puts everything in a broader context and mentions some future research possibilities of XAI in healthcare.

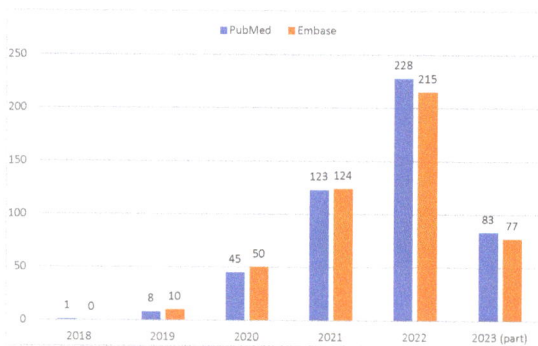

Figure 1. Number of publications containing the term "explainable artificial intelligence" in the titles, abstracts, and keywords of the PubMed and Embase databases per year. Queries performed on 26 March 2023.

2. Central Concepts of XAI

2.1. From "Black Box" to "(Translucent) Glass Box"

With explainable AI, we try to progress from a "black box" to a transparent "glass box" [16] (sometimes also referred to as a "white box" [17]). In a glass box model (such as a decision tree or linear regression model), all parameters are known, and we know exactly how the model comes to its conclusion, giving full transparency. In the ideal situation, the model is fully transparent, but in many situations (e.g., deep learning models), the model might be explainable only to a certain degree, which could be described as a "translucent glass box" with an opacity level somewhere between 0% and 100%. A low opacity of the translucent glass box (or high transparency of the model) can lead to a better understanding of the model, which, in turn, could increase trust. This trust can exist on two levels, trust in the model versus trust in the prediction, as explained by Ribeiro et al. [18]. In healthcare, there are many different stakeholders who have different explanation needs [19]. For example, data scientists are usually mostly interested in the model itself, whereas users (often clinicians, but sometimes patients) are mostly interested in the predictions based on that model. Therefore, trust for data scientists generally means trust in the model itself, while trust for clinicians and patients means trust in its predictions. The "trusting a prediction" problem can be solved by providing explanations for individual predictions, whereas the "trusting the model" problem can be solved by selecting multiple such predictions (and explanations) [18]. Future research could determine in which context either of these two approaches should be applied.

2.2. Explainability: Transparent or Post-Hoc

Arrieta et al. [20] classified studies on XAI into two approaches—some works focus on creating transparent models, while most works wrap black-box models with a layer of explainability, the so-called post-hoc models (Figure 2). The transparent models are based on linear or logistic regression, decision trees, k-nearest neighbors, rule-based learning, general additive models, and Bayesian models. These models are considered to be transparent because they are understandable by themselves. The post-hoc models (such as neural networks, random forest, and deep learning) need to be explained by resorting to diverse means to enhance their interpretability, such as text explanations, visual explanations, local explanations, explanations by example, explanations by simplification, and feature relevance explanations techniques. Phillips et al. [21] define four principles for explainable AI systems: (1) explanation: explainable AI systems deliver accompanying evidence or reasons for outcomes and processes; (2) meaningful: provide explanations that are understandable to individual users; (3) explanation accuracy: provide explanations that correctly reflect the system's process for generating the output; and (4) knowledge limits: a system only operates under conditions for which it was designed and when it reaches sufficient confidence in its output. Vale et al. [22] state that machine learning post-hoc explanation methods cannot guarantee the insights they generate, which means that they cannot be relied upon as the only mechanism to guarantee the fairness of model outcomes in high-stake decision-making, such as in healthcare.

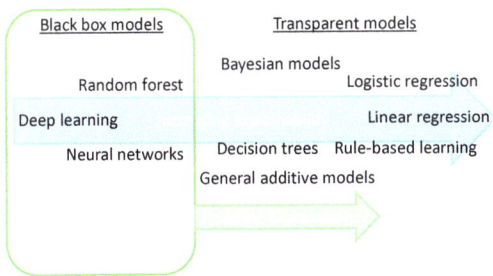

Figure 2. Black box models (needing post-hoc explanations) vs. inherently transparent models.

2.3. Collaboration between Humans and AI

It is important for clinicians (but also patients, researchers, etc.) to realize that humans can and should not be replaced by an AI algorithm [23]. An AI algorithm could outscore humans in specific tasks, but humans (at this moment in time) still have added value with their domain expertise, broad experience, and creative thinking skills. It might be the case that when the accuracy of an AI algorithm on a specific task is compared to the accuracy of the clinician, the AI gets better results. However, the AI model should not be compared to the human alone but to the combination of the AI model and a human because, in clinical practice, they will almost always work together. In most cases, the combination (also known as "AI-assisted decision making") will obtain the best results [24]. The combination of an AI model with human expertise also makes the decision more explainable: the clinician can combine the explainable AI with his/her own domain knowledge. In CDS, explainability allows developers to identify shortcomings in a system and allows clinicians to be confident in the decisions they make with the support of AI. [25]. Amann et al. state that if we would move in the opposite direction toward opaque algorithms in CDSS, this may inadvertently lead to patients being passive spectators in the medical decision-making process [26]. Figure 3 shows what qualities a human and an AI model can offer in clinical decision-making, with the combination offering the best results. In the future, there might be a shift to the right side of the figure, but the specific qualities of humans will likely ensure that combined decision-making will still be the best option for years to come.

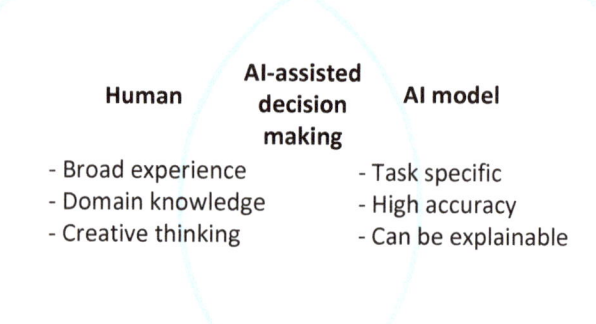

Figure 3. The combination of human and AI models can create powerful AI-assisted decision-making.

2.4. Scientific Explainable Artificial Intelligence (sXAI)

Durán (2021) [27] differentiates scientific XAI (sXAI) from other forms of XAI. He states that the current approach for XAI is a bottom-up model: it consists of structuring all forms of XAI, attending to the current technology and available computational methodologies, which could lead to confounding classifications (or "how-explanations") with explanations. Instead, he proposes a bona fide scientific explanation in medical AI. This explanation addresses three core components: (1) the structure of sXAI, consisting of the "explanans" (the unit that carries out an explanation), the "explanandum" (the unit that will be explained), and the "explanatory relation" (the objective relation of dependency that links the explanans and the explanandum); (2) the role of human agents and non-epistemic beliefs in sXAI; and (3) how human agents can meaningfully assess the merits of an explanation. This concludes by proposing a shift from standard XAI to sXAI, together with substantial changes in the way medical XAI is constructed and interpreted. Cabitza et al. [28] discuss this approach and conclude that existing XAI methods fail to be bona fide explanations, which is why their framework cannot be applied to current XAI work. For sXAI to work, it needs to be integrated into future medical AI algorithms in a top–down manner. This means that algorithms should not be explained by simply describing "how" a decision has been reached, but we should also look at what other scientific disciplines, such as philosophy of science, epistemology, and cognitive science, can add to the discussion [27]. For each medical AI algorithm, the explanans, explanandum, and explanatory relation should be defined.

2.5. Explanation Methods: Granular Computing (GrC) and Fuzzy Modeling (FM)

Many methods exist to explain AI algorithms, as described in detail by Holzinger et al. [29]. There is one technique that is particularly useful in XAI because it is motivated by the need to approach AI through human-centric information processing [30], Granular Computing (GrC), which was introduced by Zadeh in 1979 [31]. GrC is an "emerging paradigm in computing and applied mathematics to process data and information, where the data or information are divided into so-called information granules that come about through the process of granulation" [32]. GrC can help make models more interpretable and explainable by bridging the gap between abstract concepts and concrete data through these granules. Another useful technique related to GrC is Fuzzy Modeling (FM), a methodology oriented toward the design of explanatory and predictive models. FM is a technique through which a linguistic description can be transformed into an algorithm whose result is an action [33]. Fuzzy modeling can help explain the reasoning behind the output of an AI system by representing the decision-making process in a way that is more intuitive and interpretable. Although FM was originally conceived to provide easily understandable models to users, this property cannot be taken for granted, but it requires careful design choices [34]. Much research in this area is still ongoing. Zhang et al. [35] discuss the multi-granularity three-way decisions paradigm [36] and how this acts as a part of granular computing models, playing a significant role in explainable decision-making. Zhang et al. [37] adopt a GrC framework named "multigranulation probabilistic models" to enrich semantic interpretations for GrC-based multi-attribute group decision-making (MAGDM) approaches.

In healthcare, GrC could, for example, help break down a CDS algorithm into smaller components, such as the symptoms, patient history, test results, and treatment options. This can help the clinician understand how the algorithm arrived at its diagnosis and determine if it is reliable and accurate. FM could, for example, be used in a CDS system to represent the uncertainty and imprecision in the input data, such as patient symptoms, and the decision-making process, such as the rules that are used to arrive at a diagnosis. This can help to provide a more transparent and understandable explanation of how the algorithm arrived at its output. Recent examples of the application of GrC and FM in healthcare are in the disease areas of Parkinson's disease [38], COVID-19 [39], and Alzheimer's disease [40].

3. Challenges of XAI in Healthcare

3.1. Legal and Regulatory Compliance

Another advantage of XAI is that it can help organizations comply with laws and regulations that require transparency and explainability in AI systems. Within the General Data Protection Regulation (GDPR) of the European Union, transparency is a fundamental principle for data processing [41]. However, transparency is difficult to adhere to because of the complexity of AI. Felzmann et al. [42] propose that transparency, as required by the GDPR in itself, may be insufficient to achieve an increase in trust or any other positive goal associated with transparency. Instead, they recommend a relational understanding of transparency, in which the provision of information is viewed as a sort of interaction between users and technology providers, and the value of transparency messages is mediated by trustworthiness assessments based on the context. Schneeberger et al. [43] discussed the European framework regulating medical AI based on White Paper on AI from 2020 by the European Commission [44] and concluded that this framework, by endorsing a human-centric approach, will fundamentally influence how medical AI and AI, in general, will be used in Europe in the future. The EU is currently working on the Artificial Intelligence Act [45], which will make a distinction between non-high-risk and high-risk AI systems. On non-high-risk systems, only limited transparency obligations are imposed, while for high-risk systems, many restrictions are imposed on quality, documentation, traceability, transparency, human oversight, accuracy, and robustness. Bell et al. [46] state that transparency is left to the technologists to achieve and propose a stakeholder-first approach that assists technologists in designing transparent, regulatory-compliant systems, which is a useful initiative. Besides GDPR, there are other privacy laws for which XAI might be an interesting development. In the USA, there is the Health Insurance Portability and Accountability Act (HIPAA) privacy rule [47], which is related to the Openness and Transparency Principle in the Privacy and Security Framework. This Openness and Transparency Principle stresses that it is "important for people to understand what individually identifiable health information exists about them, how that information is collected, used, and disclosed, and how reasonable choices can be exercised with respect to that information" [48]. The transparency of the usage of health information might point to a need for explainability of algorithms. In China, article 7 of the Personal Information Protective Law (PIPL) prescribes that "the principles of openness and transparency shall be observed in the handling of personal information, disclosing the rules for handling personal information and clearly indicating the purpose, method, and scope of handling" [49], which also points to a need for transparency in data handling and AI algorithms. Since new, more AI-specific privacy laws are being introduced around the world, regulatory compliance with AI algorithms is gaining relevance and will be an important area for research in the future.

3.2. Privacy and Security: A Mixed Bag

On the one hand, XAI can help to improve the safety and security of AI systems by making it easier to detect and prevent errors and malicious behavior [50]. On the other hand, XAI can also raise privacy and security concerns, as providing explanations for AI decisions may reveal sensitive information or show how to manipulate the system, for example, by reverse engineering [51]. A fully transparent model can make a hacker feel as if they have endless possibilities. Therefore, it is important to carefully consider the privacy and security implications of XAI and to take appropriate risk mitigation measures, certainly in healthcare, where the protection of sensitive personal data is an important issue. Combining the explainability of algorithms with privacy-preserving methods such as federated learning [52] might help. Saifullah et al. [53] argue that XAI and privacy-preserving machine learning (PPML) are both crucial research fields, but no attention has yet been paid to their interaction. They investigated the impact of private learning techniques on generated explanations for deep learning-based models and concluded that federated learning should be considered before differential privacy. If an application requires both privacy and explainability, they recommend differential private federated learning [54] as well as perturbation-based XAI methods [55]. The importance of privacy in relation to medical XAI is shown in Figure 4 of Albahri et al. [56], with keywords such as "ethics", "privacy", "security", and "trust" being the most often-occurring keywords in papers around XAI in healthcare. Some research on security in combination with XAI has been carried out as well. Viganò and Magazzeni [57] propose the term "Explainable Security" (XSec) as an extension of XAI to the security domain. According to the authors, XSec has unique and complex characteristics: it involves several different stakeholders and is multi-faceted by nature. Kuppa and Le-Khac [58] designed a novel black box attack for analyzing the security properties (consistency, correctness, and confidence) of gradient-based XAI methods, which could help in designing secure and robust XAI methods. Kiener [59] looked specifically at security in healthcare and identified three types of security risks related to AI: cyber-attacks; systematic bias; and mismatches, all of which can have serious consequences for medical systems. Explainability can be part of the solution for all of these risks. The author specifically mentions input attacks as a type of cyber-attack that is of high risk to AI systems. Input attacks manipulate the input data (e.g., make some small changes to an MR image) so that the AI algorithm will deliver an incorrect result [60]. In an explainable model, the clinician can look at the reasoning behind the incorrect result and possibly, detect the manipulation. Systematic bias can be brought to light as well by explaining the workings of the AI algorithm. For example, it can become clearly visible that an algorithm was only trained on data from people from one ethnic background. Mismatches can occur when the AI algorithm recommends courses of action that do not match the background situation of the individual patient. The algorithm can mistake correlation for causation and suggest, for example, an incorrect treatment. In a black-box AI, such a mismatch might be undetectable, but in a transparent, explainable AI, it might be much easier to detect or at least indicate the risk of such a mismatch.

3.3. Do Explanations Always Raise Trust?

The goal of explainability to end users of AI models is ultimately to increase trust in the model. However, even with a good understanding of an AI model, end users may not necessarily trust the model. Druce et al. [61] show that a statistically significant increase in user trust and acceptance of an AI model can be reached by using a three-fold explanation: (1) a graphical depiction of the model's generalization and performance in the current game state; (2) how well the agent would play in semantically similar environments; and (3) a narrative explanation of what the graphical information implies. Le Merrer and Trédan [62] argue that explainability might be promising in a local context but that it cannot simply be transposed to a different (remote) context, where a model trained by a service provider is only accessible to a user through a network and its application programming interface (API). They show that providing explanations cannot prevent a remote service from lying about the true reasons leading to its decisions (similar to what humans could do), undermining the very concept of remote explainability in general. Within healthcare, trust is a fundamental issue because important decisions might be taken based on the output of the AI algorithm. Mistrust might result in humans discarding accurate predictions, while overtrust could lead to over-reliance on possibly inaccurate predictions. Therefore, it would be good to take all necessary actions described here to reach the correct level of trust in AI algorithms in healthcare. One of the key actions here is to create open and honest education to end users on the strengths and weaknesses of AI algorithms. For example, people should be trained to understand the difference between local context and remote context.

3.4. "Glass Box" vs. "Crystal Ball": Balance between Explainability and Accuracy/Performance

In some cases, the need for explainability can come at the cost of reduced performance of the model. For example, in order to make a model fully explainable (a "glass box"), it might need to be simplified. A very accurate prediction model (a "crystal ball") might lose part of its accuracy because of this simplification. Or it needs to introduce some extra, more simple steps to make it more transparent, causing a reduction in performance. Linear models and rule-based models are very transparent but usually have lower performance than deep learning algorithms (Figure 5 [63]). Therefore, in a real-world situation, it might not be possible to achieve full explainability because accuracy and performance are usually considered to be more important. A balance needs to be maintained between the two, as shown in Figure 4. In healthcare, this balance might shift more to the "crystal ball" as accuracy might be considered more important than transparency and explainability. Van der Veer et al. [64] concluded that citizens might indeed value the explainability of AI systems in healthcare less than in non-healthcare domains, especially when weighed against system accuracy. When developing policy on the explainability of (medical) AI, citizens should be actively consulted, as they might have a different opinion than assumed by healthcare professionals. This trade-off between accuracy and transparency could be different for each context, however, depending on the implications of a wrong decision based on the AI algorithm. Future research could be carried out on the context-specific need for explainability.

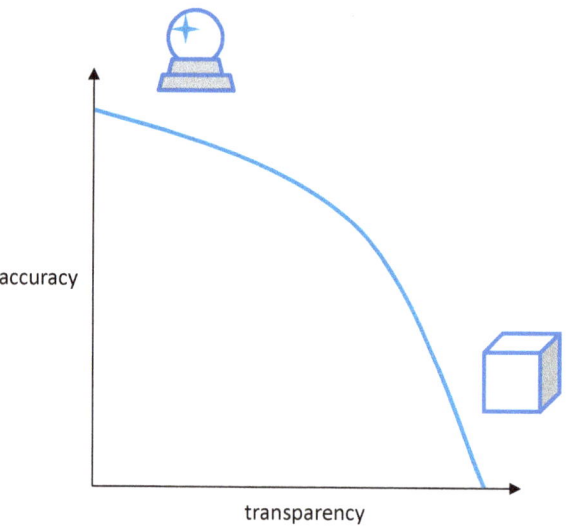

Figure 4. Increasing transparency of a (prediction) model might cause a decrease in accuracy, going from a "crystal ball" to a "glass box" and vice versa.

3.5. How to Measure Explainability?

Accuracy and performance can be measured easily by metrics such as specificity, selectivity, and area under the Receiver Operating Characteristic (ROC) curve (AUC). Explainability is much more difficult to be measured because the quality of an explanation is somewhat subjective. Multiple researchers have tried to come up with an assessment of explainability. Table 1 shows an overview of the most widely used explainability metrics from the recent literature. The four publications that introduced these metrics all look at explainability from a different angle. Sokol and Flach [65], for example, have created "explainability fact sheets" to assess explainable approaches along five dimensions: functional; operational; usability; safety; and validation. This is quite an extensive approach. Most researchers measure explainability simply by evaluating how well an explanation is understood by the end user. Lipton [66] identifies three measures: (1) simulatability: can the user recreate or repeat (simulate) the computational process based on provided explanations of a system; (2) decomposability: can the user comprehend individual parts (and their functionality) of a predictive model; (3) algorithmic transparency: can the user fully understand the predictive algorithm? Hoffman et al. [67] use "mental models", representations or expressions of how a person understands some sort of event, process, or system [68], as a user's understanding of the AI system. This mental model can be evaluated on criteria such as correctness, comprehensiveness, coherence, and usefulness. Fauvel et al. [69] present a framework that assesses and benchmarks machine learning methods on both performance and explainability. Performance is measured compared to the state-of-the-art, best, similar, or below. For measuring explainability, they look at model comprehensibility, explanation granularity, information type, faithfulness, and user category. For model comprehensibility, only two categories are defined, "black-box" and "white-box" models, suggesting that these components could be further elaborated in future work. For the granularity of the explanation, they use three categories: "global"; "local"; and "global and local" explainability. They propose a generic assessment of the information type in three categories from the least to the most informative: (1) importance: the explanations reveal the relative importance of each dataset variable on predictions; (2) patterns: the explanations provide the small conjunctions of symbols with a predefined semantic (patterns) associated with the predictions; (3) causal: the most informative category corresponds to explanations under the form of causal rules. The faithfulness of the explanation shows if the user can trust the explanation, with the two categories, "imperfect" and "perfect". Finally, the user category shows the target user at which the explanation is aimed: "machine learning expert", "domain expert", and "broad audience". This user category is important because it defines the level of background knowledge they have. As suggested by the authors, all these metrics and categories can be defined in more detail in future XAI research.

Table 1. Methods for assessing explainability.

Manuscript	Measures
Sokol and Flach (2020) [65]	- Functional - Operational - Usability - Safety - Validation
Lipton (2018) [66]	- Simulatability - Decomposability - Algorithmic transparency
Hoffman et al. (2018) [67]	- Correctness - Comprehensiveness - Coherence - Usefulness

Fauvel et al. (2020) [69]	- Performance:
	  o Best
	  o Similar
	  o Below
	- Explainability:
	  o Model comprehensibility:
	    ▪ Black box models
	    ▪ White box models
	  o Explanation granularity:
	    ▪ Global
	    ▪ Local
	    ▪ Global and local
	  o Information type:
	    ▪ Importance
	    ▪ Patterns
	    ▪ Causal
	  o Faithfulness:
	    ▪ Imperfect
	    ▪ Perfect
	  o User category:
	    ▪ Machine learning expert
	    ▪ Domain expert
	    ▪ Broad audience

3.6. Increasing Complexity in the Future

The first neural networks (using a single layer) were relatively easy to understand. With the advent of deep learning (using multiple layers) and new types of algorithms such as Deep Belief Networks (DBNs) [70] and Generative Adversarial Networks (GANs) [71], made possible by the increasing computer power, artificial intelligence algorithms are gaining complexity. In the future, this trend will likely continue, with Moore's law still continuing to proceed. With algorithms becoming more complex, it might also be more difficult to make them explainable. Ongoing research in the field of XAI might make it possible that new techniques will be developed that make it easier to explain and understand complex AI models. For example, Explainability-by-Design [72] takes proactive measures to include explanation capability in the design of decision-making systems so that no post-hoc explanations are needed. However, there is also the possibility that the complexity of AI models will overtake our ability to understand and explain them. Sarkar [73] even talks about an "explainability crisis", which will be defined by the point at which our desire for explanations of machine intelligence will eclipse our ability to obtain them, and uses the "five stages of grief" (denial, anger, bargaining, depression, and acceptance) to describe the several phases of this crisis. The author's conclusion is that XAI is probably in a race against model complexity, but also that this may not be such a big issue as it seems, as there are several ways to either improve explanations or reduce AI complexity. Ultimately, it all will depend on the trajectory of AI development and the progress made in the field of XAI.

4. Application Examples

XAI has been applied to healthcare in medicine in a number of ways already. AI has been very successful in improving medical image analysis, and recently, researchers have also been trying to combine this success (through high accuracy) with an increased explainability and interpretability of the models created. Van der Velden et al. [74] identified over 200 papers using XAI in deep learning-based medical image analysis and concluded that most papers in this area used a visual explanation (mostly through saliency maps [75]) as opposed to textual explanations and example-based explanations. These saliency maps highlight the most important features which can distinguish between diseased and non-diseased tissue [76]. Manresa-Yee et al. [77] describe explanation interfaces that are being used in healthcare, mostly by clinicians. They identified three main application areas for these interfaces: prediction tasks; diagnosis tasks; and automated tasks. One example of a clinician-facing explanation interface is the dashboard presented by Khodabandehloo et al. [78], which uses data from sensorized smart homes to detect a decline in the cognitive functions of the elderly in order to promptly alert practitioners.

Joyce et al. [79] studied the use of XAI in psychiatry and mental health, where the need for explainability and understandability is higher than in other areas because of the probabilistic relationships between the data describing the syndromes, outcomes, disorders, and signs/symptoms. They introduced the TIFU (Transparency and Interpretability For Understandability) framework, which focuses on how a model can be made understandable (to a user) as a function of transparency and interpretability. They conclude that the main applications of XAI in mental health are prediction and discovery, that XAI in mental health requires understandability because clinical applications are high-stakes, and that AI tools should assist clinicians and not introduce further complexity.

5. Discussion

Current privacy laws such as GDPR, HIPAA, and PIPL include clauses that state that the handling of healthcare data should be transparent, which means that AI algorithms that work with these data should be transparent and explainable as well. Future privacy laws will likely be even more strict on AI explainability. However, making AI explainable is a difficult task, and it will be even more difficult when the complexity of AI algorithms continues to increase. This increasing complexity might make it almost impossible for end users in healthcare (clinicians as well as patients) to understand and trust the algorithms. Therefore, perhaps we should not aim to explain AI to the end users but to the researchers and developers deploying them, as they are mostly interested in the model itself. End users, especially patients, mostly want to be sure that the predictions made by the algorithm are accurate, which can be proven by showing them correct predictions from the past. Another important issue is the balance between explainability and accuracy or performance. Especially in healthcare, accuracy (and, to a lesser extent, performance) is crucial as it could be a matter of life and death. Therefore, explainability might be considered of less importance in healthcare compared to accuracy. If an algorithm's accuracy is lowered because of post-hoc explanations, it would be good to consider other methods to increase trust. For example, trust in algorithms could also be raised by ensuring robustness and by encouraging fairness [80]. Robustness of an algorithm in healthcare can be proven by presenting good results based on long-term use in different patient populations. When a model is robust, its explanation will not change much when minor changes are made to the model [81]. The fairness of an AI algorithm is concurrent with bias minimization. A bias could be introduced by having a training dataset with low diversity or by subjective responses of clinicians to a questionnaire. XAI can help find these biases as well as mitigate them [82]. These biases can be addressed during the validation and verification of the algorithm. Finally, algorithms (scripts, but also underlying data) should be made available for reuse when possible [83] so that the results can be reproduced, increasing trust in the algorithm. GrC and FM can help increase trust as well by making models more interpretable and explainable. Another solution to the explainability–accuracy trade-off might lie in the adoption of sXAI, in which explainability is integrated into a top–down manner into future medical AI algorithms, and Explainability-by-Design, which includes explanation capability in the design of decision-making systems. GrC, FM, sXAI, and Explainability-by-Design could be combined with ongoing research in privacy and security in AI (such as XSec) to create future-proof explainable artificial intelligence for healthcare. In any case, explainability should be considered as important as other metrics, such as accuracy and robustness, as they all raise trust in AI. Future endeavors to make AI explainable should be personalized, as different end users need different levels of explanations. The explanations should be communicated to the end user in an understandable manner, for example, through an easy-to-use user interface. Explainability should also not compromise the privacy rights of the patients [84]. For XAI in healthcare to fully reach its potential, it should be embedded in clinical workflows, and explainability should be included in AI development from the start instead of adding post-hoc explanations as an afterthought.

Supplementary Materials: The following supporting information can be downloaded at: https://www.mdpi.com/article/10.3390/ai4030034/s1, Table S1: PubMed publications with the search term "explainable artificial intelligence"; Table S2: Embase publications with the search term "explainable artificial intelligence".

Funding: This research received no external funding.

Institutional Review Board Statement: Not applicable.

Informed Consent Statement: Not applicable.

Data Availability Statement: No new data were created or analyzed in this study. Data sharing is not applicable to this article.

Conflicts of Interest: Tim Hulsen is an employee of Philips Research.

Abbreviations

AI	Artificial Intelligence
API	Application Programming Interface
AUC	Area Under the Curve
CDS	Clinical Decision Support
ChatGPT	Chat Generative Pre-trained Transformer

DBN	Deep Belief Network
DL	Deep Learning
FM	Fuzzy Modeling
GAN	Generative Adversarial Network
GDPR	General Data Protection Regulation
GrC	Granular Computing
HIPAA	Health Insurance Portability and Accountability Act
MAGDM	Multi-Attribute Group Decision Making
ML	Machine Learning
MR	Magnetic Resonance
NLP	Natural Language Processing
NN	Neural Networks
PIPL	Personal Information Protective Law
PPML	Privacy-Preserving Machine Learning
ROC	Receiver Operating Characteristic
sXAI	Scientific Explainable Artificial Intelligence
XAI	Explainable Artificial Intelligence
XSec	Explainable Security

References

1. Joiner, I.A. Chapter 1—Artificial intelligence: AI is nearby. In *Emerging Library Technologies*; Joiner, I.A., Ed.; Chandos Publishing: Oxford, UK, 2018; pp. 1–22.
2. Hulsen, T. Literature analysis of artificial intelligence in biomedicine. *Ann. Transl. Med.* **2022**, *10*, 1284. [CrossRef] [PubMed]
3. Yu, K.-H.; Beam, A.L.; Kohane, I.S. Artificial intelligence in healthcare. *Nat. Biomed. Eng.* **2018**, *2*, 719–731. [CrossRef] [PubMed]
4. Hulsen, T.; Jamuar, S.S.; Moody, A.; Karnes, J.H.; Orsolya, V.; Hedensted, S.; Spreafico, R.; Hafler, D.A.; McKinney, E. From Big Data to Precision Medicine. *Front. Med.* **2019**, *6*, 34. [CrossRef]
5. Hulsen, T.; Friedecký, D.; Renz, H.; Melis, E.; Vermeersch, P.; Fernandez-Calle, P. From big data to better patient outcomes. *Clin. Chem. Lab. Med. (CCLM)* **2022**, *61*, 580–586. [CrossRef] [PubMed]
6. Biswas, S. ChatGPT and the Future of Medical Writing. *Radiology* **2023**, *307*, e223312. [CrossRef] [PubMed]
7. Celi, L.A.; Cellini, J.; Charpignon, M.-L.; Dee, E.C.; Dernoncourt, F.; Eber, R.; Mitchell, W.G.; Moukheiber, L.; Schirmer, J.; Situ, J. Sources of bias in artificial intelligence that perpetuate healthcare disparities—A global review. *PLoS Digit. Health* **2022**, *1*, e0000022. [CrossRef]
8. Hulsen, T. Sharing Is Caring-Data Sharing Initiatives in Healthcare. *Int. J. Environ. Res. Public Health* **2020**, *17*, 3046. [CrossRef]
9. Vega-Márquez, B.; Rubio-Escudero, C.; Riquelme, J.C.; Nepomuceno-Chamorro, I. Creation of synthetic data with conditional generative adversarial networks. In Proceedings of the 14th International Conference on Soft Computing Models in Industrial and Environmental Applications (SOCO 2019), Seville, Spain, 13–15 May 2019; Springer: Cham, Switzerlnad, 2020; pp. 231–240.
10. Gunning, D.; Stefik, M.; Choi, J.; Miller, T.; Stumpf, S.; Yang, G.Z. XAI-Explainable artificial intelligence. *Sci. Robot.* **2019**, *4*, eaay7120. [CrossRef]
11. Vu, M.T.; Adalı, T.; Ba, D.; Buzsáki, G.; Carlson, D.; Heller, K.; Liston, C.; Rudin, C.; Sohal, V.S.; Widge, A.S.; et al. A Shared Vision for Machine Learning in Neuroscience. *J. Neurosci.* **2018**, *38*, 1601–1607. [CrossRef]
12. Bharati, S.; Mondal, M.R.H.; Podder, P. A Review on Explainable Artificial Intelligence for Healthcare: Why, How, and When? *IEEE Trans. Artif. Intell.* **2023**. [CrossRef]
13. Sheu, R.-K.; Pardeshi, M.S. A Survey on Medical Explainable AI (XAI): Recent Progress, Explainability Approach, Human Interaction and Scoring System. *Sensors* **2022**, *22*, 8068. [CrossRef] [PubMed]
14. Tjoa, E.; Guan, C. A survey on explainable artificial intelligence (xai): Toward medical xai. *IEEE Trans. Neural Netw. Learn. Syst.* **2020**, *32*, 4793–4813. [CrossRef] [PubMed]
15. Jung, J.; Lee, H.; Jung, H.; Kim, H. Essential properties and explanation effectiveness of explainable artificial intelligence in healthcare: A systematic review. *Heliyon* **2023**, *9*, e16110. [CrossRef] [PubMed]
16. Rai, A. Explainable AI: From black box to glass box. *J. Acad. Mark. Sci.* **2020**, *48*, 137–141. [CrossRef]
17. Loyola-Gonzalez, O. Black-box vs. white-box: Understanding their advantages and weaknesses from a practical point of view. *IEEE Access* **2019**, *7*, 154096–154113. [CrossRef]
18. Ribeiro, M.T.; Singh, S.; Guestrin, C. Why should I trust you?: Explaining the predictions of any classifier. In Proceedings of the 22nd ACM SIGKDD International Conference on Knowledge Discovery and Data Mining, San Francisco, CA, USA, 13–17 August 2016; pp. 1135–1144. [CrossRef]
19. Gerlings, J.; Jensen, M.S.; Shollo, A. Explainable AI, but explainable to whom? An exploratory case study of xAI in healthcare. In *Handbook of Artificial Intelligence in Healthcare: Practicalities and Prospects*; Lim, C.-P., Chen, Y.-W., Vaidya, A., Mahorkar, C., Jain, L.C., Eds.; Springer International Publishing: Cham, Switzerlnad, 2022; Volume 2, pp. 169–198.

20. Arrieta, A.B.; Díaz-Rodríguez, N.; Del Ser, J.; Bennetot, A.; Tabik, S.; Barbado, A.; García, S.; Gil-López, S.; Molina, D.; Benjamins, R. Explainable Artificial Intelligence (XAI): Concepts, taxonomies, opportunities and challenges toward responsible AI. *Inf. Fusion* **2020**, *58*, 82–115. [CrossRef]
21. Phillips, P.J.; Hahn, C.A.; Fontana, P.C.; Broniatowski, D.A.; Przybocki, M.A. *Four Principles of Explainable Artificial Intelligence*; National Institute of Standards and Technology: Gaithersburg, MD, USA, 2020; Volume 18.
22. Vale, D.; El-Sharif, A.; Ali, M. Explainable artificial intelligence (XAI) post-hoc explainability methods: Risks and limitations in non-discrimination law. *AI Ethics* **2022**, *2*, 815–826. [CrossRef]
23. Bhattacharya, S.; Pradhan, K.B.; Bashar, M.A.; Tripathi, S.; Semwal, J.; Marzo, R.R.; Bhattacharya, S.; Singh, A. Artificial intelligence enabled healthcare: A hype, hope or harm. *J. Fam. Med. Prim. Care* **2019**, *8*, 3461–3464. [CrossRef]
24. Zhang, Y.; Liao, Q.V.; Bellamy, R.K.E. Effect of Confidence and Explanation on Accuracy and Trust Calibration in AI-Assisted Decision Making. In Proceedings of the 2020 Conference on Fairness, Accountability, and Transparency, Barcelona, Spain, 27–30 January 2020; pp. 295–305. [CrossRef]
25. Antoniadi, A.M.; Du, Y.; Guendouz, Y.; Wei, L.; Mazo, C.; Becker, B.A.; Mooney, C. Current Challenges and Future Opportunities for XAI in Machine Learning-Based Clinical Decision Support Systems: A Systematic Review. *Appl. Sci.* **2021**, *11*, 5088. [CrossRef]
26. Amann, J.; Blasimme, A.; Vayena, E.; Frey, D.; Madai, V.I.; the Precise, Q.c. Explainability for artificial intelligence in healthcare: A multidisciplinary perspective. *BMC Med. Inform. Decis. Mak.* **2020**, *20*, 310. [CrossRef]
27. Durán, J.M. Dissecting scientific explanation in AI (sXAI): A case for medicine and healthcare. *Artif. Intell.* **2021**, *297*, 103498. [CrossRef]
28. Cabitza, F.; Campagner, A.; Malgieri, G.; Natali, C.; Schneeberger, D.; Stoeger, K.; Holzinger, A. Quod erat demonstrandum?—Towards a typology of the concept of explanation for the design of explainable AI. *Expert Syst. Appl.* **2023**, *213*, 118888. [CrossRef]
29. Holzinger, A.; Saranti, A.; Molnar, C.; Biecek, P.; Samek, W. Explainable AI methods—A brief overview. In Proceedings of the xxAI—Beyond Explainable AI: International Workshop, Held in Conjunction with ICML 2020, Vienna, Austria, 12–18 July 2020; Holzinger, A., Goebel, R., Fong, R., Moon, T., Müller, K.-R., Samek, W., Eds.; Springer International Publishing: Cham, Switzerland, 2022; pp. 13–38.
30. Bargiela, A.; Pedrycz, W. *Human-Centric Information Processing through Granular Modelling*; Springer Science & Business Media: Dordrecht, The Netherlands, 2009; Volume 182.
31. Zadeh, L.A. Fuzzy sets and information granularity. In *Fuzzy Sets, Fuzzy Logic, and Fuzzy Systems: Selected Papers*; World Scientific: Singapore, 1979; pp. 433–448.
32. Keet, C.M. Granular computing. In *Encyclopedia of Systems Biology*; Dubitzky, W., Wolkenhauer, O., Cho, K.-H., Yokota, H., Eds.; Springer: New York, NY, USA, 2013; p. 849.
33. Novák, V.; Perfilieva, I.; Dvořák, A. What is fuzzy modeling. In *Insight into Fuzzy Modeling*; John Wiley & Sons: Hoboken, NJ, USA, 2016; pp. 3–10.
34. Mencar, C.; Alonso, J.M. Paving the way to explainable artificial intelligence with fuzzy modeling: Tutorial. In Proceedings of the Fuzzy Logic and Applications: 12th International Workshop (WILF 2018), Genoa, Italy, 6–7 September 2018; Springer International Publishing: Cham, Switzerland, 2019; pp. 215–227.
35. Zhang, C.; Li, D.; Liang, J. Multi-granularity three-way decisions with adjustable hesitant fuzzy linguistic multigranulation decision-theoretic rough sets over two universes. *Inf. Sci.* **2020**, *507*, 665–683. [CrossRef]
36. Zadeh, L.A. Toward a theory of fuzzy information granulation and its centrality in human reasoning and fuzzy logic. *Fuzzy Sets Syst.* **1997**, *90*, 111–127. [CrossRef]
37. Zhang, C.; Li, D.; Liang, J.; Wang, B. MAGDM-oriented dual hesitant fuzzy multigranulation probabilistic models based on MULTIMOORA. *Int. J. Mach. Learn. Cybern.* **2021**, *12*, 1219–1241. [CrossRef]
38. Zhang, C.; Ding, J.; Zhan, J.; Sangaiah, A.K.; Li, D. Fuzzy Intelligence Learning Based on Bounded Rationality in IoMT Systems: A Case Study in Parkinson's Disease. *IEEE Trans. Comput. Soc. Syst.* **2022**, *10*, 1607–1621. [CrossRef]
39. Solayman, S.; Aumi, S.A.; Mery, C.S.; Mubassir, M.; Khan, R. Automatic COVID-19 prediction using explainable machine learning techniques. *Int. J. Cogn. Comput. Eng.* **2023**, *4*, 36–46. [CrossRef]
40. Gao, S.; Lima, D. A review of the application of deep learning in the detection of Alzheimer's disease. *Int. J. Cogn. Comput. Eng.* **2022**, *3*, 1–8. [CrossRef]
41. Intersoft Consulting. Recital 58—The Principle of Transparency. Available online: https://gdpr-info.eu/recitals/no-58/ (accessed on 26 March 2023).
42. Felzmann, H.; Villaronga, E.F.; Lutz, C.; Tamò-Larrieux, A. Transparency you can trust: Transparency requirements for artificial intelligence between legal norms and contextual concerns. *Big Data Soc.* **2019**, *6*, 2053951719860542. [CrossRef]
43. Schneeberger, D.; Stöger, K.; Holzinger, A. The European legal framework for medical AI. In Proceedings of the International Cross-Domain Conference for Machine Learning and Knowledge Extraction, Dublin, Ireland, 25–28 August 2020; Springer: Cham, Switzerland, 2020; pp. 209–226.
44. European Commission. *On Artificial Intelligence—A European Approach to Excellence and Trust*; European Commission: Brussels, Belgium, 2020.
45. European Commission. Proposal for a Regulation of the European Parliament and of the Council Laying Down Harmonised Rules on Artificial Intelligence (Artificial Intelligence Act) and Amending Certain Union Legislative Acts. Available online: https://eur-lex.europa.eu/legal-content/EN/TXT/?uri=celex%3A52021PC0206 (accessed on 26 March 2023).

46. Bell, A.; Nov, O.; Stoyanovich, J. Think about the Stakeholders First! Towards an Algorithmic Transparency Playbook for Regulatory Compliance. *arXiv* **2022**, arXiv:2207.01482. [CrossRef]
47. HHS Office for Civil Rights. Standards for privacy of individually identifiable health information—Final rule. *Fed. Regist.* **2002**, *67*, 53181–53273.
48. HHS Office for Civil Rights. The HIPAA Privacy Rule and Electronic Health Information Exchange in a Networked Environment—Openness and Transparency. Available online: https://www.hhs.gov/sites/default/files/ocr/privacy/hipaa/understanding/special/healthit/opennesstransparency.pdf (accessed on 26 March 2023).
49. Creemers, R.; Webster, G. Translation: Personal Information Protection Law of the People's Republic of China—Effective 1 November 2021. Available online: https://digichina.stanford.edu/work/translation-personal-information-protection-law-of-the-peoples-republic-of-china-effective-nov-1-2021/ (accessed on 26 March 2023).
50. Charmet, F.; Tanuwidjaja, H.C.; Ayoubi, S.; Gimenez, P.-F.; Han, Y.; Jmila, H.; Blanc, G.; Takahashi, T.; Zhang, Z. Explainable artificial intelligence for cybersecurity: A literature survey. *Ann. Telecommun.* **2022**, *77*, 789–812. [CrossRef]
51. Tramèr, F.; Zhang, F.; Juels, A.; Reiter, M.K.; Ristenpart, T. Stealing machine learning models via prediction APIs. In Proceedings of the USENIX Security Symposium, Austin, TX, USA, 10–12 August 2016; pp. 601–618.
52. Kaissis, G.A.; Makowski, M.R.; Rückert, D.; Braren, R.F. Secure, privacy-preserving and federated machine learning in medical imaging. *Nat. Mach. Intell.* **2020**, *2*, 305–311. [CrossRef]
53. Saifullah, S.; Mercier, D.; Lucieri, A.; Dengel, A.; Ahmed, S. Privacy Meets Explainability: A Comprehensive Impact Benchmark. *arXiv* **2022**, arXiv:2211.04110.
54. Geyer, R.C.; Klein, T.; Nabi, M. Differentially private federated learning: A client level perspective. *arXiv* **2017**, arXiv:1712.07557.
55. Ivanovs, M.; Kadikis, R.; Ozols, K. Perturbation-based methods for explaining deep neural networks: A survey. *Pattern Recognit. Lett.* **2021**, *150*, 228–234. [CrossRef]
56. Albahri, A.S.; Duhaim, A.M.; Fadhel, M.A.; Alnoor, A.; Baqer, N.S.; Alzubaidi, L.; Albahri, O.S.; Alamoodi, A.H.; Bai, J.; Salhi, A.; et al. A systematic review of trustworthy and explainable artificial intelligence in healthcare: Assessment of quality, bias risk, and data fusion. *Inf. Fusion* **2023**, *96*, 156–191. [CrossRef]
57. Viganò, L.; Magazzeni, D. Explainable security. In Proceedings of the 2020 IEEE European Symposium on Security and Privacy Workshops (EuroS&PW), Genoa, Italy, 7–11 September 2020; pp. 293–300.
58. Kuppa, A.; Le-Khac, N.A. Black Box Attacks on Explainable Artificial Intelligence(XAI) methods in Cyber Security. In Proceedings of the 2020 International Joint Conference on Neural Networks (IJCNN), Glasgow, UK, 19–24 July 2020; pp. 1–8.
59. Kiener, M. Artificial intelligence in medicine and the disclosure of risks. *AI Soc.* **2021**, *36*, 705–713. [CrossRef]
60. Comiter, M. *Attacking Artificial Intelligence AI's Security Vulnerability and What Policymakers Can Do about It*; Belfer Center for Science and International Affairs: Cambridge, MA, USA, 2019.
61. Druce, J.; Harradon, M.; Tittle, J. Explainable artificial intelligence (XAI) for increasing user trust in deep reinforcement learning driven autonomous systems. *arXiv* **2021**, arXiv:2106.03775.
62. Le Merrer, E.; Trédan, G. Remote explainability faces the bouncer problem. *Nat. Mach. Intell.* **2020**, *2*, 529–539. [CrossRef]
63. Guang, Y.; Qinghao, Y.; Jun, X. Unbox the black-box for the medical explainable AI via multi-modal and multi-centre data fusion: A mini-review, two showcases and beyond. *Inf. Fusion* **2022**, *77*, 29–52. [CrossRef]
64. van der Veer, S.N.; Riste, L.; Cheraghi-Sohi, S.; Phipps, D.L.; Tully, M.P.; Bozentko, K.; Atwood, S.; Hubbard, A.; Wiper, C.; Oswald, M.; et al. Trading off accuracy and explainability in AI decision-making: Findings from 2 citizens' juries. *J. Am. Med. Inform. Assoc.* **2021**, *28*, 2128–2138. [CrossRef]
65. Sokol, K.; Flach, P. Explainability fact sheets: A framework for systematic assessment of explainable approaches. In Proceedings of the 2020 Conference on Fairness, Accountability, and Transparency, Barcelona, Spain, 27–30 January 2020; pp. 56–67.
66. Lipton, Z.C. The Mythos of Model Interpretability: In Machine Learning, the Concept of Interpretability is Both Important and Slippery. *Queue* **2018**, *16*, 31–57. [CrossRef]
67. Hoffman, R.R.; Mueller, S.T.; Klein, G.; Litman, J. Metrics for explainable AI: Challenges and prospects. *arXiv* **2018**, arXiv:1812.04608.
68. Klein, G.; Hoffman, R.R. Macrocognition, mental models, and cognitive task analysis methodology. In *Naturalistic Decision Making and Macrocognition*; Ashgate Publishing: Farnham, UK, 2008; pp. 57–80.
69. Fauvel, K.; Masson, V.; Fromont, E. A performance-explainability framework to benchmark machine learning methods: Application to multivariate time series classifiers. *arXiv* **2020**, arXiv:2005.14501.
70. Larochelle, H.; Erhan, D.; Courville, A.; Bergstra, J.; Bengio, Y. An empirical evaluation of deep architectures on problems with many factors of variation. In Proceedings of the International Conference on Machine Learning (ICML '07), Corvallis, OR, USA, 20–24 June 2007; pp. 473–480. [CrossRef]
71. Goodfellow, I.; Pouget-Abadie, J.; Mirza, M.; Xu, B.; Warde-Farley, D.; Ozair, S.; Courville, A.; Bengio, Y. Generative adversarial networks. *Commun. ACM* **2020**, *63*, 139–144. [CrossRef]
72. Huynh, T.D.; Tsakalakis, N.; Helal, A.; Stalla-Bourdillon, S.; Moreau, L. Explainability-by-Design: A Methodology to Support Explanations in Decision-Making Systems. *arXiv* **2022**, arXiv:2206.06251.
73. Sarkar, A. Is explainable AI a race against model complexity? *arXiv* **2022**, arXiv:2205.10119.
74. van der Velden, B.H.M.; Kuijf, H.J.; Gilhuijs, K.G.A.; Viergever, M.A. Explainable artificial intelligence (XAI) in deep learning-based medical image analysis. *Med. Image Anal.* **2022**, *79*, 102470. [CrossRef] [PubMed]

75. Simonyan, K.; Vedaldi, A.; Zisserman, A. Deep inside convolutional networks: Visualising image classification models and saliency maps. *arXiv* **2013**, arXiv:1312.6034.
76. Chaddad, A.; Peng, J.; Xu, J.; Bouridane, A. Survey of Explainable AI Techniques in Healthcare. *Sensors* **2023**, *23*, 634. [CrossRef] [PubMed]
77. Manresa-Yee, C.; Roig-Maimó, M.F.; Ramis, S.; Mas-Sansó, R. Advances in XAI: Explanation Interfaces in Healthcare. In *Handbook of Artificial Intelligence in Healthcare: Practicalities and Prospects*; Lim, C.-P., Chen, Y.-W., Vaidya, A., Mahorkar, C., Jain, L.C., Eds.; Springer International Publishing: Cham, Switzerland, 2022; Volume 2, pp. 357–369.
78. Khodabandehloo, E.; Riboni, D.; Alimohammadi, A. HealthXAI: Collaborative and explainable AI for supporting early diagnosis of cognitive decline. *Future Gener. Comput. Syst.* **2021**, *116*, 168–189. [CrossRef]
79. Joyce, D.W.; Kormilitzin, A.; Smith, K.A.; Cipriani, A. Explainable artificial intelligence for mental health through transparency and interpretability for understandability. *NPJ Digit. Med.* **2023**, *6*, 6. [CrossRef] [PubMed]
80. Asan, O.; Bayrak, A.E.; Choudhury, A. Artificial Intelligence and Human Trust in Healthcare: Focus on Clinicians. *J. Med. Internet Res.* **2020**, *22*, e15154. [CrossRef] [PubMed]
81. Marcus, G. The next decade in AI: Four steps towards robust artificial intelligence. *arXiv* **2020**, arXiv:2002.06177.
82. Das, A.; Rad, P. Opportunities and challenges in explainable artificial intelligence (xai): A survey. *arXiv* **2020**, arXiv:2006.11371.
83. Hulsen, T. The ten commandments of translational research informatics. *Data Sci.* **2019**, *2*, 341–352. [CrossRef]
84. Harder, F.; Bauer, M.; Park, M. Interpretable and differentially private predictions. In Proceedings of the AAAI Conference on Artificial Intelligence, New York, NY, USA, 7–12 February 2020; pp. 4083–4090.

Disclaimer/Publisher's Note: The statements, opinions and data contained in all publications are solely those of the individual author(s) and contributor(s) and not of MDPI and/or the editor(s). MDPI and/or the editor(s) disclaim responsibility for any injury to people or property resulting from any ideas, methods, instructions or products referred to in the content.

Disclaimer/Publisher's Note: The statements, opinions and data contained in all publications are solely those of the individual authors(s) and contributor(s) and not of MDPI and/or the editor(s). MDPI and/or the editor(s) disclaim responsibility for any injury to people or property resulting from any ideas, methods, instructions or products referred to in the content.

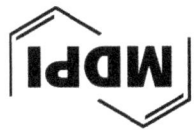

AI Editorial Office
E-mail: ai@mdpi.com
www.mdpi.com/journal/ai

MDPI
St. Alban-Anlage 66
4052 Basel
Switzerland
www.mdpi.com

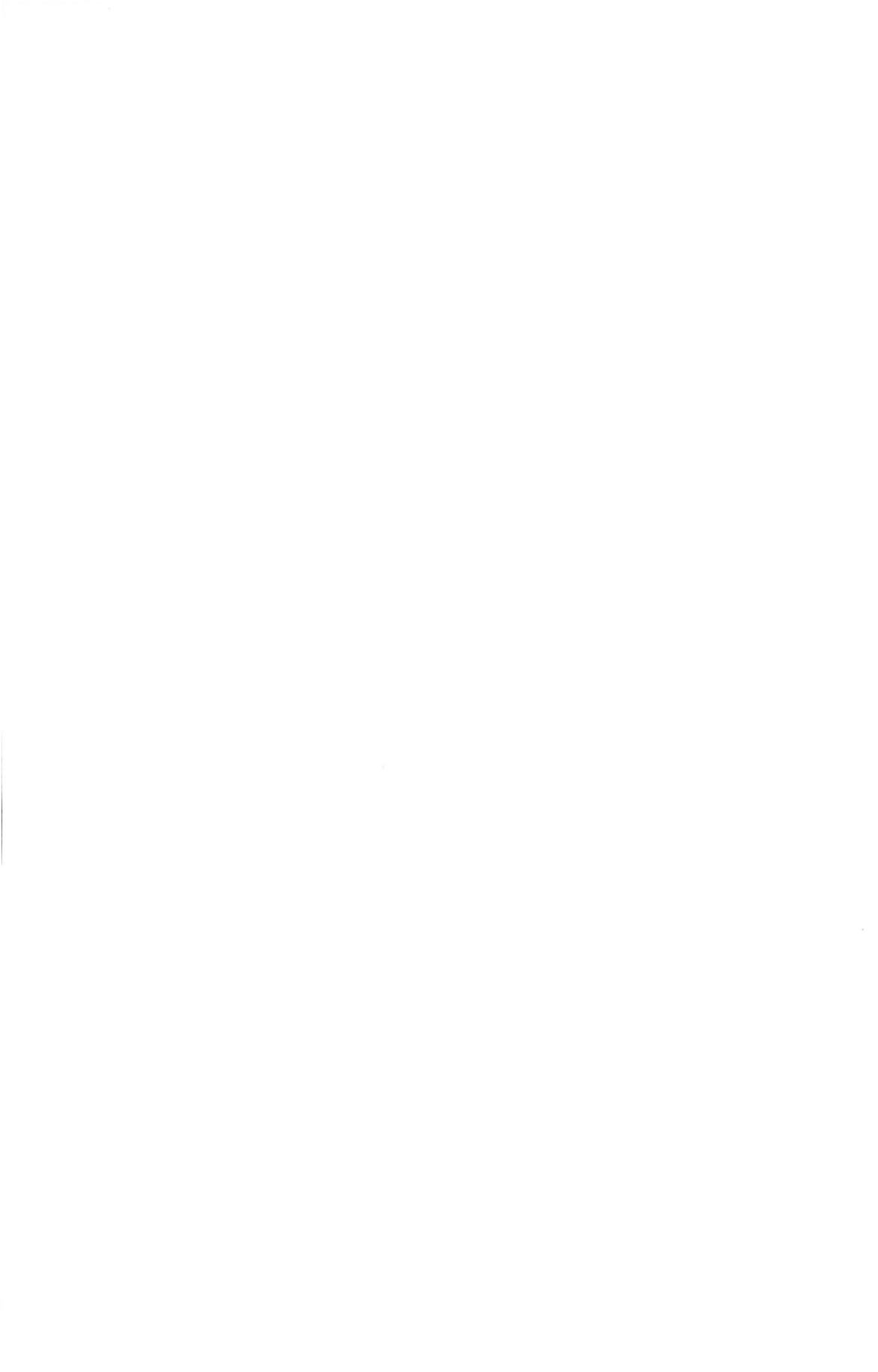